# The Adolescent and Mood Disturbance

# The Adolescent and Mood Disturbance

Edited by

## Harvey Golombek

and

## Barry D. Garfinkel

INTERNATIONAL UNIVERSITIES PRESS, INC.

New York

Library of Congress Cataloging in Publication Data

Main entry under title:

The Adolescent and mood disturbance.

    Includes bibliographies and index.
    1. Adolescent psychopathology.  2. Affective
disorders.  3. Depression, Mental.  I. Golombek,
Harvey.  II. Garfinkel, Barry D.  [DNLM:
1. Affective symptoms — In adolescence — Congresses.
WS 463 A23902 1979]
RJ506.D4A36  1983     616.89′022     82-13112
ISBN 0-8236-0085-8

Manufactured in the United States of America

# CONTENTS

# PART TWO
## CLINICAL SYNDROMES

# PART THREE
## DEPRESSION AND SUICIDE

# PART FOUR
# FORMS OF INTERVENTION

# ACKNOWLEDGMENTS

The C. M. Hincks Treatment Centre, in response to a United Nations declaration designating 1979 as the International Year of the Child, invited a distinguished group of scholars to explore the important topic of mood disturbance in the adolescent. A condensed version of each contribution was then presented at an International Symposium in Toronto, November 1 and 2, 1979. *The Adolescent and Mood Disturbance* represents the culmination of these efforts.

First, we would like to thank the authors for the serious and highly professional manner in which they responded to our invitations; we thank them for their promptness and their graceful response to our editorial suggestions.

We express our sincerest appreciation to the Director of the C. M. Hincks Treatment Centre, Dr. Angus Hood, who embraced the project enthusiastically and assumed the heavy burden of administrative work which made possible this undertaking. He is a man of exceptional talent who comprehended with ease the complexity of the task and worked diligently on one aspect after another, always retaining a sense of humor, projecting a sense of much appreciated confidence, and expressing continual optimism and support.

Special thanks are also offered to Mrs. Audrey Wilson, secretary and administrative assistant to Dr. Hood, for her constant help with a project that could only have compounded an already overtaxed schedule.

We thank the members of the local organizing committee — Morris Godel, chairman, Harvey Golombek, program chairman, Michael Hasley, Angus M. Hood, Annette Kussin, Alex Macrae, Sandra Morch, Harley Wideman, and Gordon Wolfe — and the Board of Directors of the C. M.

Hincks Treatment Centre for their support, useful suggestions and practical help. The Board unanimously supported every aspect of this project, assumed complete financial responsibility, and helped raise much appreciated funds from the community.

We are grateful to the Upjohn Pharmaceutical Company, the Canadian Imperial Bank of Commerce, and the C. M. Hincks Treatment Centre for their financial assistance.

We also wish to thank the Department of Psychiatry at the University of Toronto for its support of this project, especially Dr. Frederick H. Lowy, former Chairman of the Department of Psychiatry and current Dean of Medicine at the University of Toronto, for his personal backing and help in arranging and sponsoring our audiovisual and recording requirements.

Our gratitude goes to the many other persons who read the manuscripts and kindly offered their suggestions; in particular, our thanks to Dr. Elliot Markson for his review and editorial recommendations regarding the paper "Psychotherapy of Narcissistic Disorder in Adolescence." Also, special thanks to Dr. Michael Eleff for his constructive criticisms and proofreading, and to Mr. Russell Westkirk for his assistance in the preparation of Chapter One.

We are indebted to our subeditor, Miss Ursula Matthews, for her meticulous review of the entire manuscript and for bringing a unifying style to the complete text. She brought to the task a wealth of experience, great personal integrity, dedication, and remarkable perseverance and interest. She checked and rechecked every item in the bibliography, a task for which no "thank you" is sufficient.

We are grateful to Mrs. Betty Mair, Librarian at the C. M. Hincks Treatment Centre, who generously contributed her efforts to the time-consuming task of proofreading. Thanks also to Ms. Terry Frechette and Mrs. Isabel MacNaught for their secretarial help.

And finally, we thank Mrs. Carol Kehm who typed (and retyped and retyped) the manuscript, for her interest, enthusiasm, and continuous support. She approached each revision with good humor and with a sustained feeling that we were always making progress, and that the ultimate goal was just in sight.

# CONTRIBUTORS

E. JAMES ANTHONY, M.D.
Blanche F. Ittleson Professor of Child Psychiatry; Director, William Greenleaf Eliot Division, and Director, Edison Child Development Research Center, Washington University School of Medicine, St. Louis, Missouri.

CLIVE G. CHAMBERLAIN, M.D.
Director, Thistletown Regional Centre, Rexdale, Ontario; Associate Professor, Department of Psychiatry, University of Toronto.

NORMAN L. FARBEROW, Ph.D.
Co-Director, Suicide Prevention Center and Institute for Studies of Self-Destructive Behaviors, Los Angeles, California; Principal Investigator, Central Research Unit for Studies of Unpredicted Death, Wadsworth Medical Center, Veterans Administration, Los Angeles.

SUSAN A. FRANZEN, Ph.D.
Formerly, Adolescent Fellow, Department of Psychiatry, Michael Reese Hospital and Medical Center and Committee on Human Development, University of Chicago.

BARRY D. GARFINKEL, M.D.
Director of Research Unit and Undergraduate and Graduate Medical Education in Child Psychiatry, Bradley Hospital, East Providence, Rhode Island; Assistant Professor of Psychiatry, Brown University, Faculty of Medicine.

## HARVEY GOLOMBEK, M.D.

Head of Preventive Studies, C. M. Hincks Treatment Centre; Associate Professor, Department of Psychiatry, University of Toronto; Faculty, Toronto Institute of Psychoanalysis; Senior Psychiatric Consultant, Etobicoke Board of Education; Member of Active Teaching Medical Staff, Toronto Western Hospital.

## HERTA A. GUTTMAN, M.D.

Former Director, Family Therapy Training, and Director, Psychiatric Consultation Service, Jewish General Hospital, Montreal, Quebec; Associate Professor of Psychiatry, McGill University.

## LIONEL HERSOV, M.D.

Consultant Psychiatrist, The Bethlem Royal Hospital and The Maudsley Hospital; Senior Lecturer and Honorary Consultant in Psychological Medicine, The Royal Postgraduate Medical School and Hammersmith Hospital, London, England.

## ANGUS M. HOOD, M.D.

Director, C. M. Hincks Treatment Centre, Toronto, Ontario; Associate Professor, Department of Psychiatry, University of Toronto.

## DONALD F. KLEIN, M.D.

Director of Research, New York State Psychiatric Institute, New York; Professor of Psychiatry, Columbia University.

## SAUL V. LEVINE, M.D.

Head, Department of Psychiatry, Sunnybrook Medical Centre, Toronto; Professor of Psychiatry, University of Toronto.

## JAMES F. MASTERSON, M.D.

Clinical Professor of Psychiatry, Cornell University Medical College; Attending Psychiatrist, The New York Hospital (Payne Whitney Clinic), New York; Director of The Masterson Group for the Study and Treatment of the Character Disorders: Adolescent and Adult.

## KLAUS K. MINDE, M.D.

Director of Psychiatric Research, The Hospital for Sick Children, Toronto; Professor of Psychiatry, University of Toronto.

## KENNETH NEWMAN, M.D.

Faculty, Chicago Psychoanalytic Institute and Institute for Psychosomatic and Psychiatric Research and Training, Chicago, Illinois; Associate Clinical Professor of Psychiatry, Pritzker School of Medicine, University of Chicago.

GERHARDT NISSEN, M.D.
Professor of Child and Adolescent Psychiatry, and Director of the Hospital for Child and Adolescent Psychiatry, Julius-Maximilian University, Würzburg, Germany.

DANIEL OFFER, M.D.
Chairman, Department of Psychiatry, Michael Reese Hospital and Medical Center, Chicago, Illinois; Professor of Psychiatry, Pritzker School of Medicine, University of Chicago; Editor-in-Chief, *Journal of Youth and Adolescence.*

RAYMOND PRINCE, M.D.
Research Director, Mental Hygiene Institute, Montreal, Quebec; Associate Dean, Post-Graduate Education, Faculty of Medicine, and Professor of Psychiatry, McGill University.

QUENTIN RAE-GRANT, M.D.
Psychiatrist-in-Chief, The Hospital for Sick Children, Toronto; Professor and Vice-Chairman, Department of Psychiatry, University of Toronto.

VIVIAN M. RAKOFF, M.D., F.R.C.P. (C)
Chairman, Department of Psychiatry, University of Toronto; Professor, Psychiatric Education, University of Toronto.

JOHN E. SCHOWALTER, M.D.
Director of Training and Professor of Pediatrics and Psychiatry, Yale University Child Study Center, New Haven, Connecticut.

PAUL H. WENDER, M.D.
Professor of Psychiatry, University of Utah College of Medicine, Salt Lake City, Utah.

EDWARD A. WOLPERT, M.D., Ph.D.
Director of the Hospital, Psychosomatic and Psychiatric Institute, Michael Reese Hospital and Medical Center; Clinical Professor of Psychiatry, Pritzker School of Medicine; Consultant, Sonia Shankman Orthogenic School, University of Chicago.

# PREFACE

The purpose of this book is to integrate a broad base of investigational information to provide clinicians with background knowledge for the effective management of mood disorders in adolescents. The choice of the topic, *The Adolescent and Mood Disturbance*, was relatively simple: this area is a subject of worldwide concern. However, it has not been extensively detailed in the clinical literature; clinicians, allied health workers, correctional officers, educators, and others concerned with the care of disturbed adolescents have expressed an urgent need for clarification of specific developmental issues, assessment protocols, and therapeutic and preventive strategies.

Some of the contributors to this book describe clinical problems of adolescence that may begin before puberty and persist into adulthood. Thus the topics chosen, although focusing on adolescents, also serve to amplify and extend knowledge about children and young adults.

Does adolescence herald the arrival of new problems, disorders, and disturbances, or does it simply color an existing typography with features associated with pubescent development? Sadly, symptoms that often present in a preclinical form in childhood can become the severe manifestations of mental illness in adolescence. They can, for example, be precursors of primary affective disorders and schizophrenia. The tears and irritability of childhood may anticipate the depression of adolescence; suspicion and withdrawal may precede serious schizoid disorders; and dare-devil bravado may anticipate lethal, self-inflicted injury. The authors of this book, working from various perspectives, trace the origins and course of conditions that surface in adolescence and often persist into adulthood.

The expression of clinical features during adolescence is dramatically influenced by the epoch (as noted by Vivian Rakoff), the culture (as described by Raymond Prince), and the belief system (as studied by Saul Levine). The individual's ability to navigate adolescence successfully speaks to the necessity for a qualitative transformation from being a child into being an adult, and the capacity for the maturation of effective adaptive processes.

The developmental tasks of adolescence are made more difficult if existing clinical states continue from childhood. Physical illness, attentional deficits, phobias, primary affective disorders, character disorders, and borderline states are described by John Schowalter, Paul Wender, Edward Wolpert, Donald Klein, and James Masterson. Resolution of developmental demands is less likely if the adaptive functions are impaired or severely stressed.

The collapse of an adolescent's ability to cope with his immediate environment can result in suicidal behavior. The adolescent who exhibits an excessive inability to manage stress and conflict as he struggles with independence, and who demonstrates an excessive reluctance to be guided by others or use the support and direction of adults, can be overwhelmed by dysphoric affect, and may attempt suicide.

Mood disorders should be treated comprehensively. The treatment of suicidal behavior and mood disorders, and the prevention of suicide are discussed in detail by Donald Klein, Kenneth Newman, Herta Guttman, and Norman Farberow, all of whom have demonstrated versatility and skill in selecting varied forms of intervention. Therapy is no longer a selection of one approach alone, having become a combination of organic and psychosocial methods of intervention.

This compilation of studies has been designed to assist all who are interested in more fully understanding adolescent mood disturbance. It is hoped that these contributions will promote further research and improved clinical care.

CHAPTER ONE

# PERSONALITY DEVELOPMENT DURING ADOLESCENCE: IMPLICATIONS FOR TREATMENT

HARVEY GOLOMBEK

*The rotations of the Universe are the same, up and down, from age to age.... In a moment earth will cover us all, then earth, too, will change and what ensues will change to eternity and that again to eternity. A man who thinks of the continuous waves of change and alterations, and the swift passage of all mortal things, will hold them in disdain.*

—Marcus Aurelius (121–180 A.D.)
*Meditations*, Book 9, Chapter 28

How does adolescent personality grow? What is the nature of its baseline, mid-childhood? What external and internal influences promote the changes of adolescence and what kind of theoretical models can be developed to explain evolving identity? Are all of the changes necessary, or inevitable; are they evolutionary, revolutionary, or cathartic? How rigid and predetermined is the adolescent's personality structure; to what degree is there flexibility and freedom for self-direction?

These and other major questions still puzzle us, but clear answers are hopefully forthcoming. To understand the adolescent we must pay attention to historical, social, familial, cognitive, and emotional as well as biological forces; systems theory teaches us that all of these components influence each other, and that a change in one part of the system affects all others (1).

Adolescence is an intriguing age, chiefly because of the multiplicity of changes that occur during an abbreviated span. For this dissertation, ado-

1

lescence is defined as the period of development that begins with a physical event—the height of the pubescent crest, and ends with an intrapsychic event, the firm formation of a restructured identity (2-5).

A child's physical growth begins to show an upturn from the plateau of early latency at about 8 years in girls and 10 in boys (6); this marks the beginning of pubescence, which proceeds for about 9 years, and is complete at approximately 17 years of age in girls and 19 in boys. During this time of physiological growth there is a period in which children "shoot up" rapidly, the maximal growth age (MGA). It is as if the groundwork necessary for the development of the adolescent phase is fertilized and tilled by the early stages of pubescence. But it is the rapid and intense physiological changes (7) induced by the MGA (6), combining with the intense social pressures for differentiation generated by the familial and cultural environment (8-10), that disrupt the homeostasis of the psychological stage of latency (11) and herald the onset of adolescence proper.

Paradoxically, latency (middle childhood) is an active period for most children; youngsters on the threshold of adolescence tend to be busy, inquisitive, searching, and experimental; they admire adults, emulate them, and readily identify with them; and, if circumstances permit, love to learn and acquire skills. But latency is also a period of quiescence for the internalized sense of self or internalized object, i.e., the accumulation of representations of other persons. The self, built up in early childhood through a series of incorporations, introjections, internalizations, and identifications, generally remains strong and stable: most children of about 10 years of age enjoy a sense of security and the strong feeling that their beliefs about most subjects are true. If asked, many latency-age children will confidently share their opinions and values about religion, education, finance, politics, or entertainment—all presented as their own individual points of view. However, on meeting their parents, teachers, or neighbors, one is unlikely to be surprised; much of the secure internalized self is built up by taking in values and beliefs from significant figures in the child's immediate environment. Although secure, the child appears undifferentiated, a composite reflection of his upbringing and circumstances.

Soon, however, as in all phases of human development, there is a disruption of progress before the onset of the subsequent stage. At the MGA, the rapid changes induced by the pubertal spurt, coupled with strong social pressures from the child's external world, interrupt the stability, security, and assuredness of the internalized object (12).

During the 9 years of pubescence, height increases by 25% and weight doubles; growth is centered in the extremities—neck, arms, and legs (thus the long-legged, gawky, or coltish look) (6); and there are changes in the appearance and distribution of hair, increased activity in sebaceous glands, and increases in blood pressure, basal metabolic rate and pulse rate (5-7). At the endocrine level, changes in pituitary gland activity influence secretions in the thyroid, adrenal, and sex glands (6, 7), which contribute to the development of secondary sexual characteristics: changes in breasts, vagina, penis, and testes, the most obvious indicators of sexual maturity. There is also an upsurge of sexual and aggressive instinctual forces (11, 13) that are experienced in a new and therefore alien way, and are intensely felt (12, 14-16).

At the environmental level, the pubertal child is bombarded with changing expectations from his parents, friends, teachers, and—an area not to be minimized—the marketplace (1). The 12- or 13-year-old is expected to show heterosexual interest, give up childish hobbies, prefer the company of peers, and become involved in a separate (sub)culture; he is told what records to buy, what restaurants to prefer, how to dress, what make-up to use, and how long hair should be (17).

At puberty, therefore, interaction between the multitude of internal changes (12, 16, 18) and considerable external pressures have extensive effects on personality structure and content. Offer's studies of modal suburban adolescent boys (19-21) led him to conclude that, unlike populations seen in mental-health clinics, his samples demonstrated little external turmoil or rebellion. I suspect that all adolescents undergo considerable internal personality shift (although in the majority, as in Offer's group, the upheaval and restratification may not be externally evident) (22-24). Certainly my experience in working with teachers from junior and senior high schools supports this. Over the course of a year or two, teachers witness considerable shifts in ego functioning (5, 25-28) in their adolescent students, the majority of whom nevertheless stay out of major trouble and do not display serious antisocial activity; such students continue to perform and achieve well. This transformation, which can be described as a period of accelerated evolution (4, 19-22, 24, 29-33) is in direct contrast with the highly visible minority of adolescents who seem to undergo revolutionary change. These latter adolescents have been exhaustively described in the psychiatric, psychoanalytic, and social-science literature; they are portrayed as excessively rebellious toward adults, and at war within themselves. This internal struggle is variously described as between ego and id (11, 16, 34) or between neurotic defenses and strong opposing impulses or instincts (35, 36). Anna Freud (37) has championed the position that revolutionary change is normal and expected in adolescence.

Whether experiencing evolution or revolution, most adolescents demonstrate changes in personality. Internal and external forces seem to weaken the ego's boundaries and reorganize internal structural components (12, 16, 38). Physiologically intensified drives induce a surge of aggressive and sexual feelings (15, 39). Peter Blos has provided a useful conceptual framework for understanding intrapsychic changes in adolescence (40). He proposes that this stage of development be divided into three distinct phases — early, middle, and late — each with its own characteristics. Application of this thesis, augmented by concepts developed by Laufer (13, 41-43), Erikson (3), and Jacobson (12, 16), enables one to develop a conceptual model that describes the process of normal adolescent intrapsychic growth. Such a schema can provide a useful guide around which one can organize observations, judge the degree of maturity, and assess deviation, psychopathology, and transference during therapy. (It should be realized, of course, that no adolescent follows any schema exactly; one rarely, if ever, meets the prototypical adolescent.)

The onset of the pubertal thrust subjects the structure of the child's personality to considerable stress. The boundaries of the personality tend to become fluid and diffuse (3, 35). The youngster's presentation to the outer world changes: in latency, he appeared as an integrated person with his own specific interests, values, and skills, and was active and inquisitive; but with the onslaught of the external and internal stresses associated with the MGA he begins to appear inconsistent and confused (38). Youngsters 12 or 13 years old seem fidgety and "on the go"; they feel mixed up and unsure of themselves (15, 39, 40). Beliefs and values that previously went unquestioned, and about which they felt strongly, now seem less worthwhile and are held less tenaciously. These children often describe feeling that they are coming apart.

The next stage — early adolescence — for most children lasts from 13 until 14½ years of age. The personality boundaries remain weakened, and the incompleteness is compounded by the loss of many major components inculcated during childhood. The internalized object breaks down, becoming impoverished and fragmented (15, 16, 40). It is a paradox that the self suffers this serious loss of internal resources at a time when stresses are great and increasing. Previous incorporations, introjections, internalizations, and identifications are extruded (15, 40); there is a tendency toward a general poverty of defense mechanisms (40); and the use of very early defenses such as denial seems to predominate. The young adolescent is again preoccupied with oral needs, wishes, and conflicts. They seem to be constantly demanding, viewing adults in unambivalent terms as either all-good or all-bad providers.

During this phase there is a tendency for large-group friendships: the young teenager likes to roam with groups of six to ten, and friends are looked to primarily for satisfaction of specific needs. Parents often quizzically report that their previously satisfied, self-assured, sublimated latency-age youngster has become narcissistic, needy, voraciously demanding, unsatisfied, and somewhat unsettled.

At the age of about 14½ or 15 years, this early phase usually gives way to the next — middle adolescence (40, 41). A process begins to emerge that allows the inner self to become reconstituted. New growth and resynthesis occur, rebuilding the impoverished, weakened, internalized self. A new personality evolves through what can be viewed as a repetition of the processes of incorporation, introjection, internalization, and identification. New values, beliefs, ideals, and prohibitions are taken into the self as the reconstruction of identity proceeds. This phase presents yet another paradox: even as the youngster refashions his internalized object by taking into himself important new representations of heroes in the environment (entertainers, athletes, teachers, religious leaders) he tends to deny their significance or value. This stems from his wish to believe and to make others believe that he is independent, and can look after himself completely if circumstances allow. Contrary to appearances, however, adults are very much needed and depended upon, both to act as sources for new identifications (40, 41) and as foils for the clarification of what parts of themselves they will permanently give up.

The mid-adolescent's behavior is designed to demonstrate separateness. It is somewhat exaggerated and flamboyant, conveying an air (usually tolerated and ambivalently enjoyed by adults) of superiority, of knowing-it-all, and of striving toward omnipotence. Teenagers at this stage find it convenient to argue, which accomplishes two tasks: on the surface, it communicates opposition and independence; underneath, it allows for the secret discovery and subsequent incorporation of new ideas from adult figures, without giving any overt evidence of the personality-rebuilding process. For mid-adolescents to admit openly that they are dependent, needy, and seek instruction would be to lose face; therefore they have enormous difficulty showing appreciation directly, or expressing gratitude, especially to persons in authority.

During this middle phase, teenagers tend to split their feelings about peers, associating with those they identify as "great" and staying away from those who are viewed as "useless." This kind of extreme demarcation results from the fluctuating state of the internalized object (5, 16). Qualities in friends are sought that conform to those being re-internalized. Fear and panic can result from contact with values, ideals, and beliefs from which the adolescents are escaping or which they have recently ejected. In this phase there is little capacity for tolerating ambivalent feelings toward others.

Thus the mid-adolescent is most susceptible to hero-worshipping. As he is involved in a continuing process of internal reconstruction, it is not surprising that there are frequent shifts in the objects of his idealization and what he internalizes (41, 43). Idols of one month are denigrated a few months later and replaced by new heroes, new pictures, new record albums, and new buttons.

At about the age of 17 years, the teenager enters the final stage of adolescent development. Entry into late adolescence is demarcated by reconstitution of the self: a new homeostasis is established, and becomes consolidated (40); a new identity is formed, and crystallizes in time (3). Thus the internalized self is whole again (16). The late adolescent regains many characteristics he had as a latency-age child (36), but this time with greater complexity and significant individuation (44). Once again, but now to a higher level, he is able to employ, to a greater extent, mental mechanisms such as intellectualization, sublimation, and rationalization (45). (Through early and middle adolescence he had progressed to a new individuation, achieving significant differentiation for himself, from his family and immediate community, and thus from the world of his early childhood.) During late adolescence the relative completeness of this internalized self allows for true intimacy (3). Because he has become a renewed and whole person on the inside, he is able to search for and value whole-person alliances on the outside; in other words, he has changed from a stage of predominantly taking-in from others to giving of himself to others.

The late adolescent begins to experience and understand that he is a separate, somewhat autonomous human being, with his own unique complement of values, beliefs, ideals, and prohibitions; he can thus begin to recognize that others are different. Mature, ambivalent relationships can be established with persons who share some similar values and needs, but are not identical. Other human beings are sought who can value both similarities and differences and who can thus reciprocate. Characteristically, late adolescents become involved in problems of the heart, wanting to love and be loved by another. Unlike the early adolescent, who approaches adults with excessive demands, or the middle adolescent, who is preoccupied with independence, the late adolescent predominantly relates to adults with wishes to be understood and appreciated (3, 40).

## ON THE NATURE OF THE PSYCHOTHERAPEUTIC
## RELATIONSHIP WITH ADOLESCENTS

Knowledge of the phases of adolescence sheds light on the nature of the relationship an adolescent in each phase can establish with a psychotherapist (2, 34, 37, 40, 46, 47).

Fenichel (48), writing about transference, stated:

The analytic situation induces the development of derivatives of the repressed, and at the same time a resistance is operative against it. The derivatives may make their appearance as highly concrete emotional needs directed toward the person who happens to be present. Resistance distorts the true connections. The patient misunderstands the present in terms of the past; and then instead of remembering the past, he strives, without recognizing the nature of his action, to relive the past and live it more satisfactorily than he did in childhood. He "transfers" past attitudes to the present.

In analysis, transference has a twofold aspect. Fundamentally it must be considered as a form of resistance. The patient defends himself against remembering and discussing his infantile conflicts by reliving them. . . . On the other hand, the transference offers the analyst a unique opportunity to observe directly the past of his patient and thereby to understand the development of his conflicts [pp. 29–30].

Fenichel's (48) description, derived from psychoanalysis, is accurate and useful for the treatment of the neurotic, post-oedipal late adolescent, or the adult who has mastered the psychological vicissitudes of adolescence, yet unconsciously retains serious, anxiety-provoking internal conflicts. Such a patient has established a relatively complete internalized self-representation (the internalized object); but because of maladaptive defenses, he experiences anxiety or depression resulting from unresolved conflicts that find expression in everyday life. Classical transference neuroses can occur only after a significant number of the gaps in self-identity have been filled.

In contrast, a different kind of psychotherapeutic relationship develops with an early or middle adolescent who is going through the characteristic changes induced by the breakdown and reintegration of personality. Clearly, the patient brings to the relationship, existentially, a sense of who he is and what he is experiencing. He also presents to the therapist the incompleteness of his personality and the conflicts associated with its current stage of dissolution or reconstruction (46, 47, 49). The latter problem, that of structure, predominates. Early and middle adolescents tend to live in the present, bringing into therapy problems that relate to the life-substance they are experiencing at the current level of their development (28); only in a secondary sense is the material colored by the vicissitudes of childhood, such as the adequacy of caretaking received or the degree of serious frustration suffered. As with older patients, the therapeutic relationship is affected most by the developmental state of personality (whether construction or reconstruction), and is influenced by the quality and quantity of the remains of original internalizations, incorporations, and identifications (2, 49).

It is fundamental that one cannot regard another person as whole unless one feels whole and integrated within oneself. Therefore, because of his own internal incompleteness, an early or middle adolescent cannot relate as a whole person to another person, and thus cannot view a therapist as a whole object (16). His personality boundaries are weak and elements of his internalized self have been ejected, impoverishing his personality. For ex-

ample, sitting in therapy with a 13- or 14-year-old, one senses an intense
newly created emptiness and the adolescent's pressing need to be given to
(15, 46). This condition is greatly accentuated in patients who have been
overindulged or excessively frustrated.

The early adolescent's state of need leads him to expect that he will be
responded to as he was when he was a young, dependent, and needy child.
During therapy the young adolescent patient not only relives this unconscious state of neediness, but also in a developmental (structural) sense,
experiences a state of personality breakdown and internal impoverishment
(15, 16, 40). Thus the therapist must be able to allow himself to be perceived, and used, as a provider. Great demands are made upon him; within
the context of treatment, he must provide interest, warmth, understanding,
and a reassuring attitude, without giving in to pressures to smother the
patient with excessive gratification.

TREATING THE EARLY ADOLESCENT

Parents of early adolescents repeatedly describe youngsters who seem
to them excessively at loose ends, fidgety and restless. If they ask such a
child what they can do to help, typically the youngster will request some
material object as the solution to his problems (e.g., the volume of 10-speed
bicycles sold to the families of early adolescents is staggering). However,
most parents find that although a gift is highly appreciated and reduces the
youngster's anxiety at the time, the effects are extremely short-lived. Many
such trials of giving may be required before the parents recognize that this
state of exaggerated need is internal and developmental. Similarly, middle-
school principals lament the pressures of the vast volume of demands made
by their early adolescent population: to change teachers, change classes, re-
allocate subject material, and so on. Like the parents, principals who sense
the teenager's enormous need, and agree to requests only court disappointment; the hoped-for long-term remedial effects are not forthcoming. Ultimately, they too realize that this pressure to receive derives from the internal
needs of the adolescent and not simply from deficiencies in the youngster's
environment.

Treating a patient who is going through early adolescence gives rise to
particular countertransference problems. Therapists are likely to be made
anxious by patients who appear clinging, demanding, needy, and continually frustrated; they may complain of not being treated as whole persons
but as filling-stations or cows—simply as providers. They feel a lack of
empathy coming from the teenager, who seems under no obligation to give
in return for what he is receiving. They also become concerned with the
repetitive nature of the demands, and begin to question how growth can be
promoted.

The psychotherapist must be able to present himself to his patients as a firm, stable, strong, consistent, permanent, and not-easily-flappable human being. Treatment can provide the patient with a feeling of being supported through a difficult developmental phase, of sharing the stability and consistency provided by a human being who is not overwhelmed, and does not panic (34). The therapist must be able to listen repetitively to his patients' needs, demands, and wishes, while trying to understand the nature of these requests. Within the developing therapeutic alliance he must help his patients understand more clearly what it is they want, identify the realities that would allow them to secure whatever is possible, and clarify limits. For weeks or months on end, therapy may revolve around the clarification of these needs and their realistic possibility for satisfaction. Helping a youngster to accomplish this usually starts the process of reinternalization, reincorporation, and reidentification that is so necessary for advancement to the next stage of adolescence.

TREATING THE MIDDLE ADOLESCENT

With entry into the second stage of adolescence, a new identity begins to emerge. The presentation is dramatically different: the 15-year-old swaggers into the consulting room, appears omnipotent, is arrogant and insolent, and knows everything. This stage is characterized by a tendency to use therapists as duelling partners to test out newly acquired components (values, beliefs, and ideals) of a reconstituting internalized self. The new attitudes and convictions are brandished about to test whether they will stand up to scrutiny.

The mid-adolescent patient uses his therapist as a rich source of new identification, taking in many of the values and beliefs he observes (41). In addition, through the process of projective identification, he projects onto and takes back from the therapist qualities that arise from his own idiosyncratic needs. Middle adolescence seems to generate a need for responsive sparring partners. How a patient fights, what he fights about, and the kind of response and retaliation he expects from his therapist are colored by early childhood experiences. However, although the patient's developmental history influences the content and form of the fighting, the basic behavior is not predominantly an anachronistic response stemming from early unresolved conflicts; rather, the predilection for excessive challenging and sparring represents an important characteristic of his current stage of psychological development.

For these patients, the therapist must deviate from the orthodox insight-oriented, nondirective stance so useful with adult patients. He must be willing to share some of his own ideas, beliefs, and values with his patients, recognizing their need for identification. In addition, he must be willing to participate in healthy phase-specific sparring, while remembering that he is being used as a part-object, and that empathy is seldom reciprocated.

Here too, many therapists experience considerable pain in the countertransference. Being drawn into a relationship that demands aggression, confrontation, and challenge, they feel that such activity violates a highly valued personal image of the ideal therapist. Through training or reading or personal need, they wish to present themselves as caring and concerned, nondirective, interpretive, intuitive, nonthreatening, and extremely accepting. But mid-adolescents will not, and cannot, accept such a posture: if they feel a therapist is unable to stand up to their bravado, they become frightened; if their omnipotence is not challenged, they fear their own destructive impulses; and if their ideas are not confronted, they cannot experience the necessary and comforting sense of differentiation.

Above all, while demonstrating interest in his patient's developing uniqueness, the therapist must convey a sense of his own individuality and separateness. He must be able to tolerate differences of opinion and to convey respect for others' values, even if he does not subscribe to them himself. Such an attitude helps the patient achieve more comfortably the resynthesis of his personality, and allows movement into the third stage of adolescence.

### TREATING THE LATE ADOLESCENT

It is in this last phase that the adolescent comes to feel a newly created state of internal completeness. He enters relationships willing to demonstrate his own uniqueness, which he values and trusts will be valued by others. He is curious, and more able to accept and respect others' unique abilities, despite their differences. He can begin to acknowledge ambivalent feelings, even though he still may feel uncomfortable with them.

Psychotherapeutic relationships of the type established with adults can be achieved during late adolescence. The patient has acquired a capacity for whole-person relationships with significant others, and thereby has also acquired the ability to develop a classical transference neurosis. Although these patients have the capacity for empathy, intimacy, and whole-object relationships, at appropriate moments in their treatment they can regress to allow unresolved conflicts to come to the fore for examination and interpretation. Regression in the service of the ego is possible because the ego has been reconstructed as a cohesive whole.

The major difficulty in treatment is the tendency for therapists to forget that these patients have just reached the brink of adulthood; they are infantile adults (40, 50). Because the patients' problems seem so similar to those of adults in their twenties or thirties, undue credit is often given to their experience in using a recently evolved personality structure. Although the self has been reconstituted, a person who is traversing late adolescence has little or no practice with his newly created self; he needs a considerable time for experimentation to discover who and what he is, and how he can best apply himself in everyday life. As Shakespeare put it,

*I know you all, and will awhile uphold*
*The unyok'd humour of your idleness:*
*Yet herein will I imitate the sun,*
*Who doth permit the base contagious clouds*
*To smother up his beauty from the world,*
*That when he please again to be himself,*
*Being wanted, he may be more wonder'd at,*
*By breaking through the foul and ugly mists*
*Of vapours that did seem to strangle him.*
*If all the year were playing holidays,*
*To sport would be as tedious as to work;*
*But when they seldom come, they wish'd for come,*
*And nothing pleaseth but rare accidents.*
*So, when this loose behaviour I throw off,*
*And pay the debt I never promised,*
*By how much better than my word I am,*
*By so much shall I falsify men's hopes;*
*And like bright metal on a sullen ground,*
*My reformation, glittering o'er my fault,*
*Shall show more goodly and attract more eyes*
*Than that which hath no foil to set it off.*
*I'll so offend to make offence a skill;*
*Redeeming time when men think least I will.*

—William Shakespeare,
*King Henry the Fourth*

## SUMMARY

Adolescence represents a special stage of human development; it is not more important than other stages of life, but is different and possesses its own unique characteristics.

Serious consideration of adolescence requires a multidimensional probe, its focus ranging from wide-angle, low-power observation to microscopic, high-power investigation. Changes occur at biological, intrapsychic, inter-personal, familial, and cultural levels; and changes at one level affect all others.

Psychoanalytic contributions to our knowledge have deepened our understanding of intrapsychic development during adolescence, and have described three distinctly separate phases: early, middle, and late adolescence. It is held that each phase represents a different state of dissolution and reconstruction of the character, and that each encompasses a specific state of ego-structure, a characteristic organization of defenses, and a recognizable theme of a verbal and behavioral nature.

The state of the internalized self determines the quality of relationships, and in particular the nature of the relationship between patient and therapist with its attendant transference and countertransference reactions. Therefore, therapeutic intervention requires an understanding of changing personality organization, and must be tailored to meet the patients' changing needs during passage through the different phases of adolescence.

## REFERENCES

1. Nesselroade, J. R. & Baltes, P. B. (1974), *Adolescent Personality Development and Historical Change: 1970–1972.* Soc. Res. Child Dev. Monograph, Serial No. 154, Vol. 39(1).
2. Bernfeld, S. (1938), Types of adolescence. *Psychoanal. Q.,* 7:243–253.
3. Erikson, E. H. (1956), The problem of ego identity. *J. Am. Psychoanal. Assoc.,* 4: 56–121.
4. Green, M. R. (1966), The problem of identity crisis. In: *Science and Psychoanalysis,* Vol. 9: *Adolescence, Dreams and Training,* ed. J. H. Masserman. New York: Grune & Stratton, pp. 69–79.
5. Group for the Advancement of Psychiatry, Committee on Adolescence (1968), *Normal Adolescence: Its Dynamics and Impact.* Report No. 68, Vol. 6, pp. 747–858. New York: Scribner's.
6. Stone, L. J. & Church, J. (1973), *Childhood and Adolescence: A Psychology of the Growing Person,* 3rd ed. New York: Random House, pp. 417–477.
7. Boutourline Young, H. (1971), The physiology of adolescence (including puberty and growth). In: *Modern Perspectives in Adolescent Psychiatry,* ed. J. G. Howells. Edinburgh: Oliver & Boyd, pp. 3–27.
8. Friedman, R. (1975), The vicissitudes of adolescent development and what it activates in adults. *Adolescence,* 10:520–526.
9. Hurlock, E. B. (1973), *Adolescent Development,* 4th ed. New York: McGraw-Hill.
10. Langsley, D. G., Fairbairn, R. H. & DeYoung, C. D. (1968), Adolescence and family crises. *Can. Psychiatr. Assoc. J.,* 13:125–133.
11. Freud, S. (1905), Three essays on the theory of sexuality. *Standard Edition,* 7: 130–243. London: Hogarth Press, 1953.
12. Jacobson, E. (1961), Adolescent moods and the remodeling of psychic structures in adolescence. *Psychoanal. Study Child,* 16:164–183.
13. Laufer, M. (1968), The body image, the function of masturbation, and adolescence: problems of the ownership of the body. *Psychoanal. Study Child,* 23: 114–137.
14. Ausubel, D. P. (1952), *Ego Development and the Personality Disorders: A Developmental Approach to Psychopathology.* New York: Grune & Stratton.
15. Blos, P. (1965), The initial stage of male adolescence. *Psychoanal. Study Child,* 20:145–164.

16. Jacobson, E. (1964), *The Self and the Object World.* (J. Am. Psychoanal. Assoc. Monograph Series No. 2.) New York: International Universities Press.
17. U.S. President's Science Advisory Committee, Report of the Panel on Youth (1974), *Youth: Transition to Adulthood.* Chicago: University of Chicago Press.
18. Speigel, L. A. (1951), A review of contributions to a psychoanalytic theory of adolescence: individual aspects. *Psychoanal. Study Child,* 6:375-393.
19. Offer, D. (1969), *The Psychological World of the Teenager: A Study of Normal Adolescent Boys.* New York: Basic Books.
20. Offer, D. & Offer, J. B. (1975), *From Teenage to Young Manhood: A Psychological Study.* New York: Basic Books.
21. Offer, D. (1975), Adolescent turmoil. In: *The Psychology of Adolescence: Essential Readings,* ed. A. H. Esman. New York: International Universities Press, pp. 141-155.
22. Douvan, E. & Adelson, J. (1966), *The Adolescent Experience.* New York: Wiley.
23. Mead, M. (1958), Adolescence in primitive and modern society. In: *Readings in Social Psychology,* 3rd ed., ed. G. E. Swanson. New York: Holt, pp. 341-349.
24. Rutter, M., Graham, P., Chadwick, O. F. D., & Yule, W. (1976), Adolescent turmoil: fact or fiction? *J. Child Psychol. Psychiatry,* 17:35-56.
25. Elkind, D. (1975), Recent research on cognitive development in adolescence. In: *Adolescence in the Life Cycle: Psychological Change and Social Context,* ed. S. E. Dragastin & G. H. Elder, Jr. New York: Wiley, pp. 49-61.
26. Inhelder, B. & Piaget, J. (1958), *The Growth of Logical Thinking from Childhood to Adolescence: An Essay on the Construction of Formal Operational Structures,* trans. A. Parsons & S. Milgram. New York: Basic Books.
27. Piaget, J. (1975), The intellectual development of the adolescent. In: *The Psychology of Adolescence: Essential Readings,* ed. A. H. Esman. New York: International Universities Press, pp. 104-108.
28. Shapiro, R. L. (1966), Identity and ego autonomy in adolescence. In: *Science and Psychoanalysis,* Vol. 9: *Adolescence, Dreams and Training,* ed. J. H. Masserman. New York: Grune & Stratton, pp. 16-24.
29. Grinker, Sr., R. R., Grinker, Jr., R. R., & Timberlake, J. (1962), "Mentally healthy" young males (homoclites): a study. *Arch. Gen. Psychiatry,* 6:405-453.
30. Grinker, Sr., R. R. & Werble, B. (1974), Mentally healthy young males homoclites) 14 years later. *Arch. Gen. Psychiatry,* 30:701-704.
31. Holmström, R. (1972), On the picture of mental health: a psychiatric approach. *Acta Psychiatr. Scand.,* Suppl. 231.
32. King, S. H. (1972), Coping and growth in adolescence. *Sem. Psychiatry,* 4:355-366.
33. Offer, D. & Offer, J. (1971), Four issues in the developmental psychology of adolescence. In: *Modern Perspectives in Adolescent Psychiatry,* ed. J. G. Howells. Edinburgh: Oliver & Boyd, pp. 28-44.
34. Geleerd, E. R. (1961), Some aspects of ego vicissitudes in adolescence. *J. Am. Psychoanal. Assoc.,* 9:394-405.
35. Beres, D. (1961), Character formation. In: *Adolescents: Psychoanalytic Approach to Problems and Therapy,* ed. S. Lorand & H. I. Schneer. New York: Hoeber, pp. 1-9.

36. Jones, E. (1922), Some problems of adolescence. In: *Papers on Psycho-analysis,* 5th ed. London: Baillière, Tindall & Cox, 1948, pp. 389–406.
37. Freud, A. (1958), Adolescence. *Psychoanal. Study Child,* 13:255–278.
38. Spiegel, L. A. (1961), Disorder and consolidation in adolescence. *J. Am. Psychoanal. Assoc.,* 9:406–416.
39. Blos, P. (1958), Preadolescent drive organization. *J. Am. Psychoanal. Assoc.,* 6: 47–56.
40. Blos, P. (1962), *On Adolescence: A Psychoanalytic Interpretation.* Glencoe: Free Press.
41. Laufer, M. (1964), Ego ideal and pseudo ego ideal in adolescence. *Psychoanal. Study Child,* 19:196–221.
42. Laufer, M. (1965), Assessment of adolescent disturbances: the application of Anna Freud's profile. *Psychoanal. Study Child,* 20:99–123.
43. Laufer, M. (1966), Object loss and mourning during adolescence. *Psychoanal. Study Child,* 21:269–293.
44. Schafer, R. (1973), Concepts of self and identity and the experience of separation-individuation in adolescence. *Psychoanal. Q.,* 42:42–59.
45. Freud, A. (1946), *The Ego and the Mechanisms of Defense.* New York: International Universities Press.
46. Bryt, A. (1966), Modifications of psychoanalysis in the treatment of adolescents. In: *Science and Psychoanalysis,* Vol. 9: *Adolescence, Dreams and Training,* ed. J. H. Masserman. New York: Grune & Stratton, pp. 80–90.
47. Eissler, K. R. (1958), Notes on problems of technique in the psychoanalytic treatment of adolescents, with some remarks on perversions. *Psychoanal. Study Child,* 13:223–254.
48. Fenichel, O. (1945), *The Psychoanalytic Theory of Neurosis.* New York: Norton.
49. Geleerd, E. (1958), Some aspects of psychoanalytic technique in the treatment of adolescents. In: Panel Report, The Psychology of Adolescence, by E. Buxbaum. *J. Am. Psychoanal. Assoc.,* 6:112–117, 119.
50. Deutsch, H. (1967), *Selected Problems of Adolescence, with Special Emphasis on Group Formation.* New York: International Universities Press.

# PART ONE

# PERSPECTIVES

# INTRODUCTION

# PART ONE:
# PERSPECTIVES

## Angus M. Hood

The examination of *The Adolescent and Mood Disturbance* begins within a nonclinical context; the four papers of Part One are designed to provide "perspectives" for the later chapters, which have a predominantly clinical orientation. Important here is the understanding of how mood is experienced and expressed, and what ego functions it serves during normal adolescent development.

Although these authors recognize intrapsychic and interpersonal parameters, the effect of the environment on the adolescent is emphasized; the adolescent is an actor and reactor within his cultural milieu. As the adolescent struggles with the task of identity formation, society either helps or hinders in the transmission of supportive beliefs, values, and a sense of belonging. Why do some adolescents accept and others reject what is offered, and what role does cultural conflict play in the creation of affective disturbances? These questions are addressed in this section.

The papers in Part One are expositions regarding both normal and abnormal adolescence. Daniel Offer is renowned for his extensive studies of normal adolescent development, and he and Susan Franzen begin their opening chapter "Mood Development in Normal Adolescents" by reviewing and contesting the romantic statement of G. Stanley Hall that adolescents are, by nature, "moody individuals." They distinguish affect from mood: affects are the specific feeling representations of psychic impulses, whereas moods are multiply determined, the result of intense stimulation which produces psychic tension too strong to find relief in specific affective discharge. The function of moods is defensive, allowing the gradual discharge of such tension.

In their discussion of the role of mood in adolescent development, Offer and Franzen advance formulations from ego psychology. In Jacobson's (1) opinion, "During all of adolescence the psychic organization is in a state of fluidity as never before or since" (p. 177). It is this reorganization which makes the psychic structure particularly vulnerable to regression and overstimulation. Mood discharge is then seen to represent normal defensive regulation.

Recognizing that most contributions on adolescent mood states (such as Jacobson's) are clinically based, Offer and his colleagues have undertaken a study of mood in normal adolescents. A "mood scale" was constructed by selecting items from the Offer Self-Image Questionnaire that best exemplified good or bad feelings about the self, and four groups each of adolescents in the 1960s and the late 1970s — all middle-class, midwestern males and females — were compared. The results are reviewed in depth. The most striking finding was the relative stability of mood among these teenagers. (However, the adolescents in the later sample described greater awareness of internal feelings and more problems relating to mood.) Based on these findings, the authors contend that psychic reorganization takes place unconsciously in mentally healthy adolescents, without spilling into antisocial behavior or causing serious mood swings.

Vivian Rakoff, in keeping with his interests in social history and philosophy, presents "Historical Forces in the Etiology of Psychiatric Disorders in Adolescence." A master of metaphor, he takes as his task "the problem of how the great ship of history gets into the bottle of the individual psyche." His panoramic view of process, enlivened by case histories, attests to the success of this undertaking.

In his preamble, he traces the development of extended adolescence as part of the new mythology of the post-revolutionary Western world with its emphasis on pluralism, freedom, and self-definition. With the decline of social oppression and fixed roles came the right to express and define one's true self. But the search for identity involves constant conflict in an ever-changing unpredictable society. Thus, social alienation and loss of moral significance are dangers inherent in the journey through adolescence.

Setting the stage for a wider exploration of his theme, the author begins with three clinical vignettes of adolescents who have grown up in families that are detached from contexts of place, history, religion, and even communal customs. It is in this climate that these patients develop profound feelings of alienation and depressive mood. In developing his thesis, Rakoff leans on the theoretical formulations of Winnicott, for whom the "transitional object" is the foundation of security in the personal world — the security of the "unclothed" person. Rakoff extends this concept to objects, language, history, ethical norms, and myths as essential for the process of functioning in the "clothed" world; these are the transitional structures necessary to the ego for development of a public self.

Many adolescents who are psychiatrically disturbed have experienced elements of historical or ethical rootlessness. They are adrift with no historical context in a society they cannot appreciate or even comprehend. Thus cults can fill their void and restore a sense of personal significance; however, such a prosthesis does not allow the adolescent to cope with the difficulties of moral choice and personal growth within the community.

Therefore, Rakoff ends by warning that the renewed awareness of these needs for context, sense-making mythologies, ethical standards, and shared cultural symbols may erode hard-won rights to self-determination and individuation.

Raymond Prince, whose career in transcultural psychiatry has included work in Nigeria, offers his study of the "brain-fag syndrome" in African students. It gives us another dimension of the impact of cultural transition on adolescent functioning, quite different in its genesis and manifestations from the affective disorders and alienation of North American youth.

The brain-fag syndrome, which has been widely reported (20–40%) especially among male students in emerging African countries, is characterized by unpleasant head symptoms, difficulties with vision, loss of ability to grasp the meaning of printed or spoken words, poor retention of information, and fatigue and sleepiness. Although components of both depression and anxiety are noted, it is generally held to be a depressive equivalent, often responding to antidepressant medication.

In the exploration of the etiology of this condition, the author takes us into interesting areas of observation and conjecture. He points out that Western high school students, with scholastic problems and study-inhibitions, usually are depressed over an unhappy home life, or their difficulties are part of a more profound neurosis or character problem; but such conditions are uncommon in African students whose symptoms seem to result simply from excessive studying. An intriguing thesis, the "forbidden-knowledge theory," is advanced; it suggests that these students unconsciously see themselves as betraying their ancestors by delving into alien lore and worshipping foreign gods. In support of this formulation, Prince cites both dream material and the fact that the lowest incidence of brain-fag occurs in students whose families have the highest level of identification with Western education and values.

Another possibility presented is that the African student suffers a basic lack of ego energy to accomplish the task of education. The ego is depleted of energy by the tasks of acculturation — not by neurotic conflict and defensive maneuvers. Thus Prince gives us a fascinating glimpse into the world of transcultural psychiatry.

Lastly, Saul Levine pursues a major area of personal academic interest in studying adolescent alternative life styles; "Alienation as an Affect in Adolescence" is a distillation of his clinical and research experience.

Recognizing the imprecision with which the words "alienation" and "affect" are used, Levine begins by clearly defining his terms. Alienation is set in the framework of Seaman and Keniston to include a sense of isolation, meaninglessness, normlessness, powerlessness, and self-estrangement; it is not synonymous with psychiatric disturbance, but is a delineated affect. (Affect is defined as the "feeling-tone" accompaniment of an idea or mental representation or symbol.) Alienation, like other affective experiences, is a continuum both in degree and kind. Leighton's concept of psychosocial disintegration, the reaction by individuals to rapid change in their social system, is also considered relevant to this view.

The author emphasizes that adolescence, as an age of rapid explosive change and unpredictability, provides fertile soil for the development of alienation. However, he also points out that it is not a universal phenomenon; rather, it profoundly engulfs young people who are vulnerable, pessimistic, possess poor adaptive skills, and experience low self-esteem. In short, this particular affect is but one possible answer to the existential questions of life, as the adolescent attempts to solve the dichotomy between "identity-related issues" and "alienation-related feelings."

Believing and belonging are then suggested as powerful psychosocial needs of adolescents; if achieved, they are effective antidotes to alienation. It is just these needs that the family and society have not been able to meet, which alternative life styles, religious and cult groups are able to fulfill. As his case illustrations suggest, the results for the individual who chooses these solutions are a lessening of negative affects and an increased sense of well-being.

Though membership in such groups may help the adolescent toward positive changes in self-feeling and behavior, Levine expresses deep concern that we have been unable to instill in many young people a sense of purpose from which both they and society would benefit. He challenges us as mental health professionals to continually seek ways to capture the adolescent's inherent need for an ideology and group identity.

These four papers confirm that the majority of young people traverse the adolescent developmental stage without pathological mood disturbance. However, there is a significant group—be they in the third world or urban North America—for whom cultural pressures or instability create serious problems; for some it leads to disabling symptom formation, for others to a state of alienation from the mainstream of society.

In our role as clinicians, adolescents test our therapeutic skills. As members of society, they stimulate our concern about problems created for this generation by a culture fraught with change and unpredictability. As adults, we too are enmeshed by forces in society that often seem beyond our capacity to modify. Our own experience and understanding emphasize the need to develop coping mechanisms for what we cannot readily change. In working with vulnerable adolescents who are wrestling with these same challenges, we require a thorough appreciation of the existential problems they face as well as their intrapsychic dynamics. Only then shall we be able to help them to live in the real world. The papers that follow are a start in this direction.

## REFERENCE

1. Jacobson, E. (1961), Adolescent moods and the remodeling of psychic structures in adolescence. *Psychoanal. Study Child*, 16:164–183.

CHAPTER TWO

# MOOD DEVELOPMENT
# IN NORMAL ADOLESCENTS

DANIEL OFFER

and

SUSAN A. FRANZEN

## INTRODUCTION

It has long been held that the subject of moods is particularly relevant to the adolescent phase of development. Many are of the opinion that adolescents are by nature extremely moody individuals, and the following statement by G. Stanley Hall in 1904 (1), although quite romantic in style, is still representative of current views (2-5).

> Youth cannot be temperate, in the philosophical sense. Now it is prone to laughter, hearty and perhaps almost convulsive, and is abandoned to pleasure, the field of which ought gradually to widen with perhaps the pain field, although more. There is gaiety, irrepressible levity, an euphoria that overflows in every absurd manifestation of excess of animal spirits, that cannot be repressed, that danger and affliction, appeals to responsibility and to the future, cannot daunt nor temper. To have a good time is felt to be an inalienable right. The joys of life are never felt with so keen a relish; youth lives for pleasure, whether of an epicurean or an esthetic type. It must and ought to enjoy life without

This work was supported in part by the Judith Baskin Offer Research Fund of the Department of Psychiatry, Michael Reese Hospital and Medical Center.

The authors are grateful to E. Ostrov, Ph.D., and K. I. Howard, Ph.D., for their help in the study reported here.

alloy. Every day seems to bring passionate love of just being alive, and the genius for extracting pleasure and gratification from everything is never so great.

But this, too, reacts into pain and dysphoria, as surely as the thesis of the Hegelian logic passes over to its antithesis. Young people weep and sigh, they know not why; depressive are almost as characteristic as expansive states of consciousness. The sad Thanatopsis mood of gloom paints the world in black. Far-off anticipations of death come in a foreboding way, as it is dimly felt, though not realized, that life is not all joy and that the individual must be subordinated and eventually die [p.77].

Moods, and fluctuations in mood, can be explained in terms of how adolescent development is regarded. If adolescent development is viewed as being basically discontinuous with childhood, the age of the growing adolescent is tested to its limits. Any internal or external stimulus or crisis would have a greater impact on the adolescent. In this situation, the adolescent would react with mood fluctuation in reaction to either internal or external situations. The ego of the adolescent would simply not be strong enough to withstand even minor fluctuations. However, if adolescent development is viewed as being continuous with that of childhood, the ego strength of the adolescent can easily cope with the everyday trauma which the adolescent has to face. It is the purpose of this paper to empirically discover which of these does really take place among normal adolescents.

This paper includes the description of a study in which moods were defined and their psychologic function examined. Data were obtained on the distribution of certain mood states among younger and older normal adolescents of both sexes at two points in time, the 1960s and the late 1970s.

DEFINITION OF MOODS

*Webster's New International Dictionary,* Second Edition, defines a mood as "temper of mind; humor; esp. the sum of those mental dispositions which give the dominant emotional character or cast of mind; as, a man of somber mood." As a sum of mental dispositions, moods are distinguishable from affects, which are traditionally defined as specific representations of psychic impulses. According to Freud (6), an affect is the recognizable derivative of a simple (unconscious) idea. Underlying the affect of gaiety, for example, might be the need for instinctual gratification, whereas underlying the affect of anger might be murderous rage. In his paper "Repression" (7), discussing the fate of the instincts, Freud wrote: "Either the instinct is altogether suppressed, so that no trace of it is found, *or it appears as an affect* which is in some way or other qualitatively coloured, or it is changed into anxiety" (p. 153, author's italics).

Moods, in contrast to affects, have multiple determinants. Moods are the result of intense stimulation that produces degrees of psychic tension too strong to find relief in specific affective discharge. The underlying stimulation is channeled more broadly throughout the total personality and its various psychic components. According to Jacobson (8), a mood represents "a cross-section through the entire state of the ego, lending a particular, uniform coloring to all its manifestations for a longer or shorter period of time" (p. 75).

## FUNCTION OF MOODS

If moods are a means of discharging psychic tension, their function is defensive. Moods allow for gradual discharge, protecting the ego from the overwhelming effects of explosive reactions, even though, as Jacobson has pointed out, dramatic outbursts may be a feature of a particular mood state. The prolonged depressed mood state of normal mourning, for example, is an adaptive alternative to complete fragmentation in the face of object loss. While extreme grief and even panic-like reactions are occurring during the normal mourning process, the prevailing aura of sadness facilitates gradual resolution of the pain of loss, and concomitant withdrawal from the outside world permits narcissistic replenishment and the redistribution of object cathexes.

Whereas mood states, as in the above example, may serve an advanced psychologic function, mood swings represent a more primitive attempt to achieve psychologic equilibrium. According to Jacobson, it is an immature ego that attempts to regulate all stimulation through diffuse and global mood channels. In such cases, the ego may be said to function as the servant of psychic imbalance and not as the master of internal stability.

Kohut (9) explained extremes of mood in terms of self-psychology, i.e., reflecting a lack of integration of the split-off, primitive, grandiose self into the total psychic apparatus. In individuals with this psychopathology, moods fluctuate depending on the extent to which infantile grandiosity is allowed expression versus the extent to which it is defensively denied. For example, one of his patient suffered from mood swings:

> Which were associated with a pervasive uncertainty about the reality of her feelings and thoughts. [She tended to swing between] (1) states of anxious excitement and elation over a secret "preciousness" which made her vastly better than anyone else (during times when the ego came close to giving way to the grandiose substructure, i.e., the strongly cathected grandiose self); and (2) states of emotional depletion, blandness, and immobility (which reflected the ego's periodic enfeeblement when it used all its strength to wall itself off from its unrealistic, grandiose substructure) [p. 283].

Thus, as in the ego psychology model proposed by Jacobson, extreme fluctuation in moods indicates immature functioning. Sustained and less extreme moods, however, are an option for a relatively mature ego or self to vent internal stimuli in ways that minimize psychologic disruption; at the same time they may be increasing a person's range of expression.

## MOOD STATES IN ADOLESCENCE

Although writers on the subject of adolescence unanimously agree that adolescents are moody individuals, there has been surprisingly little empirical research demonstrating this. Similarly, no studies have examined the kind of mood states adolescents are likely to experience, and why such moods particularly characterize the teenage years. We could trace only one study, by Larson (10), in which adolescents and adults were compared in regard to mood variability. Larson found that adolescents do experience wider extremes of mood, a variation not related to lower well-being. Rather, in Larson's opinion, it simply reflects the increased openness of adolescents to life experiences in contrast to adults' more predictable and stereotyped responses.

Most of the writings on adolescent moods, then, are theoretical; and most of the theoretical works on mood states in adolescents are clinically based. Our current theories are drawn by inference from patient populations, and thus biased in terms of an exaggerated view of the degree of psychopathology in adolescents. Jacobson (3, 4, 8), widely considered an authority on psychic development and moods in adolescents, is clearly a member of the clinical-inference school of thought. As her work is considered pioneering and is so widely referred to, the following discussion of the psychic structural substrate of moods in adolescents is extrapolated principally from her work.

Jacobson's major contribution to the theory of adolescent development is her view of the changes in psychic structure, especially changes in the superego. She stated (3) that with puberty comes an increased demand on the ego and superego to regulate drive. In this regard, Blos (11) also has written of the disruptive effect of the "resurgence of infantile drive positions" on the psychic balance achieved in the latency years. In the face of increased drive pressure, the superego must become stronger; however, it must also become less rigid, more flexible. Whereas the superego of a pre-latency child deals with infantile sexual demands by requiring that they be repressed entirely, the adolescent superego must continue to prohibit incestuous demands, yet allow for the possible expression of adult sexuality. Jacobson (3) wrote:

This confronts the adolescent with the complex and confusing task of toning down the idealized sexually prohibiting parental images, of reconciling them with realistic concepts of sexually active and increasingly permissive parents, and at the same time of building up new sets of goals and values based on a firm re-establishment of the incest taboo [pp. 170–171].

Described thus, growth of the superego implicates both the ego and the self and object representations in the process. To the ego falls the task of regulating increased id and superego pressures. The ego must become more autonomous and learn how to distinguish between incestuous and nonincestuous object relationships. According to Jacobson (3):

> During this struggle [the] ego. . . may alternately yield to [the superego] or rebel actively against it, and in overthrowing it join forces with the id [pp. 170–171].

These changes in the strength and functioning of the superego and ego are based at least partly on changes in the representational system. Both structures are based originally on the internalization of parental strictures and parental functions (12). As quoted above, superego growth requires toning down of parental idealizations. Similarly, ego growth requires a certain degree of internalized object loss as the regulating aspects of the parents are relinquished, and the child's independence develops in accord with new internalized representations of parental autonomy.

In summary, in Jacobson's (3) opinion: "During all of adolescence the psychic organization is in a state of fluidity as never before or since" (p. 177). This makes the adolescent psychic structure particularly vulnerable to regression and overstimulation, which may very well be dealt with via defensive regulation by mood discharge, as described above. It is Jacobson's view that hyperactive moods may be stimulated by the increased sexual and aggressive tensions, and that asceticism and repentance may follow this. Narcissistic inflation may result from the resurgence of feelings of infantile grandiosity; but, alternatively, states of emptiness, inferiority, and depression may reflect feelings of object loss and isolation. "Evidently," Jacobson further wrote, "the adolescent's erratic emotional vacillations mirror his swings from temporary disorganization, drive deneutralization and regression causing a partial dissolution of old psychic structures, to dramatic mental progression leading to drive reneutralization and to a restructuring and reorganization of the psychic systems" (p. 180).

## THE STUDY

In earlier studies (1960s) we obtained a self-description by adolescents of their psychological world (13). Subsequently (in the late 1970s), we applied the previously developed self-descriptive personality test—the Offer Self-Image Questionnaire (OSIQ) (14, 15) to measure the self-system of adolescent males and females between the ages of 13 and 18 years.

The OSIQ is a useful tool for the following reasons: Self-concept is a particularly crucial personality dimension for adolescents (5, 16-18) and has been directly correlated empirically with the mental health and adjustment of adolescents (19, 20); it is also a relatively stable personality trait from adolescence onward (21, 22).

Because it has often been observed clinically that adolescents who can master one aspect of their environment may fail to adjust in other areas, the OSIQ was constructed to evaluate adolescents' functioning in all areas considered important in their psychological world. This questionnaire was originally developed to provide a reliable means for selecting a representative group of modal or "normal" adolescents from a larger group of high-school students (23). It has been used in many studies, and has been administered to over 20,000 teenagers in Australia, India, Ireland, Israel, and Mexico, as well as the U.S.A. The populations sampled include both sexes, younger and older teenagers, the "normal" and psychiatrically disturbed, physically ill, and delinquent, in rural, urban, and suburban areas, in about 90 metropolises.

The OSIQ's reliability and validity have been established (23). It contains 130 items, grouped into 11 scales that describe the important areas in the adolescent's psychological world (e.g., impulse control and family relationship). The scales were theoretically constructed; therefore, their internal validity is high.

METHOD

The original OSIQ did not include a mood scale; therefore, we reassessed its 130 items to determine which could be theoretically grouped under a "mood scale." We selected items which we believed belonged together conceptually, and chose the 10 that best exemplify good or bad feelings about the self (Table 1). Obviously, we were limited in our selection by the original 130 items; we believe that certain aspects of mood (such as dysphoric/euphoric) are rather well covered, but the moods of guilt and anger, for example, are not.

To eliminate as many intervening variables as possible (such as social class), we studied only "normal" middle-class midwestern males and females. Our main interest was to compare two indices: age: younger (13 to 15 years) *versus* older (16 to 18 years); and gender. Each subject was asked to score for each item. Scores for each of the 10 items were subjected to chi-square analysis and ANOVA (analysis of variance), with five degrees of freedom: $\chi^2 = 11.07 = p < 0.05$, and $\chi^2 = 15.08 = p < 0.01$. The first four samples had been studied during 1962–1969 (Table 2). Analysis across time was undertaken by study in the late 1970s of four additional samples from a midwest suburb (samples 5–8 in Table 2).*

* We are grateful to Drs. A. C. Petersen and I. Gitelson, who shared their data with us.

## TABLE 1

## THE MOOD SCALE*

1.  Most of the time I am happy. (#32)
2.  Sometimes I feel so ashamed of myself that I just want to hide in a corner and cry. (#36) Reversed
3.  I feel relaxed under normal circumstances. (#44)
4.  I feel so very lonely. (#66) Reversed
5.  I enjoy life. (#68)
6.  I keep an even temper most of the time. (#69)
7.  A job well done gives me pleasure. (#70)
8.  My parents are ashamed of me. (#95) Reversed
9.  Even when I am sad I can enjoy a good joke. (#100)
10. I frequently feel sad. (#130) Reversed

* Items for this scale were selected from the 130 included in the Offer Self-Image Questionnaire (23) (the number in parentheses is the item's number in the questionnaire). Each item is scored in the range 1 to 6; the lower the score the better the mood. For the reversed (negative) items, the score is reversed before it is computed.

## TABLE 2

## STUDY POPULATIONS OF "NORMAL" MIDDLE-CLASS ADOLESCENTS FROM MIDWEST SUBURBS

| Sample No. | Data Collected | Description of Sample* |
| --- | --- | --- |
| 1 | 1962 | 326 younger males |
| 2 | 1966 | 141 older males |
| 3 | 1969 | 278 younger females |
| 4 | 1966 | 154 older females |
| 5 | late 1970s | 40 younger males |
| 6 | late 1970s | 126 older males |
| 7 | late 1970s | 80 younger females |
| 8 | late 1970s | 1280 older females |

* "Younger" = aged 13–15 years; "older" = aged 16–18 years

As part of the construction of the mood scale we performed alphas (24) on the 10 items on each of the four samples from the 1960s. This showed acceptable internal reliability for each sample, though somewhat low for the young males (Table 3).

Discriminate analysis was applied to the items for both groups of samples to determine which item(s) correlated best with changes in time (13).

RESULTS

The most significant finding was the stability of mood recorded by the subjects overall (Table 4), although there was a trend for the girls, but not the boys, to consider themselves less moody as they grew older (i.e., the younger females described themselves as having more negative affect).

Investigation of the adolescents' self-description across time (Table 5) showed no significant difference in interaction with the 10-item set tested. However, for both sexes the generation effect was very significant ($p < 0.001$), indicating that today's adolescents do not feel quite as good about themselves as they did in the 1960s. Adolescent girls describe themselves as being sadder, lonelier, and easier to hurt. They are more sensitive to their internal affective world than the boys. This finding is true for young as well as old adolescents. Girls have a lower self-image than boys do. The difference between boys and girls was consistent throughout the years of our investigation. In general, we should stress again that the vast majority of normal adolescents tested were happy individuals who believed that they could cope adequately with their emotional world.

## DISCUSSION

The OSIQ differentiates significantly between normal, psychiatrically disturbed, and delinquent adolescents of both sexes at all ages. The standard deviation (SD) of the items is low, eliminating the possibility that subjects answer by alternately choosing extreme responses (the latter would yield the same means but higher SDs). Furthermore, 95% of all the adolescents we tested chose a score of 3 or 4 for all 10 of the items of the mood scale. These responses are on the positive end of the continuum. Had the respondents been experiencing mood swings, their answers should have fluctuated more between the positive and negative ends of the six-point scale.

The mood scale derived for this study is reliable and valid; its 10 items constitute an important part of the adolescent's psychological world as he or she perceives it. However, it has some limitations. The scale contains only 10 items and these relate to specific moods; certain affects, such as anxiety and guilt, are missing. A further drawback is the use of different cohorts; a developmental design where each group of adolescents was studied for 4 years and compared across time, would give more exact data.

## TABLE 3
## INTERNAL RELIABILITY* OF ADOLESCENT SAMPLES

| Sample | Age (years) | Alpha |
|---|---|---|
| 1. Younger males | 13–15 | .56 |
| 2. Older males | 16–18 | .75 |
| 3. Younger females | 13–15 | .76 |
| 4. Older females | 16–18 | .79 |

* Applying alpha testing (24).

## TABLE 4
## COMPARISON OF ADOLESCENT MOOD-SCALE SCORES*
## BY AGE, SEX, AND TIME

| | A: Samples 1–4 (1960s) | | | | B: Samples 5–8 (late 1970s) | | | |
|---|---|---|---|---|---|---|---|---|
| | Male | | Female | | Male | | Female | |
| Age Group | Mean | SD | Mean | SD | Mean | SD | Mean | SD |
| Younger | 2.04 | 0.58 | 2.13 | 0.69 | 2.12 | 1.57 | 2.27 | 0.68 |
| Older | 2.06 | 0.64 | 1.96 | 0.66 | 2.16 | 0.59 | 2.14 | 0.70 |

* The lower the score, the better the mood.
Two-way ANOVA: For A: Main effects not significant. Interaction effect significant at 0.03 level. For B: No significant effect.

## TABLE 5
## COMPARISON OF ADOLESCENT MOOD-SCALE SCORES*
## IN THE 1960s AND LATE 1970s

| | A: Younger Adolescents (13–15 yrs) | | | | B: Older Adolescents (16–18 yrs) | | | |
|---|---|---|---|---|---|---|---|---|
| | Male | | Female | | Male | | Female | |
| Time | Mean | SD | Mean | SD | Mean | SD | Mean | SD |
| Samples 1-4 (1960s) | 2.04 | 0.58 | 2.13 | 0.69 | 2.06 | 0.64 | 1.96 | 0.66 |
| Samples 5-8 (late 1970s) | 2.12 | 0.57 | 2.27 | 0.68 | 2.16 | 0.59 | 2.14 | 0.70 |

* The lower the score, the better the mood.
Two-way ANOVA: A and B: Time effect significant ($p < 0.001$). Sex effect and interaction effect not significant.

We are, of course, very aware that asking adolescents to respond to specific items concerning their selves, as opposed to letting them talk freely about themselves, limits the scope and nature of investigation. However, the use of specific items enhances the reliability of the data and permits group comparison of individual scores. In addition, we have found that adolescents in particular are psychologically aware; our studies of normal adolescents (23, 25) have shown significant correlations between the adolescents' self-image and the mental-health-professional assessment of them. We therefore consider it valid to use their self-description in this type of study.

The most significant finding was that mood as described by these normal adolescents was much more stable across developmental time-span than has been found in studies of psychiatrically disturbed or socially deviant populations; mood swings just were not part of the life experience of our subjects. There was a trend for the girls, but not the boys, to describe themselves as less moody with increasing age (Table 4). To put our finding in different words, if one were to come to know a young adolescent boy and girl well and to follow him or her through the teenage years, it ought to be possible to maintain a rather stable impression of the pattern of mood throughout that period. This would not be so in the case of psychiatrically disturbed or socially deviant adolescents.

Comparison of findings in the two sets of samples with time indicated that, in the 1960s, an adolescent got more pleasure from "a job well done" than he or she received from it a decade or more later. This difference showed up as a trend, but was not significant statistically. Items 3 and 10 were significant when the results of the 1960s and 1970s were compared. These items represent the affect of depression and the feeling of tension. The adolescent of the 1960s described himself as being happier and more relaxed. The differences were not dramatic, but they were consistent.

Returning to the main finding of our research, mood is a more stable part of the psychic apparatus among *normal* adolescents than studies of patients have led us to believe. Obviously, there are great differences between the self-image of psychiatrically and socially disturbed adolescents and that of normal ones. According to the psychodynamic literature, the onset of "moodiness" in adolescence reflects the re-emergence of infantile drives and increased demands on the ego for psychic regulation. Moods function as a means of controlled discharge of psychic tension; they are associated with adjustment, with a capacity to integrate and balance intrapsychic stimulation. Therefore, changes in mood patterns indicate a response to changing internal conditions. According to Jacobson (3):

> They [changes in the adolescent's moods] mirror his swings from temporary disorganization, drive deneutralization and regression, causing a partial dissolution of old psychic structures, to dramatic mental pro-

gression leading to drive reneutralization and to a restructuring and reorganization of the psychic systems [p. 180].

By contrast, the inability to experience mood shifts and changes is seen by Jacobson as a sign of psychopathology; i.e., a person with a weakened defensive organization is incapable of the variety of mood changes found in normal persons. This seems to be upside-down reasoning, as Jacobson and her colleagues have not studied normal adolescents; she is generalizing from experiences with patients. The findings in the present study necessitate a different theory (from Jacobson's) of the developmental psychology in normal adolescence. It seems to us that the self-system is formed earlier than previously assumed. In the mentally healthy, adolescence is not a second individuation process because this is not needed; any psychic reorganization that is necessary takes place unconsciously, without spilling into behavior or causing mood swings.

The finding that the adolescents in the later samples described more problems relating to mood can be explained in two ways: First, that today's teenagers indeed have more problems than did their peers in the 1960s; second, a hypothesis we tend to favor, that there is more acceptance today of psychiatry and mental health. The stigma formerly attached to personal problems or pathology is reduced, and therefore adolescents are willing to be more open than before about their feelings. This is particularly relevant when one studies the mood-scale items (see Table 1); they do not represent gross or even moderately severe psychopathology. In addition, in a parallel study (26) we found no change in the self-image of delinquent inpatients across 1969 to 1976. We stated:

> Given the range of different components of self-image assessed by the OSIQ, it may be somewhat surprising that a temporal trend was not observed. Despite certain limitations of sample size and the inherent individual variability of delinquent self-image scores, a robust effect of social change would be expected to manifest at least a diminutive effect in these data. We are led, therefore, to a consideration of the expectations regarding social change and delinquent self-image generated by differing theoretical positions [p. 99].

Thus the self-image of socially deviant adolescents stayed the same over the past decade. We believe that the self-image of mentally healthy adolescents also remained stable, and showed no significant sex-related differences through developmental time; it moved, though, to a psychologic position of greater awareness of internal feelings.

## SUMMARY AND CONCLUSIONS

In an attempt to learn more about the nature of normal mood development in adolescence, we examined data from our studies of the self-image of normal, middle-class American adolescents of both sexes. We compared the findings in younger and older age groups (13 to 15 and 16 to 18 years) in relation to gender, and in relation to time (data collected in the 1960s and late 1970s). Comparisons were also made with findings in psychiatrically disturbed and delinquent adolescents. Limitations of our method were reviewed.

The most striking finding was the relative stability of moods among the adolescents. The only significant difference was between subjects studied in the 1960s and late 1970s. Discussion focused on the relevance of our findings to theories of the psychological development of mood in adolescence. Finally, we tried to explain why the adolescents studied in the two periods described different mood states.

## REFERENCES

1. Hall, G. S. (1904), *Adolescence: Its Psychology and Its Relations to Physiology, Anthropology, Sociology, Sex, Crime, Religion, and Education,* reprint ed. Vol. 2, 1916. New York: Appleton.
2. Freud, A. (1958), Adolescence. *Psychoanal. Study Child,* 13:255–278.
3. Jacobson, E. (1961), Adolescent moods and the remodeling of psychic structures in adolescence. *Psychoanal. Study Child,* 16:164–183.
4. Jacobson, E. (1964), *The Self and the Object World.* New York: International Universities Press.
5. Blos, P. (1962), *On Adolescence: A Psychoanalytic Interpretation.* New York: Free Press.
6. Freud, S. (1915), The unconscious. *Standard Edition,* 14: 166–215. London: Hogarth Press, 1957.
7. Freud, S. (1915), Repression. *Standard Edition,* 14:146–158. London: Hogarth Press, 1957.
8. Jacobson, E. (1957), Normal and pathological moods: their nature and function. *Psychoanal. Study Child,* 12:73–113.
9. Kohut, H. (1971), *The Analysis of the Self: A Systematic Approach to the Psychoanalytic Treatment of Narcissistic Personality Disorders.* New York: International Universities Press.
10. Larson, R. (1979), *Adolescent Experience: Riding the Roller Coaster of Emotions.* Chicago: Michael Reese Hospital. (Manuscript)
11. Blos, P. (1970), *The Young Adolescent: Clinical Studies.* New York: Free Press.
12. Freud, S. (1923), The ego and the id. *Standard Edition,* 19:12–66. London: Hogarth Press, 1961.
13. Offer, D., Ostrov, E., & Howard, K. I. (1980), *The Self-Image of Adolescents.* New York: Basic Books. (In press.)
14. Offer, D., Ostrov, E., & Howard, K. I. (1977), *The Offer Self-Image for Adolescents: A Manual.* Special publication. Chicago: Michael Reese Hospital and Medical Center.
15. Offer, D., & Howard, K. I. (1972), An empirical analysis of the Offer Self-Image Questionnaire for Adolescents. *Arch. Gen. Psychiatry,* 27:529–533.

16. Block, J. (1971), *Lives through Time.* Berkeley: Bancroft Books.
17. Erikson, E. H. (1950), *Childhood and Society.* New York: Norton.
18. Masterson, J. F., Jr. (1967), *The Psychiatric Dilemma of Adolescence.* Boston: Little, Brown.
19. Rosenberg, M. (1965), *Society and the Adolescent Self-image.* Princeton, N.J.: Princeton University Press.
20. Offer, D., Marohn, R. C., & Ostrov, E. (1979), *The Psychological World of Juvenile Delinquents.* New York: Basic Books.
21. Engel, M. (1959), The stability of the self-concept in adolescence. *J. Abnorm. Soc. Psychol.*, 58:211–215.
22. Vaillant, G. E. & McArthur, C. C. (1972), Natural history of male psychologic health. I. The adult life cycle from 18–50. *Sem. Psychiatry,* 4:415–427.
23. Offer, D. (1969), *The Psychological World of the Teenager: A Study of Normal Adolescent Boys.* New York: Basic Books.
24. Cronbach, L. J. (1970), *Essentials of Psychological Testing,* 3rd ed. New York: Harper & Row.
25. Offer, D. & Offer, J. B. (1975), *From Teenage to Young Manhood: A Psychological Study.* New York: Basic Books.
26. Welsh, J. B. & Offer, D. (1978), Delinquent self-image and social change. In: *The Child in His Family,* Vol. 5: *Children and Their Parents in a Changing World,* ed. E. J. Anthony & C. Chiland. New York: Wiley, pp. 93–106.

# CHAPTER THREE

# HISTORICAL FORCES IN THE ETIOLOGY OF PSYCHIATRIC DISORDERS IN ADOLESCENCE

VIVIAN M. RAKOFF

## PREAMBLE

In the past the privileged allowed their sons (and rarely their daughters) an extended period of education and development between puberty and the responsibilities of a career and marriage; but it was only after World War I, and more notably after World War II, that a lengthy adolescence became a democratic option. Concomitant with this social change from aristocratic privilege to an almost universal psychobiological state of the urban middle classes, there developed new ways of being adolescent, with new rites of passage. No longer were the choices restricted to the limited career of the young m'lord expected to choose between attendance at an ancient university or being a military cadet. They were extended to the entire domain of leaving home, taking political action, traveling, and "finding oneself," and rejected all notions of context and history in the process of discovering an authentic identity (1-3).

Of course, I am stating the case paradigmatically: most young people proceed somehow through puberty, high school and college, and after a few fluctuations arrive at marriage and procreation. But the familiarity of the process should not obscure the fact that this new form of life career was the product of revolutionary changes and forces that created the massive social upheavals of the French and American Revolutions.

The same historical forces that created the contemporary Western way of being adolescent may have contributed to the characteristic forms of adolescent distress — anomie, narcissism, complaints of emptiness, loneliness, and existential despair. To the degree that the mass option of extended adolescence may represent an extraordinary social achievement of the Western world during the past 200 years, an understanding of the stresses on adolescents may clarify forms of social distress not necessarily confined to this age group.

Specifically, the democratic right to individual personality and identity developed from the destruction of historical context. For centuries, the aristocratic personality and identity evolved and was expressed within the contexts of clearly defined social relationships and securely defined place ("old" families lived on specified territory and took their names from places or positions); and the landless poor took their names from their crafts or familial identity in simple patronymics.

For most people, pre-capitalist societies were confining and oppressive, holding them from full personhood. In particular, almost all Americans (including Canadians) were immigrants or the descendants of immigrants who fled the context of a defined past; they fled from emperors, kings, dictators, and religious orthodoxy. In leaving behind the external and often tyrannical definers of who they were, they embraced the opportunity to define themselves, or at least the opportunity that their children might do so. They created a new mythology, a new complex of psychological and social structures that gave shape and meaning to life. This new myth replaced nationhood, class, language, ancestral landscape, traditional culture and custom, and the graves of their fathers; on this continent it took the form of a pluralist America that offered an open frontier both to the body and the sense of self. The ultimate freedom promised was, ideally, the right to define oneself, to unleash one's energy fully, even to live dangerously, if one wished.

American society expressed these ideas most explicitly and consistently, being heir to currents of political development that in England flowed like a strong and broadening stream, and in continental Europe exploded in the French Revolution. The new post-revolutionary, capitalist-individual man prefigured in Diderot's characterization of Rameau's nephew, a man released in fantasy from the defined modes of a court personage into the exciting and dangerous territory of "sincerity and authenticity" (4). Such a social mode was defined by the revolutionary expectation that one not only existed, but had the right to express one's true self. The task involved constant conflict: in place of fixed roles and certainties of the old context and a universe of predictable and relatively certain categories, there was the constant labor of perpetual movement and redefinition in the direction of increasing self-consciousness, the Hegelian *Auf-heibung* (5). This meant elevating oneself by stages to an ideal, fully realized and fully conscious personhood.

Those of us who work with adolescents will recognize that these historical injunctions and opportunities, offered to all the freed citizens of post-revolutionary Europe and America, sound very similar to the task of adolescence defined by Erikson as establishing a sense of identity (6). Its defined opposite and failure were sensed long ago by Nietzsche and Kierkegaard, the one exultantly and the other in despair. The exciting prospect of establishing a true self, of making a personally defined journey through life, was accompanied by the twin dangers of social alienation and loss of moral significance.

## HISTORICAL DETERMINANTS OF PSYCHOPATHOLOGY

The emphasis of this paper is on history and culture and their possible relationship to clinical pathology; however, this does not deny the importance of other interpersonal and intrapersonal relationships so significant in the formation of the individual, his capacity to withstand stress and relate to others. My concern is with the problem of how the great ship of history gets into the bottle of the individual psyche. In particular, I shall define some determinants of the psychopathology of patients who are severely depressed, confused about their roles, and preoccupied with ethical and moral concerns against a background of poorly defined values; I will also consider those at the extreme who are labeled as narcissistic, borderline, or sociopathic personality disorders. The following clinical vignettes may help to focus these concerns.

### CASE 1

J., a young woman in her early 20s, was referred to me by her ex-lover. She had asked urgently for an appointment, but on arrival had made it clear she had come only because she been advised to. She had made up her mind to carry out a plan to join a major religious organization in India, and had already bought a one-way ticket. She said: "I want to do something drastic about my life."

In telling me about her plan, J. used the characteristic language of the seeker after mystical experience — she wanted to discover her true self and live on a plane above the mundane. The girl felt that her life and the lives of those around her were frivolous and insignificant. Convinced that proper training and a change in attitude would enable her to break through to a vivid spiritual experience which would make sense of her life, she said, "I want to renounce everything because there is no meaning to the physical world . . . I have to find people who are thinking of spiritual things all the time."

J. appeared unaware that her preoccupations, language, and plans were stereotypic. She was surprised I could supply phrases to describe her aspirations and experience, feeling (like many of us) that her choice and plans were completely personal, in fact, eccentric. She was not psychotic or sociopathic; she had always worked, and had used drugs sparingly. During a period with a religious sect in New York she had had some experiences that provided the model for her quest, which she described as a search for "a blissful, detached state, an inner joy."

Inquiry into J.'s family history produced a story that bewildered me. Both her parents, she said, were very loving and supportive. ("I had a very good childhood. We did lots of things together, and we lived in the family.") When I asked her what she meant by this, she elaborated, "We had to [live in the family] because we moved every 3 or 4 years." Then she described her various dwellings, all of which had been in a prosperous part of the city. Asked about the family's community attachments, such as church, political party, and social networks, she replied, "I can't think of anything. My parents were and are agnostic. They never went to church and I don't think they really were much involved in politics."

J. comes from an Anglo-Saxon family. She is not underprivileged. Her decision to go to India seems wild. Were it not for the fact that there are many like her, who go to India or some local variant of an India, it would be difficult to categorize her other than as an adventure-seeker of a curious variety.

CASE 2

M. has a completely different background. His father (A.) spent part of his childhood in a concentration camp. After the war, when his father was 14 years old, he was sent by his mother and stepfather to live on a kibbutz in Israel. Once, after his parents had visited him, A. was depressed and the kibbutz psychologist counseled him: "Don't be sad about your stepfather. He seems like a nice man." The boy had replied quite openly that he felt he had lost all connection with his parents.

M. was born in Israel, and when he was 10 years old the family moved to Canada. Here they severed ties with the past: M. and his older brother did not receive a Hebrew education, and the family did not join any identity-giving organization—synagogue, political party, or social group.

M., 16 years old, was referred to me because of difficult behavior, poor work at school, and disciplinary problems. From the parents' point of view the most significant problem was M.'s trouble with the police because of dealings in marijuana. M. himself seemed unconcerned about his difficulties, made light of them and often told lies about his drug dealing. The mother was concerned and appeared genuinely warm. The father was a bit excitable but not pathologically so, and his comments on his work were flat and direct: "I hate my work. I always say I hate my work. It's a living." M.'s older brother, who had had behavioral problems in the past, was now a hyperconforming model boy. M. was sad and lackadaisical, had flat affect, and was very casual about his problems. He said his only pleasures came from acting, music, and smoking "pot."

CASE 3

K. was 17 years old, good-looking, and an only child. In appearance, K. was a display board of the fundamental problem in today's troubled adolescents. He dressed in a style reminiscent of the 1960s, a "street crazy" costume that reflected his striving for individuality, but so clearly a fashion of a given time and place. He wore a fancy new brown fedora ("My mother gave it to me for Christmas") with a razor-blade in the hatband; his hair was long and unkempt; a tie was knotted around his neck inside his open shirt collar, and the tie pin was a short length of chain pinned with small brass safety pins; his jeans were scrawled with obscenities and the names of rock-music groups; attached to his belt was a heavy steel chain, fastened to the loop with a heavy brass lock; and pinned to his clothing were buttons advertising rock groups, and one plain blue coat-button about the size of a silver dollar, ordinary and with no inscription.

K. was not delinquent, stupid, or underprivileged. Why, then, was his clothing such a collection of aggressive, ironic references? He wasn't a "punk-rocker" (although he would have liked to look like one) or a cocaine addict. The plain blue button, taken from his mother's sewing box, seemed as significant to him as the ones bearing slogans. When I asked K. the meaning of his ornaments, chains, and deliberate inversions of conventional dressing, he professed not to know what I was talking about, and then said: "I do it because I like it." When I pressed him a bit further, asking if he couldn't see that the chains, the punk-rock safety pins, and the dirty words scrawled on his trousers were aggressive signals, he replied: "No. . . I just do it for fun."

Further discussion showed that K. did not consciously know why he was doing these things. He had adopted some of the styles of the '60s without any knowledge or interest in the ideologies of the peace movement, student rebellions, or even the drug culture; he wore the tag ends of fashions and recent mythologies without participating in them. When I asked, "Where do you see yourself 20 years from now?" the most I could get from him was a vague wish to run a rock-music band.

At 17, K. belonged to no church, no political movement, and had only a few friends with whom he was mildly rebellious against his elite private school. K. was born on the West Coast, had lived on the East Coast, and had had many moves in Toronto. His family structure was small in scope. The only consistent figure was his mother, an intelligent, troubled woman who had known loneliness and rootlessness, and felt she had no reference group. She had recently joined a church, and there found congenial people. She regarded the friendships as more important than the systems of religious belief.

The origin of K.'s lack of direction, the panoply of ironic signals he didn't understand, and his lack of any sense of shape to his life, could be construed in purely personal, psychopathologic terms. His biography contained all the necessary elements. There was no effective father; and K. and his mother had moved repeatedly, with the result they had lost all consistent community as well as their extended family. The boy's life was a classical recipe for a chaotic superego; but in fact, in most of his functioning, K. did have standards of conduct. It was as though he had been deprived of part of his existence, and in his behavior and dress was trying to satisfy this missing part.

If K. were alone, or even very unusual, he would be interesting enough; but children like K., J., and M., in their depression, lack of direction, and lack of public structure, are characteristic of an entire class of adolescents. They appear to be casualties of the same great historical forces that bequeathed us many of our most valued freedoms and opportunities.

These adolescent patients are typically depressed, restless, and apathetic, wanting creative jobs without applying themselves to disciplined preparation or study. They are hungry for authority, meaning, and belief. On close examination, one finds distortions of communication, oddities of personality, and some sadistic behavior; but none of these seems sufficient cause for the degree of presenting symptoms.

I believe there is a common thread in the distress evidenced by the three young people I have described. I shall try to unravel it to show how it may contribute to the complex and varied pathologies presented by such adolescents. It should be borne in mind, however, that this is only one contributory factor; it does not invalidate other factors of crucial importance in psychiatric disorder, such as the subtle entanglements of distorted family functioning, the sad tyranny of genetic predisposition or organic diathesis, and the major contribution of economics.

J. and M. came from families which seemed to provide everything for human growth — affection, food, education, and money. Further, the families encouraged creativity. For example, J. described her brother as a very creative person in film photography, and M.'s mother, while threatening to throw him out of the house, pleaded with him to go to a theater school: "To develop his great talent as an actor."

All three children share one other important characteristic: their families, like thousands of others in our culture, are restless movers, detached from the contexts of place, history, religion, and even communal customs. M.'s father was repeatedly detached during his lifetime—from country, family, personal and group history; the one piece of information he gave repeatedly was how much he hated his work. J. moved within her language and within one city, and her disruption was less obvious than M.'s, but her family had moved frequently and had no group attachments. Perhaps it is also significant that J.'s father is president of an advertising agency. J.'s very name is cute and fashionable, detached from history and any mythical structure, reflecting only an ephemeral fashion. She was named by whim, like actresses are named or soap is labeled—to be appealing in the marketplace. In this she is unlike the boys, who also have become alienated, but were named for figures important in the shared myths of their society.

Although these three adolescents are representative of our contemporary clinic populations, in their curious social detachment they are reminiscent of Durkheim's descriptions of anomic individuals at the turn of the century. A study of Durkheim's concern with the relationship of anomie to suicide (7) may shed light on some of our concerns. Whether described as detachment, alienation, or anomie, this state expresses itself in the most serious form of psychopathology—the desire to kill oneself. The absence of a nurturing community, at either the level of intimacy or for more distant social relationships, can precipitate a psychic "illness unto death."

Contemporary Canadian suicide data support this observation (8). The lowest suicide rates in Canada are in Newfoundland, where people are the poorest in the country and move least often. By contrast, the highest rates are in the big cities and the Western provinces, where prosperity is at its highest and physical movement is at its greatest: these cities and provinces attract the rootless and adventurous. But there is another group that must be considered, because it confounds some of our assumptions and supports others. Garfinkel and Golombek (9) have drawn attention to the high suicide rates of Indian adolescents in western Ontario. These young people are not alienated from place or community—they live in reservations within clearly defined community and family context. They are not poorer than their urban counterparts and, curiously, their rate of employment is higher than that of a comparable sample of urban Caucasian adolescents in Ontario. However, they are alienated, in a crucial way that relates them to Durkheim's anomic figures and migrants to British Columbia: their sense of historical continuity has been destroyed, their culture having been invalidated by the powerful patterns of the dominant society.

The above comments bring into sharp focus the human need for connectedness and for a coherent sense of the self within a culture and within history. In short, in the case histories cited, in anomic alienated suicides, and in joiners of cults, there appears to be a need for community and mythology, and for public sources of identity, guidance, and personal significance.

This need for association of the individual (and the family) with society is recognized almost universally. In modern psychiatry, however, the tendency has been to dramatize the opposition of the individual to society. Beginning with Freud's classical formulations of *Civilization and Its Discontents* (10), and epitomized in Norman Brown's (11) pronouncement that "History is the accumulated result of repression," commentators have emphasized the individual's opposition to oppression by the group and historical forces. In *Life against Death* (11) Brown wrote: "Repression transforms the timeless instinctual compulsion to repeat into the forward-moving dialectic of neurosis which is history" (p. 93). The universal association of human beings in complex societies has been defined in the language of neurosis and conflict, a language echoed by Róheim, Reich, and Marcuse (12).

Erikson unquestioningly placed the developing individual within concentric rings of relationships (6), each a required component of possible achievement during successive stages of human growth. It is now accepted that there are necessary phases of development—achievements, capacities, and skills—that need not be placed within the context of neurosis and conflict. In addition, there is a possible model, i.e., Winnicott's "transitional object" (13), for the nonconflicting relationship of the individual to a single other, which allows association as well as individuation. This refers to the class of things which are not mother *or* child, but contain the mother sufficiently to be talismans of safety and trust for the child, and are not only the child's possession, but also part of him. This mechanism permits the symbiotic mother-child entity to become the mother and child, and constructs the parent-child relationship without destroying the infant's security or basic trust.

We should also note another important aspect of these transitional objects. They exist within a transitional space, a species of psychic territory where one can play and create, and in which one is released from emergency and pure necessity. Winnicott suggested it is the space in which culture is elaborated, i.e., the source of the tradition that must be established before there can be original action. Thus the transitional objects allow the child to move from the mother's side, and range free within the ecos (e.g., the household, the family) regardless of the size of the "household" in that society.

A child is loved for itself alone. The child does nothing for its keep; its existence is sufficient cause for an entire complex of rewards. The substrate for this extraordinary altruism is the bonding that connects the helpless (dirty and noisy) infant to the receiving, responsive parent. It is this structure of mutually accepting relationship, of bonding to intimates and not strangers, of notions of family, home, "my parents," and "my siblings," which provide for the needs of intimate man as the "unclothed" person. Ultimately it provides the template for expectation of the self and others in intimate relationships. Stemming from its origins in the parent-child bonded pair, it generates the capacities for affection, erotic intimacy, and transgenerational protectiveness in the fully developed adult.

Beyond the context of the family is the universal context of a containing society, i.e., the world of the "clothed" (public) human being, which is governed by different expectations from those that operate in the intimate family cluster. In its public context, bonding is sustained by membership in a group established through shared belief systems and, crucially and commonly, by a common language. Mere existence is insufficient to generate reward in this context, which instead respects and rewards performance. Competence, power, political ability, and social graces are within this domain of the evolution of the life-career. At the most commonplace level, membership in such public groups (using a common language and respecting shared assumptions) provides an essential component of identity; it comprises the sense of self as perceived by the individual and as recognized by others. Thus, one is not only John or Jane but also a Torontonian, an Ontarian, a Canadian, a somebody defined by place and culture as well as by early and intimate experience.

Alienation is detachment from a social structure. A central life task is the ability to move back and forth between the context of family (the world of the "unclothed") and one's society or public ("clothed") existence. Structures are needed that bond the individual to the receiving group in much the same way the infant needs to be bonded not only to its initial mothering figure, but to its household. Such mechanisms must embody shared perceptions, signaling systems, and common expectations not only of immediate action; they must also embody the significance of the individual and his society in time.

## LANGUAGE, TRANSITIONAL OBJECTS, AND IDENTITY

In particular, transformations of language may reflect transition from the intimate family to the public community. A city such as Toronto provides daily confirmation that the children of immigrants speak in the accent and style of the receiving society, particularly the school, rather than those of the parents. This sharing of the common social language becomes the basis of communal empathy, much as early bonded relations within the family constitute the basis of personal empathy.*

*This is not the place to elaborate the profound effects of the use of Greek, which bonded many peoples of different races and religions into one Hellenistic civilization. In

Henry Roth's novel *Call It Sleep* (14) contains a poignant reminder of differences between the language of intimacy and that of the community. One theme concerns the relationship between a young immigrant Jewish boy in New York and his loving mother and tyrannical father. For most of the novel the mother is represented as a woman of poetic, subtle speech, never defined as being English or Yiddish. When the boy is lost and the mother goes to the police station for help, Roth transliterates her speech into her actual language, broken English. She is no longer subtle and poetic, but is diminished into a primitive user of English as a lingua franca. At that moment she is obviously a lesser human being both in her own perception, and as perceived by the Irish policemen who hear her within the framework of ethnic comedy and stereotype.

Kohut stated (15): "The capacity for empathy belongs, therefore, to the innate equipment of the human psyche and remains to some extent associated with the primary process." However, this formulation fails to recognize the empathic sharing of public affective experience, which becomes the substrate for the powerful emotions of group identity. Although a common language is a primary vehicle in adults as well as children for the specific bondedness of the nonintimate world, it is only one of the factors (albeit an early and necessary one) for the development of a sufficient sense of social security.

Rather, the history of the communal context permits projection of the self into the future because it establishes continuity with the past, a shared sense of ethical values, and an elaborate compendium of social rituals involving games, art forms, and visual symbols (such as flags, national colors, and badges); all of these are necessary to the self's identity within the world.

In this regard, Winnicott elaborated his concept of the transitional object as follows (16): "In favourable circumstances the potential space (between mother and child) becomes filled with the products of the baby's own creative imagination. . . . Given the chance, the baby begins to live creatively and to use actual objects to be creative into. If the baby is not given this chance, then there is no area in which the baby may have play or cultural experience; then there is no link with the cultural inheritance and there will be no connection with the cultural pool." He went on to say: "It is these cultural experiences that provide the continuity in the human race which transcends personal existence. I am assuming that cultural experiences are

---

Canada, the use of a common language may be a more powerful definer of identity than almost any other social structure, including class, religion, and country of origin. Furthermore, when the language is used to create a literate culture, and to record the group's mythology, it becomes a central survival mechanism for group-identity capable of resisting the onslaught of other powerful cultures.

in direct continuity with play, the play of those who have not yet heard of games." For Winnicott, the transitional object—the thing that is "not me, not mother, but which is between us"—embodies the child's trust that if his mother leaves him, she will return. It is the foundation of security in the personal world.

This extremely important concept can be extended readily to objects that define our personal space and security in the world—mementos and ornaments, the walls of our homes, furniture—although these may represent second- or third-order elaborations of initial transitional objects. It seems to me that the concept as outlined by Winnicott can be extended even further to explain the painful effects of loss of history, and the yearning for history that is so common in psychiatrically disturbed patients. Winnicott's concept accounts for the growth of personal security and for the object-seeking patterns of personal, emotional, and intimate development. It accounts for the development of security for the "unclothed" person, and most clearly for mechanisms that allow a growing infant to move away from his mother. Although Winnicott's concept did not account for the similar but separate process of functioning in the "clothed" (public) world, I believe it is possible to take the thought a stage further, into the second sphere of human relating beyond the family—the world of the public social identity, the great complex of experiences shared by the individual with others in his society.

Is there in fact a separate sphere of relating that requires a separate set of transitional structures? Why should the maternal-child interspace not contain enough potential elaboration to satisfy both the object-hunger (seeking) of the intimate personal life and that of the sphere beyond the family? Simply citing the case histories and the cultural pathology referred to above only begs the question. Further, it could be claimed that rootless fathers and historical severance are insufficient basis for a new elaboration of a profound and respected concept. It may be more useful to consider again the mechanism of language. Géza Róheim (17) reduced language to: "The word used to summon the mother when the child is hungry" (p. 169). And Freud (18) said: "When someone speaks it is as though a light goes on." Language may be these things, but it is also another: it links the individual to his community. The transformation of language into an instrument of intricate social communication suggests a series of ego-necessities specifically developed for nonintimate relating—a genetic anlage for an expected community, analogous to the genetic behavioral structures that anticipate the nurturing mother. These ego-necessities, which are essential for the development of the public self, but have been neglected in psychiatry, are perhaps best perceived as essential when they are lacking, as in the K.s of our day.

If we accept this hypothesis, we can understand the yearning for history that takes the form of searching for roots, real or imagined; or it may express itself in the current fad for places of entertainment that pretend to be somewhere else in time or space (such as old-time music halls, and restaurants styled as Italian trattoriae or English pubs). The latter is not a frivolity, but also relates to the painful sense of rootlessness that afflicted the adolescents described above. Furthermore, the need for ethical norms or, at its most elaborate, membership within a religious community, is no longer perceived as "comparable to a childhood neurosis" (19) but as the expression of a fundamental need, deprivation of which will lead to neurosis. Fortunately, an understanding that myths are necessary sense-making structures and are indeed essential "manifestations of mental functioning" (20) has replaced earlier excessively simple perceptions of the role of the religious life for the individual.

The development of a secure sense of reality within the context of family appears to relate to the maternal function, whereas movement into society may be mediated by what Mahler (21) called "the first stranger" (the father), and relate to the paternal function. In most societies the males have been responsible for defense and preservation of religious continuity, and have been the principal political heroes. The loss of paternal authority, commented on by Marcuse (22) and more recently by Lasch (23), has accompanied a growing failure to recognize the distinction between the domains of intimacy and public existence, and in some cases has led to Sennett's (24) "tyrannies of intimacy." Sennett specifically regrets the loss of social forms of behavior and the decreased energy expended on public concerns, when working for what one wants is not differentiated from loving. Furthermore, both Sennett and Lasch have emphasized that failure to recognize the area of public action as different from that of intimate action does not increase a sense of social security. Rather, it leads to an increase in (what is now fashionably labeled) narcissism, particularly the terror of death, solipsistic evaluation of events, vacillation between feelings of omnipotence and all-pervading weakness, and an incapacity for complex and formal modes of public behavior.

## HISTORY AND TODAY'S ADOLESCENTS

Why are there so many adolescents today whose disorders contain some element of historical or ethical rootlessness? A sense of social connectedness and a sharing of structures of language and history constitute ego-needs of maturing individuals, and are the basis for a feeling of security and the development of a realistic career. For a long time the pluralism of democratic societies in North America and Western Europe provided their own mythology; immigrants did not need to continue their subscription to an identity determined by religion or country of origin. In the post-war years, however, the myth of American liberalism faltered, and all the shared institutions of patriotism and social forms were threatened, eroding supports necessary for maintaining the psyche. It is significant that many who were leaders of student rebellions and political movements in the 1960s are now among the most vocal subscribers to new endeavors that promise rediscovery of the self. For example, Jerry Rubin (a leader in the Chicago riots a decade ago) has reported adherence to one therapeutic enterprise after another (25); and Rennie Davis (a student activist when at Columbia University) became a leading supporter of the Maharaj Ji. It seems that when there is a social void, the hunger for belief will embrace any form that is offered.

Young people such as J. who join cults are probably the most serious victims of failure to receive social values. Saul Levine has reported (26) that many very disturbed adolescents seem to benefit by joining fringe religious groups. Those who before their conversion could not work, get up in the morning, or wash themselves, or were drug addicts, suddenly are able to get up. They scrub floors, beg in the streets, and labor for little money, in return for certainty.

Cults, as opposed to established religions, are ethical groups that declare their rejection of a society they consider bankrupt and empty. They represent a historical discontinuity with the life of the individual and group; therefore they cannot be tainted by the loss of values that may have determined the convert's pathology in the first place. (Hinduism is not a cult in India because it is part of the history of that society; but in North America it lacks historical basis and therefore may take on the characteristics of a cult.) Thus a cult separates an individual from his embedding society; it does not enhance his function within his society or help him return to it. A cult promotes an intense group identity via explicit authoritarian rules for action, elaborate rituals of behavior, and even in some instances, a uniform or mode of dress that separates the individual from his former context; and it is usually ensured by denial of freedom to discuss the community's precepts or the leader's right to authority.

Today's disturbed adolescents, adrift with no historical context in a society they cannot appreciate or even comprehend, are seeking beliefs and meaning in life that will satisfy their ego-needs. A cult acts as a prosthesis; it fills the void in the convert's life, and restores the sense of personal significance that derives from history, public behavior, and myth. Thus context, albeit changed, is restored. But such surrender of historical and personal privileges does not allow the individual to cope with the unremitting and difficult, but necessary, task of moral choice and personal growth within the community.

## CONCLUSIONS

Acceptance of the right to individual liberty and personal identity, coupled with economic and social opportunity previously confined to young upper-class males, has extended the option of a lengthy adolescence to the middle classes. This has had many positive results, but the negative components are beginning to emerge. Thus, particularly in North America, the right of self-expression has enjoined suspicion and rejection of historical (usually oppressive) contexts and beliefs; this distrust has resulted in uncritical dismissal of public values and community connectedness. For many, individual freedom and the right to self-determination have shaded into anomie and a sense of purposelessness.

Psychiatric theory, perhaps unwittingly, has aided this devaluation of history and public life. Theoretical and clinical concern has focused almost exclusively on the individual's experiences within the narrow domain of the family and erotic life; and young persons, particularly adolescents, have been viewed as constantly in opposition to an oppressive society.

The need for ethical norms and social connectedness does not arise from infantile neuroses; these components are as psychologically necessary as satisfactory intimate relationships. Furthermore, Winnicott's concept of the transitional object can be extended. As conceived, it leads to an understanding of the process whereby the infant gains sufficient support and security to move from the mother's side into the household and the family. But it is now postulated that a secondary set of transitional structures, i.e., language and factors stemming from the group's history, may mediate the necessary move from the family (the community of intimacy) to the public community (the general culture), without which the individual is incomplete.

Unfortunately, renewed awareness of the need for context, sense-making mythologies, ethical standards, and shared cultural symbols, also brings the danger of devaluation and discredit of hard-won rights of individual self-determination. We need to remind ourselves that there have been times when "the world of the clothed" has been too dominant, and that it was a world of repression, intense social conformity, and gross hypocrisy. Thus both elements are necessary: our increasing awareness of the need for the development of the public person should not displace equally relevant concerns for intrapsychic and interpersonal individuation.

## REFERENCES

1. Ariès, P. (1962), *Centuries of Childhood: A Social History of Family Life.* New York: Knopf.
2. Hall, G. S. (1904), *Adolescence: Its Psychology and Its Relations to Physiology, Anthropology, Sociology, Sex, Crime, Religion, and Education,* New York: Appleton, 1916, Vol. 2, reprint ed.

3. Rakoff, V. M. (1978), The illusion of detachment. *Ann. Am. Soc. Adolesc. Psychiatry*, 6:119–129.
4. Trilling, L. (1972), *Sincerity and Authenticity*. (Charles Eliot Norton Lecture Series, 1969–70.) Cambridge, Mass.: Harvard University Press.
5. Weisberg, P. (1979), Adolescence, *Auf-heibung*; dream's end and dream's beginning. Presentation to the Canadian Eastern Seaboard Conference, American Society of Adolescent Psychiatry, Winnipeg, Man.
6. Erikson, E. H. (1963), *Childhood and Society*, 2nd ed. New York: Norton.
7. Durkheim, E. (1897), *Suicide: A Study in Society*. Trans. J. A. Spaulding & G. Simpson. Glencoe: Free Press, 1951.
8. Sakinofsky, I., Roberts, R., & Van Hauten, A. (1975), The end of the journey: a study of suicide across Canada. Presentation to the 8th International Congress on Suicide Prevention, Jerusalem, Israel.
9. Garfinkel, B. D. & Golombek, H. (1980), Suicidal behavior in adolescence. *This Book*.
10. Freud, S. (1929–1930), Civilization and its discontents. *Standard Edition*, 21: 64–145. London: Hogarth Press, 1961.
11. Brown, N. O. (1959), *Life against Death: The Psychoanalytical Meaning of History*. Middletown, Conn.: Wesleyan University Press.
12. Robinson, P. A. (1970), *The Freudian Left: Wilhelm Reich, Geza Róheim, Herbert Marcuse*. New York: Harper & Row.
13. Winnicott, D. W. (1958), *Collected Papers: Through Paediatrics to Psycho-analysis*. London: Tavistock Publications, pp. 229–231.
14. Roth, H. (1934), *Call It Sleep*. New York: Cooper Square, 1970. Reprint ed.
15. Kohut, H. (1966), Forms and transformations of narcissism. *J. Am. Psychoanal. Assoc.*, 14:243–272.
16. Winnicott, D. W. (1967), The location of cultural experience. *Int. J. Psychoanal.*, 48:368–372.
17. Róheim, G. (1962), *Magic and Schizophrenia*. Bloomington: Indiana University Press.
18. Freud, S. (1905), Three essays on the theory of sexuality. *Standard Edition*, 7: 130–243. London: Hogarth Press, 1953.
19. Freud, S. (1927), The future of an illusion. *Standard Edition*, 21:5–56. London: Hogarth Press, 1961.
20. Goddard, D. (1970), Lévi-Strauss and the anthropologists. *Social Res.*, 37:366–378.
21. Mahler, M. S., Pine, F., & Bergman, A. (1975), *The Psychological Birth of the Human Infant*. New York: Basic Books.
22. Marcuse, H. (1965), Repressive tolerance. In: *A Critique of Pure Tolerance*, by R. P. Wolff, B. Moore, Jr., & H. Marcuse, 1969. Boston: Beacon, pp. 81–123.
23. Lasch, C. (1979), *Haven in a Heartless World: The Family Besieged*. New York: Basic Books.
24. Sennett, R. (1977), *The Fall of Public Man*. New York: Knopf.
25. Rubin, J. (1977), *Growing up at Thirty-Seven*. New York: Warner.
26. Levine, S. V. (1978), Youth and religious cults: a societal and clinical dilemma. *Ann. Am. Soc. Adolesc. Psychiatry*, 6:75–89.

# CHAPTER FOUR

# TRANSCULTURAL ASPECTS OF AFFECTIVE DISORDERS IN ADOLESCENTS: THE BRAIN-FAG SYNDROME IN AFRICAN STUDENTS

RAYMOND PRINCE

> *Les étudiants africains étudient d'une façon formelle, quasi littérale, et aboutissent, après un surmenage journalier constant, à une fatigue telle qu'une réaction dépressive aiguë les guette.*
>
> —R. van Eeckhoutte (1), (pp. 157–158)

The time is not yet ripe for a review article on transcultural aspects of affective disorders in adolescence since the data are not available. However, it is generally agreed that many problems (e.g., depression, rebelliousness) that are encountered in Western youth are not necessarily the result of biological changes, but spring rather from social and cultural factors. Mead (2, 3) found this to be the case in her pioneering studies in Samoa and New Guinea; Swift and Asuni (4) expressed the same opinion about village adolescents in Africa:

> Adolescence in the village appears to be a relatively uneventful phase of development, so psychological problems rarely come to the atten-

tion of the doctor. Traditional systems seem to provide considerable security for these youths; their transition from childhood to adolescence to adulthood takes place without much distress. "Passage rites" are helpful and identity develops naturally and easily with the assistance of customary practices [pp. 113–114].

Whether this generalization is valid for all African cultures seems highly questionable, and information about adolescents in parts of the world not subject to Western influences is scattered and fragmentary (5, 6). In any case it is clear that most non-Western cultures today increasingly involve their adolescents in Western types of schooling, which often requires massive cultural change resulting in profound alienation (7, 8).

I shall focus on one type of affective disorder in adolescence that has received considerable attention in the past 20 years, and is intimately linked with the imposition of Western education systems upon non-Western adolescents, the "brain-fag syndrome." It is exceedingly common and often incapacitating among students in Africa south of the Sahara, as though a black depressive cloud descends upon perhaps one-quarter to one-half of the adolescent high-school and university populations, blocking their progress in education. I shall describe the nature of this syndrome and its epidemiology, and discuss theories of its etiology.

## CHANGES IN PSYCHIATRY IN AFRICA

The late 1950s and early 1960s saw sweeping developments in psychiatry in Africa, where many countries were gaining independence after a half century of European colonial adminstration; some 23 African countries became independent between 1957 and 1968, including Ghana, Nigeria, Kenya, Zaire, Tanzania, and Chad. African colonial psychiatry had dealt largely with patients of the "mental-hospital" type, particularly the "criminally insane." In 1953, Carothers published his controversial book, *The African Mind in Health and Disease* (9), in which he summarized writings on African personality and psychiatric disorders during the colonial era. Among his conclusions was that the Africans behaved like lobotomized Europeans!

Harbingers of the new, post-colonial approach to psychiatry in Africa were two papers by Thomas Lambo (10, 11). Lambo, trained at the Maudsley Hospital in London, England, was the first Nigerian psychiatrist, and a pioneer in the development of psychiatric outpatient clinics. He began to write about psychoneuroses as well as psychoses in Africans; he also brought a new and refreshing social and cultural approach to African psychiatry.

### BRAIN-FAG SYNDROME

I arrived at Aro Hospital, Abeokuta, in September 1957, to work in Lambo's outpatient clinics in Ibadan and Abeokuta, and after a few months became aware that the vast majority of patients attending the clinics were male adolescents.* Furthermore, it gradually dawned on me that there was a pattern of symptoms in these students different from anything I remembered treating in Canada. The following letter illustrates the characteristic complaints.

Ibadan, Jan. 19, 1959

Dear Sir:

The main reason why I am writing this letter is to complain to you sir that for some time now I have been sick and the sickness is rather mental in nature. A little before the time of the flu epidemic in 1957, I was doing a course leading to an oversea examination. I developed a severe headache and when the hospital treatment was not improving the condition I had to stop reading. This state of affairs continued for months. The headache developed unusual characteristics I never experienced before. It developed in such a way that I seemed to be tired of life. As time went on I made the following observations: it would appear as if there were something walking about in the center of my head. The aching seemed to burn me on the head and I experienced unusual heaviness of the head. The most surprising thing was that except when I slept this headache would not leave me. I also noticed that if I walked in the sun without protecting the head the headache got much more serious just within less than a minute. Life was becoming almost unbearable. . . .

When I consulted private doctors, I was told that I was suffering some sort of nervous or mental disease as a result of a worried mind. At this stage actually all that had happened to me was enough to give me a worried mind and I would not disagree with the suggestion that the state of my mind was contributing to my troubles. At one stage I visited an optician on the recommendation of a doctor. At another stage I resorted to a native cure. But all to no avail. Even at one stage my ordinary seeing of text books would scare me. Any attempt to read even newspapers made my head heavier within a few minutes.

I fervently look up to you for help. May God Almighty help you too sir. I am anxiously look for a reply.

Yours sincerely

I listened to dozens of such descriptions before I realized that this was a distinctive syndrome. In retrospect, it is puzzling, as I had gone to Nigeria specifically to study the effects of cultural factors on the forms of psychiatric

---

* I use a rather broad definition of adolescence to cover the period between childhood and the assumption of adult responsibilities, such as marriage and self-supporting work.

disorder. But the culture-related syndromes described in the earlier literature were much more flamboyant — *koro, latah, amok*, and so forth. The pattern I was seeing was not so exotic; in fact, at first I debated with myself whether or not Canadian adolescents also suffered from such symptoms. But what were these sensations of burning in the brain and of worms crawling in the head, the inability to read, the loss of meaning of words — all made worse by reading? Perhaps most important was the fact that, unlike Canadian students' study-inhibitions, which arise in the context of life stresses, the Nigerian students' symptoms seemed to result simply from studying. In fact, the students themselves referred to the condition as "brain-fag," believing that the syndrome was due to overworking the brain.

My first publications on brain-fag (12, 13) listed five major categories of symptoms: unpleasant head symptoms (pain, burning, crawling sensations, etc.); difficulties with vision (blurring, ocular pain, excessive tearing, etc.); inability to grasp the meaning of printed symbols and, sometimes, of spoken words; poor retention of information; and fatigue and sleepiness despite adequate rest. The following quotation exemplifies some of these symptoms:

> When I read I don't assimilate anything, and when they teach me my mind won't take it in. I forget the word that I am supposed to be looking up in the dictionary as I am leafing the pages. If I pick up a book, it seems as if a child of five is looking at it, the letters don't mean anything. I have forgotten all that I learned; it is as if I have no past. If someone talks to me, it doesn't go to my brain. When I talk it doesn't seem to come from my brain at all, but just from my mouth. I will sit down to read, but I am just helpless, my mind isn't there. I cannot write. I have given up writing letters and send telegrams instead. I will read several pages and realize I can't remember a thing I have read.

Many authors have essentially confirmed these components of the syndrome, not only in Nigeria (14, 15) but also in other African countries — including Uganda (16, 17), Liberia (18, 19), and the Ivory Coast (20). Boroffka and Marinho (14) further noted in a large number of their cases, deterioration in the school's language (English) during the acute phase, and its restoration to normal after recovery. Other observers have not mentioned this deterioration, but it is consistent with the illness's regressive aspects suggested by the loss of meaning of written words "as if a child of five were looking at the page." It is clear that the syndrome is a very stereotyped one which is widespread south of the Sahara (4), and may be common in other developing countries. I saw a clear-cut case in a Ugandan Indian in Montreal; and Nicholas Malleson (personal communication, 1960) reported its occurrence in Indian, Siamese, and Malayan Chinese students, but not in

Caribbean Blacks, in Britain. Edourdo E. Krapf (personal communication, 1960) reported that he had seen the syndrome in Argentinian students at Roman Catholic seminaries, and Chakraborty and Mallick (21) described cases in students in northeast India. I saw no cases among students during my two years in Jamaica as a WHO consultant, but have seen several among African students in Montreal.

The prevalence of brain-fag in adolescents is not known; no adequate epidemiologic studies have been conducted. As a preliminary approach, in April 1959 I distributed a short questionnaire to the principals of five major Nigerian secondary schools for completion by all students. The introduction to the form read as follows:

> It has been found that many students suffer to a greater or lesser extent from certain symptoms of a nervous nature which interfere with or are related to study and reading.
>
> We are at present carrying out some research on the nature and cause of this disturbance with a view to obtaining some understanding of it and arriving at suitable treatment or preventive methods. It is of importance to determine how prevalent in the student population these symptoms are and we are therefore asking you to fill out this questionnaire as completely and accurately as possible to assist us in this study.

The students were asked to state their age, tribe, and occupation of father and mother, and to answer the following questions.

1. Have you ever suffered from burning or pain or other sensation in the head associated with reading or study?
2. Have you ever suffered any other unpleasant body sensations that appear to be related to study? If so, please list them.
3. Give an estimate of the average amount of time you spend in study (apart from lectures) in hours per day.
4. Are you satisfied with your general efficiency and retentiveness in study? Please check appropriate opinion: (a) fully satisfied, (b) moderately satisfied, (c) not satisfied.

The findings (22) (see Table 1) indicated that a very high proportion (54%) of the students experienced symptoms of the brain-fag type. Furthermore, almost 90% responded that they were less than fully satisfied with their "general efficiency and retentiveness in study." Age did not seem to be a factor, as analysis of the results showed the proportion of students with symptoms to be roughly the same from 12 to 21 years (Table 2). In addition, all five schools surveyed were for boys only, so this study sheds no light on the sex factor.

TABLE 1
SELF-REPORT SURVEY OF BRAIN-FAG SYMPTOMS
STUDY OF FIVE NIGERIAN SECONDARY SCHOOLS(22)

| School | No. Students | % Students Complaining of Symptoms | % Students Fully Satisfied with Study | Mean Age (yrs.) | | Study Time (hrs.) | |
|---|---|---|---|---|---|---|---|
| | | | | With symptoms | Without symptoms | With symptoms | Without symptoms |
| A | 139 | 32 | 27 | 18.4 | 18.3 | 3.22 | 3.12 |
| B | 163 | 54 | 9 | 16.0 | 16.4 | 2.24 | 2.20 |
| C(1) | 160 | 57 | 11 | 14.2 | 14.2 | 3.14 | 3.29* |
| C(2) | 142 | 58 | 10 | 17.9 | 18.0 | 3.64 | 3.37 |
| D | 159 | 57 | 6 | 16.9 | 16.9 | 3.33 | 3.01 |
| E | 81 | 64 | 6 | 17.0 | 16.9 | 2.41 | 2.07 |
| Total/Mean | 844 | 54% | 11.5% | 16.7 yrs. | 16.7 yrs. | 3.00 hrs. | 2.84 hrs. |

* School C(1) students without symptoms reported *more* hours of study than those with symptoms. (This discrepancy was due to 6 students without symptoms who studied 7, 8, or 9 hours per day!) When correction was made, mean study time for students without symptoms was appropriately reduced.

## TABLE 2
## SELF-REPORT SURVEY OF BRAIN-FAG
## SYMPTOMS BY AGE (21)

| Age (yrs.) | No. Students | % Students with Symptoms |
|:---:|:---:|:---:|
| 12 | 17 | 41.2% |
| 13 | 39 | 59.0% |
| 14 | 73 | 64.6% |
| 15 | 116 | 56.9% |
| 16 | 121 | 62.0% |
| 17 | 168 | 52.4% |
| 18 | 151 | 53.6% |
| 19 | 79 | 46.8% |
| 20 | 54 | 37.0% |
| 21 | 13 | 69.2% |
| 22 | 4 | 50.0% |
| Total/Mean | 835* | 54.5% |

* Nine of the 844 students did not state their age.

The data in Table 1 indicated only slightly more complaints of symptoms with longer study hours. Perhaps the most striking finding was the variation between the schools. School A, a private Catholic college in Lagos, whose students were from families with a high proportion of literate parents, had a far lower frequency of reported symptoms and a much higher proportion of students fully satisfied with their studies than school E. The latter was a government secondary school in a predominantly Ibo area of Nigeria; its students had a below-average proportion of literate parents. The other three schools had roughly equal percentages of symptomatic students and, excluding D, of students satisfied with their studies. This variation could reflect differences in the school milieu or, more likely, relate to socioeconomic factors.

The only other survey relating to brain-fag that I am aware of is Wintrob's (18) systematic social/psychological interview survey of all first-year students at the University of Liberia. The author's aim was early detection of emotional disorder and referral to the students' mental-health clinic. Some 20% of the students suffered from brain-fag, and half of these were referred for treatment. On the basis of this survey we might conclude that the prevalence of such symptoms is lower among university students, at least in Liberia, than among high-school students; however, the author gave no information on his methods, so comparison of this kind is not warranted.

A final epidemiological point: brain-fag has been reported as much commoner in males than in females (13-15). This finding may simply reflect the far larger population of males in high schools and universities in all African countries at their present stage of development. However, Boroffka and Marinho (14) found that this factor alone could not account for all the difference in prevalence in their study. Although the male:female ratio for brain-fag was 34:1, at the same Lagos outpatient clinic the male:female ratio for other psychosomatic disorders in the same age range was 2.9:1, and the ratio of students attending high school in the area was much closer to 2:1. Similarly, German and Arya's study (23) of students attending Makerere University in 1966–1967 showed a prevalence of psychiatric problems (brain-fag in the majority of cases) only half as great among girls as among boys; and German, Assael, and Muhangi (16) found a somewhat similar difference among Kampala high-school students with brain-fag. German and Arya (23) attributed this to the much greater difficulty for girls to obtain higher education; they reasoned that this would weed out girls with a potential for brain-fag or other problems, leaving a healthier group of girls than boys.

It is interesting that only 3 of 23 detailed case histories of brain-fag among African students reported in the literature relate to females (19, 20), none of which describes typical brain-fag symptomatology, whereas several clear-cut cases in Hindu women have been reported from India (21). We can tentatively conclude that brain-fag affects African males disproportionally; the cultural reasons for this are not clear.

IS BRAIN-FAG A DEPRESSIVE EQUIVALENT?

Increasingly, those writing about the brain-fag syndrome have been impressed by its depressive elements. In my own first contact with the disturbance, however, I characterized it as a psychoneurotic syndrome with prominent somatization of conflict and hysterical elements (disorders of special sense and memory). I did note that "patients have an unhappy, tense facial expression," and that in 2 of the 10 original cases there were marked depressive aspects with suicidal fantasies (13). In those days there was considerable debate as to whether depressions existed in African cultures. In the colonial era, depressions were regarded as distinctly uncommon, but by the late 1950s they were being detected with increasing frequency (24, 25). During my 1959 survey of high-school students (22) the word "depression" appeared in only 1 of the 844 completed questionnaires, and depressive complaints were noted in only 2 others ("feeling of death at all times and thinking that this world is not the place for me"; and "thoughts of my dead mother, and thought of my poor condition"). By contrast, 34 students complained of fear, nervousness, anxiety, palpitation, restlessness, or uneasiness. Thus, anxiety complaints were much commoner than depressive complaints, although both types of affective complaints were quite uncommon compared with somatic and cognitive ones.

In 1961, during the three-month Cornell-Aro survey of mental health in Nigeria (26), I had the opportunity to discuss the syndrome with a psychoanalyst, Charles Savage; and he carried out brief psychotherapy with a brain-fag patient. He was strongly of the opinion that the syndrome was a depressive equivalent, an opinion with which, after a time and with some reluctance, I concurred. My earlier success in treating several intractable cases of brain-fag with electroconvulsive therapy increased my willingness to accept this conclusion.

In our later joint presentation (27), Charles Savage and I argued that brain-fag had not been considered a manifestation of depression because "an excessively narrow definition of depression had been employed which laid too much emphasis upon self-recrimination and upon verbalization of depressive feelings." It should be pointed out that a similar controversy, over whether syndromes of somatic complaints and minimal verbal expression of depressive affect and guilt should be called depressive, is occurring in regard to Chinese patients (28, 29). Indeed, in a world context, it appears that the textbook picture of depression in Western psychiatry is the exception rather than the rule, being limited to persons with high levels of Western-type education and usually a Judeo-Christian religious heritage. The African picture of depression, as manifest in brain-fag, is closer to the world norm.

Success in treating brain-fag with antidepressant drugs provides further evidence that it is a depressive condition. The first study of this type was reported by Neki and Marinho, in 1968 (15). Although both men worked in the same hospital in Lagos, Nigeria, Neki was impressed by the depressive aspects of the syndrome and treated his patients with antidepressants, whereas Marinho thought the anxiety aspect predominant and administered tranquilizers. Comparison of outcomes showed that patients treated with antidepressants responded significantly better than those treated with tranquilizers. (The therapist variable was not controlled in this study; further double-blind research is needed.)

Most later authors have emphasized the depressive aspects of brain-fag, at the same time remarking on the frequent accompaniment of a major degree of anxiety (16, 17, 19, 20, 23). The consensus is that antidepressant drug therapy is the preferred treatment, but that anxiolytics and electroconvulsive therapy provide better responses in some cases.

In recent years, Lehmann (20) and Minde (17) have found group relaxation therapies highly effective. Lehmann (20), pointing out the preponderance of somatic symptoms in many African psychiatric disorders (including the brain-fag syndrome), introduced somatic relaxation therapy, conducted with groups of four to eight students. He noted that many patients considered this form of therapy more acceptable than verbal psychotherapy, because they perceived it as approaching the problem where it resided—in the body; after time, however, the patients were able to talk about subjects of concern to them.

Minde (17), having identified 25 Ugandan high-school students with brain-fag whose symptoms had not responded to prolonged high doses of antidepressants and anxiolytics, discontinued all drugs and started group therapy. Since a major request that emerged was "to learn to relax," Minde introduced group relaxation techniques. Another major topic of discussion was the students' anger at not being given drug therapy; they found it difficult to understand that their symptoms could be due to tension and anxiety, and felt, rather, that they had a definite illness that called for medical treatment. Despite this complaint, half the students reported some relief of symptoms; of these, half experienced great relief. However, these reports of good response to group relaxation therapy probably do not help us to decide whether we are dealing with an anxiety-based or depressive illness.

## DISCUSSION

A puzzling feature of brain-fag is the usual failure to detect a precipitating factor other than excessive study (4, 13, 14). Many Western high-school students complain they are depressed or cannot study because they find the curriculum irrelevant or the teachers or subjects boring; they often skip classes, fail subjects for lack of interest, and may become high-school dropouts. African students, on the other hand, are very highly motivated, study excessively long hours, and greatly fear they may *have* to leave school. As Boroffka and Marinho noted (14): "The complaints of the teacher ever and again is never laziness of the student but his staying up late at night to read." Further exploration of the scholastic problems of Western high-school students usually reveals that the student is depressed chiefly because of an unhappy home life, or that the difficulties are part of a more profound neurosis or character problem (30). Although such interpersonal problems and neuroses are occasionally identified in African students (19, 27), they are extremely uncommon.

Thus the question remains why the reading or study of books causes African students to be depressed. Two explanations have been offered: the "forbidden-knowledge" theory and the "ego-energy" theory.

### THE FORBIDDEN-KNOWLEDGE THEORY

This theory, first advanced by Savage and Prince (27), holds that study involves the African student in an act of betrayal of his own culture. This betrayal may be more or less conscious, depending upon the degree of Westernization of his culture. Wintrob (8, 18) described four stages through which non-Western cultures may pass in their attitudes toward Western education for their young:

1. *Opposition,* during which the elders of the group strongly oppose education because it involves giving up traditional ways, and undermines their own traditional positions of power and control.

2. *Ambivalence,* during which the adults begin to see the need for some degree of Western education for their children, to enable them to act as cultural brokers between their culture and Western agents; however, they still oppose higher education.

3. *Selective valuation,* during which the adults see education of a single member of their family as an important source of income and prestige. They strongly encourage one of their brighter children to attend school or university, and by investing family money in his education, exert considerable pressure upon him to succeed.

4. *Projective identification,* when the values of the group have shifted to regard Western education as very prestigious, and there is general denigration of indigenous values.

Most African cultures today seem to be moving toward the stage of "selective valuation," or even perhaps "projective identification." Other cultures, particularly those with strong Islamic influences, remain in the "opposition" or "ambivalence" stages.

One of the overriding values of African cultures is that members should live in accordance with custom, and behave in a way acceptable to one's family, group, and ancestors. To be rejected by one's family, including one's ancestral relatives, is tantamount to social death. Even in cultures at the "projective identification" level, there still seems to be a profound unconscious need to please one's ancestors (27). The following case report of a 22-year-old Yoruban male with typical brain-fag, is illustrative. Of special relevance is the mode of onset.

> When he was about 18 years old and attending secondary school he began to have bad dreams. He had no brain-fag then, but observed that he had the bad dreams only immediately after he had been reading or studying. In the dreams he was being beaten by a crowd of unknown people. They would beat him with their hands, but he was unable to recognize exactly who they were. During the dream he would be very frightened, and when he awoke his body would be sore all over. At first he gave up reading or studying during the evening,

but when the pressure of school made it necessary for him to study at night and the dreams recurred, he consulted a native healer. After a time the dreams disappeared. The patient believed that this was the result of the medicines administered by the healer. About 6 months later, however, the symptoms of brain-fag appeared and prevented any further study. The dreams did not recur.

The dream of being beaten (often by masqueraders, called *Egunguns*, who represent the ancestors) is common in circumstances where a person is not living in accordance with custom, or is failing to abide by the wishes of the ancestors. The following life history of a diviner is illustrative.

> In 1915 I was a service man and went to East Africa. Before I went there and after my father died I became a Christian and forgot Ifa [traditional divination system] though I knew it having learned it from my father. Still though, all the time I was a Christian I used Ifa power and Ifa words but kept it secret saying I was a Christian and believed in the power of the Psalms and of Jesus Christ.... Then I returned to Nigeria and worked as a trader.... On one occasion I was trading in the bush and I came to a village where there was a small boy who had passed out. There and then I got out my Ifa equipment, uttered the right words and he woke up. The boy's parents gave me five shillings and invited me to spend the night with them.
>
> In the dead of night that night my father came to me in a dream. He taunted me saying, "Why don't you use the words of Jesus Christ?" Then my father wrestled with me all night long, used a whip and razor and cut me all over the body. When I awakened my body was sore all over.

This diviner went on to describe further dreams in which his father and Orunmila (an ancient prophet, the originator of the Ifa system) tormented him and tried to force him to relinquish Christianity and return to Ifa. Finally he became extremely ill:

> For 10 months I couldn't get up off my bed; my wife was carrying me about. I couldn't eat, but could only take snuff. I had rashes all over my body like sand. I was very thin and got two sores on my back from lying on the floor all that time.

Ultimately, he gave up Christianity. He returned to Ifa and recovered his health.

Bascom (31) reported a similar phenomenon in the case of the chief priest of a Yoruban *orisha*\* cult.

---

\* *Orisha* is a Yoruban word for an ancestral spirit which presides over a religious cult group. Each family traditionally belongs to one or more *orisha* groups. Orisha Ikire is a healing deity who is also believed to cause his followers to go mad if they do not worship him properly.

Akire was brought up as a Christian. He was taught to read and study the Bible, but during his sleep he dreamed that someone came and beat him. From the whip that his tormentor used, he knew that it was Orisha Ikire, the *orisha* of his sibling. After flogging him, and telling him to continue reading the book, Orisha Ikire would leave. But Akire knew that the *orisha* wanted him to give up Christianity and return to him.

Akire dreamed this three times at night and then a fourth time during the day when he was dozing over the book. Akire saw himself lying face down on the ground again being beaten and tormented. The *orisha* ran his middle finger into Akire's back and then went on whipping him. Afraid that he would go mad, Akire gave up studying the Bible and became a worshipper of Orisha Ikire [p. 18].

This type of pursuit by offended ancestors of deities, often associated with illness or misfortune, is not uncommon in the life histories of Yoruban traditional healers. A person engaged in Western-type activities fails to prosper or suffers illness, and is warned by dreams or through consultation with a diviner that he must return to traditional ways. When he does return, his illness disappears and he prospers. Two other examples have been reported (32, 33).

Of interest in this connection is an annual ceremony (the Itapa festival) I witnessed on February 4, 1962, in Ile Ife, the religious capital of Yorubaland. This ceremony evidently commemorates the overcoming of an ancient intrusion into the Yoruban world of some alien culture that introduced books. Early in the evening the town chief and several elders enact the ceremony of "burying the books." The next night, groups of elders go about the town inquiring: "Have you seen the book?" If the answer is "Yes, I have seen the book," that person is flogged (in earlier times he was killed). Just what alien civilization is being recalled in this ceremony has been forgotten, but clearly it long antedated the introduction of Christianity in the early 19th century.

In light of these rituals and dreams, the forbidden-knowledge hypothesis holds that the adolescent students unconsciously see themselves as betraying their ancestors by reading Western books and attending Western schools. This is true even though their families — and, indeed, contemporary Yoruban culture in general — advocate Western education. Although supported by their living kin, at a more basic level these adolescents are depressed and suffer brain-fag because they are offending their forefathers by delving into this alien lore, and worshipping foreign gods.

THE EGO-ENERGY THEORY

This explanation of brain-fag holds that a significant proportion of

African students suffers a basic lack of ego energy to accomplish the task of education. The lack may result from the tremendous amount of energy required to cope with change to a new culture, and more specifically, to overcome discontinuities (34) that occur during the shift from the collective and cooperative culture of their childhood to the highly individualistic and competitive requirements of Western education. Early travelers' anecdotes refer to such energy deficiencies in various non-Western cultures; for example, Burchell in 1822 noted of his Bushman interpreter (35):

> I have sometimes been obliged to allow Machunka to leave off the task [of explaining his language], when he had scarcely given me a dozen words, as it was evident that exertion of mind, or continued employment of the faculty of thinking, soon wore out his powers of reflection and rendered him really incapable of paying any longer attention to the subject. On such occasions he would betray by his listlessness and the vacancy of his countenance that abstract questions of the plainest kind soon exhausted all mental strength and reduced him to the state of a child whose reason was yet dormant. He would then complain that his head would begin to ache [p. 24].

Von Spix and van Martius, in 1923 (36), described a Brazilian informant in similar terms:

> No sooner have we begun to ask him questions about his language than he becomes impatient, complains of headaches, and shows that he finds sustained effort of such a kind impossible [p. 24].

And van Eeckhoutte (1) seems to be making a similar comment about university students in Zaire (see introductory quote, this chapter), which translated reads: "African students study by memorizing the text word for word, and end up, after constant daily overexertion, in a state of exhaustion bordering on an acute depressive reaction" (p. 156).

If we are to take brain-fag students at their word, the usual series of events is: first, hard intellectual work; second, the appearance of brain-fag symptoms; and third, only later, because of their inability to study, the experience of anxiety or despair over continuing their education. With the Western student, on the other hand, the order is much clearer: first, disturbing interpersonal events; second, emotional upheaval; and third, only later, "study inhibition" or an "interest disorder" (37, 38); the latter forms only one facet, and most often a rather minor one, of the overall illness.

One might in fact call the brain-fag syndrome an ego disease, a designation suggested by Dr. Savage (27). This would distinguish it from other types of psychoneuroses in which the ego is only *secondarily* crippled (the

primary manifestation being an emotional disturbance based upon unconscious conflicts). Theoretically, in such psychoneuroses the ego becomes
depleted when energies habitually employed for high-level functions (e.g.,
perception, interest, recollection, abstraction, problem-solving) are diverted
for neurotic defensive purposes. In the brain-fag syndrome, however, the
ego is depleted of energy by the tasks of acculturation, not because of neurotic conflict.

The brain-fag syndrome seems to reflect the ego's lack of sufficient energy to cathect the ego apparatus and external data necessary for the task of
education. It appears that the more abstract the intellectual task, the greater the ego energy required to accomplish it. In conditions of health, an ego
which is not called upon to make the acculturation effort seems to have a
more than adequate supply of ego libido for any intellectual task.

Research findings in alien Western-type settings provide some support
for the ego-energy hypothesis. Most authors (13, 14, 17, 20, 22) have found
that the students most prone to brain-fag are those who come from the least-
Westernized families, for whom adaptation to the alien culture is most
arduous. Lehmann (20) reported brain-fag commonest in "those who were
the first ones to leave family and village to go to high school" (p. 47).

The theory of brain-fag as an ego disease or primary ego disturbance
recapitulates earlier discussions in Western psychiatry about the etiology of
neurasthenia. This condition was first described in 1869 by Beard (39), who
considered it a functional abnormality of the nervous system. He thought
neurasthenia involved a pathologic decrease in nervous energy, and was
precipitated by all activities that lead to overexertion and exhaustion, particularly the increased pace and heavy demands of modern life. Symptoms
described by Beard included weakness, headache, backache, inability to
concentrate, insomnia, gastric disturbances, impotence, and premature
ejaculation. Some authors have emphasized the effects of mental work; for
example, in 1878 Erb wrote (40): "Mental overexertion can often. . . lead to
neurasthenia"; he singled out "very exacting professions, and difficult mental work, especially when it involves working at night" (p. 392). Most authors also implicated excessive masturbation and coitus interruptus (41).

Freud took very little interest in neurasthenia early in his career, regarding it as basically a physical illness with few psychological implications
(41); at the same time, it was thought to be resistant to psychotherapy. Later, because of his view of the importance of sexual factors in the genesis of
hysteria, and the prevailing opinion that masturbation was a major etiological factor in neurasthenia, Freud began to study the condition more closely. First, he separated neurasthenia from anxiety neurosis: he speculated
that neurasthenia resulted from excessive masturbation, and anxiety neurosis from coitus interruptus. Freud included both in his classification of

actual neuroses (i.e., illnesses resulting from current problems), in contra-
distinction to the neuropsychoses (i.e., hysteria and obsessional neurosis,
resulting from adverse childhood experiences). Furthermore, he regarded
the actual neuroses as physiological disturbances, the neuropsychoses as
basically psychological in origin (40).

At this stage in his thinking, Freud would probably have regarded
brain-fag as an "actual" neurosis akin to neurasthenia. In this connection it
is of interest to consider the sexual lives of students who experience brain-
fag; nearly all of my brain-fag patients were young unmarried males
between 15 and 25 years of age. Apart from my own early observations
(13), little attention had been paid to the subject. At that time, I noted:

> Many of them say that they have given up dealings with women to
> allow themselves to give their full energies to their studies. Impotence
> was complained of in several cases. In one case, the symptoms began
> during masturbation. Another patient reported that he experienced
> orgasm during the writing of an examination [p. 561].

Lehmann much later reported the following statement by an 18-year-old
college student (20): "While writing compositions, I passed out semen.
That happened four times. It made me very frightened" (p. 47). One of my
patients noted a dramatic relief of symptoms after he married.

Of course, Freud's early views were superseded long ago. When Jones
(42) asked Freud why no one ever saw actual neuroses anymore, Freud replied that he himself no longer saw them, but that he had seen them at the
beginning of his practice! It is of course possible that neuroses were in fact
different in the days of Beard and Erb and of Freud when he was young; it
is even possible that the trend toward industrialization in the Western world
in the latter half of the nineteenth century produced social conditions similar to those in Africa during the first half of the twentieth century. A study
of the evolution and ultimate disappearance of the concept of neurasthenia
in Western psychiatry might thus prove relevant to our understanding of
"brain-fag" and its development.

## CONCLUSIONS

Although our understanding of the brain-fag syndrome is still very incomplete, progress during the past 20 years suggests the following:

1. Brain fag is a stereotyped psychiatric syndrome, generally held to
be a depressive equivalent.

2. It affects perhaps 20–40% of high-school and university students
in very diverse cultures across Africa south of the Sahara; it also occurs,
to an unknown extent, in the Indian subcontinent and other developing
countries.

3. Its frequency is sex-related, being disproportionally high among males. It also seems to vary directly with the level of Westernization of the culture native to the student.

4. Antidepressant drugs and group relaxation therapy appear to be the most efficacious treatments.

However, much further investigation is needed, especially in relation to the following areas:

1. What is the epidemiology of brain-fag—particularly its variation in relation to gender and age or education level? Does brain-fag also occur in elementary school children, and in adults who are studying intensively to further their efforts at adjustment to an alien culture? Is school milieu a major factor when class level and the level of adjustment to a new culture are held constant?

2. What are the essential etiological or exacerbating factors of brain-fag? What constitutes the depressive nature of the syndrome? What part do interpersonal problems, as opposed to excessive study, play in the genesis of brain-fag? Does the sexual life of students with brain-fag differ from that of unaffected students? To what extent is brain-fag related to removal or change from the home environment or simple "homesickness?" How important is the forbidden-knowledge theory as manifest in dreams and fantasies, or the symbolic meaning of the stereotyped symptom pattern? What is the role of associated sleep disorders? Why does the syndrome afflict males more commonly than females?

3. What are the most effective treatment procedures? Can group education techniques be successfully introduced to prevent brain-fag in schools? Should group relaxation techniques be incorporated into the school program as a preventive measure?

These and other compelling questions about the epidemiology, etiology, and treatment of brain-fag have yet to be answered.

## REFERENCES

1. Van Eeckhoutte, R. (1958), Brève note contributive au problème de l'hygiene mentale et des étudiants. In: *Mental Disorders and Mental Health in Africa South of the Sahara.* CCTA/CSA–WFMH–WHO Meeting of Specialists on Mental Health, Bukavu, Congo, March 1958. London: Commission for Technical Co-operation in Africa South of the Sahara, pp. 156–157.
2. Mead, M. (1928), *Coming of Age in Samoa: A Psychological Study in Primitive Youth for Western Civilization.* New York: Morrow.
3. Mead, M. (1930), *Growing Up in New Guinea.* New York: Morrow.
4. Swift, C. R. & Asuni, T. (1975), *Mental Health and Disease in Africa.* Edinburgh: Churchill Livingstone.
5. Whiting, B. B., Ed. (1963), *Six Cultures: Studies of Child Rearing.* New York: Wiley.
6. Masserman, J. H., Ed. (1969), *Youth: A Transcultural Psychiatric Approach.* New York: Grune & Stratton.

7. Wintrob, R. M. (1969), Rapid socio-cultural change and student mental health. *McGill J. Educ.*, 4:174–183.

8. Wintrob, R. M. (1970), Rapid socio-cultural change and student mental health. *McGill J. Educ.*, 5:56–64.

9. Carothers, J. C. (1953), *The African Mind in Health and Disease: A Study in Ethnopsychiatry.* Geneva: World Health Organization.

10. Lambo, T. A. (1956), Neuropsychiatric observations in the western region of Nigeria. *Br. Med. J.*, 2:1388–1394.

11. Lambo, T. A. (1960), Further neuropsychiatric observations in Nigeria. *Br. Med. J.*, 2:1696–1704.

12. Prince, R. H. (1959), The brain-fag syndrome in Nigeria. *Rev. Newsletter Transcult. Res. Ment. Health Prob.*, 6:40–41.

13. Prince, R. H. (1960), The "brain-fag" syndrome in Nigerian students. *J. Ment. Sci.*, 106:559–570.

14. Boroffka, A. & Marinho, A. A. (1962), Psychoneurotic syndromes in urbanized Nigerians. (Manuscript.) Abstract: (1963), *Transcult. Psychiatr. Res.*, 1:44–46.

15. Neki, J. S. & Marinho, A. A. (1968), A reappraisal of the "brain-fag" syndrome. Presentation to the Second Pan-African Psychiatric Conference, Dakar, March 5–9, 1968. Lagos, Nigeria: Pacific Printers.

16. German, G. A., Assael, M. I., & Muhangi, J. (1970), Psychiatric disorders associated with study in the mid-adolescent years. Unpublished; presentation to the Second Pan-African Psychiatric Workshop, Mauritius, 1970, pp. 131–135.

17. Minde, K. K. (1974), Study problems in Ugandan secondary school students: a controlled evaluation. *Br. J. Psychiatry*, 125:131–137.

18. Wintrob, R. (1971), The cultural dynamics of student anxiety: a report from Liberia. In: *Report on Seminar/Workshop on Psychiatry and Mental Health Care in General Practice*, ed. A. Boroffka. Ibadan, Nigeria, pp. 1–12.

19. Thebaud, E. & Rigamer, E. F. (1976), Some considerations on student mental health in Liberia. *Afr. J. Psychiatry*, 1:227–232.

20. Lehmann, J. P. (1972), Le vécu corporel et ses interprétations en pathologie africaine. A propos des inhibitions intellectuelles en milieu scolaire. *Rev. Med. Psychosomat.*, 14:43–67. Abstract: (1973), *Transcult. Psychiatr. Res.*, 10:53–57.

21. Chakraborty, A. & Mallick, S. A. (1966), Headache (A cross cultural study). *Ind. J. Psychiatry*, 8:101–108.

22. Prince, R. H. (1962), Functional symptoms associated with study in Nigerian students. *West Afr. Med. J.*, 11:198–206.

23. German, G. A. & Arya, O. P. (1969), Psychiatric morbidity amongst a Uganda student population. *Br. J. Psychiatry*, 115:1323–1329.

24. Collomb, H. & Zwingelstein, J. (1961), Depressive states in an African community. In: *Conference Report of the First Pan-African Psychiatric Conference in Abeokuta, Nigeria*, ed. T. Lambo. Ibadan, Nigeria: Government Printer, pp. 227–234.

25. Prince, R. H. (1968), The changing picture of depressive syndromes in Africa: is it fact or diagnostic fashion? *Can. J. Afr. Studies*, 1(2):177–192.

26. Leighton, A. H., Lambo, T. A., Hughes, C. C., Murphy, J. M., & Macklin,

D. B. (1963), *Psychiatric Disorders among the Yoruba*. Ithaca: Cornell University Press.

27. Savage, C. & Prince, R. (1967), Depression among the Yoruba. In: *The Psychoanalytic Study of Society*, Vol. 4, ed. W. Muensterberger & S. Axelrad. New York: International Universities Press, pp. 83–98. Presentation to the Scientific Meeting of the American Psychoanalytic Association, St. Louis, May 1963. Also in: *Transcult. Psychiatr. Res.*, 1:46–48.

28. Singer, K. (1975), Depressive disorders from a transcultural perspective. *Social Sci. Med.*, 9:289–301.

29. Kleinman, A. M. (1977), Depression, somatization and the "new cross-cultural psychiatry." *Social Sci. Med.*, 11:3–10.

30. Zamanzadeh, D. & Prince, R. H. (1978), Dropout syndromes: a study of individual, family, and social factors, in two Montreal high schools. *McGill J. Educ.*, 13:301–318.

31. Bascom, W. R. (1944), The Sociological Role of the Yoruba Cult Group, Memoir no. 63. Washington, D.C.: Am. Anthropolog. Assoc.

32. Prince, R. H. (1961), Some notes on Yoruba native doctors and the management of mental illness. In: *Conference Report of the First Pan-African Psychiatric Conference in Abeokuta, Nigeria*, ed. T. A. Lambo. Ibadan, Nigeria: Government Printer, pp. 279–288.

33. Prince, R. H. (1964), Indigenous Yoruba psychiatry. In: *Magic, Faith, and Healing: Studies in Primitive Psychiatry Today*, ed. A. Kiev. New York: Free Press, pp. 84–120.

34. Benedict, R. (1938), Continuities and discontinuities in cultural conditioning. *Psychiatry*, 1:161–167.

35. Burchell, W. J. (1822), Travels into the Interior of Southern Africa. In: *Primitive Mentality*, by L. Levy-Bruhl, 1923. London: Allan & Unwin.

36. Von Spix, J. B. & van Martius, C. F. F. (1923), Reise in Brasilien. In: *Primitive Mentality*, by L. Levy-Bruhl, 1923. London: Allan & Unwin.

37. Prince, R. H. (1961), Interest disorders; with some comments upon similarities between the reticular activating system and the ego. *Can. Psychiatr. Assoc. J.*, 6:309–322.

38. Handforth, J. R. (1978), Study difficulty: psychiatric and psychological aspects. *Can. Psychiatr. Assoc. J.*, 23:549–556.

39. Beard, G. M. (1869), Neurasthenia or nervous exhaustion. *Boston Med. Surg. J.*, 80:217–221.

40. Erb, W. (1878), *Handbuch der Krankheiten des Nervensystems*, 2nd ed. Leipzig.

41. Levin, K. (1978), *Freud's Early Psychology of the Neuroses: A Historical Perspective*. Pittsburgh: University of Pittsburgh Press.

42. Jones, E. (1953), *The Life and Work of Sigmund Freud*, Vol. 1. New York: Basic Books.

CHAPTER FIVE

# ALIENATION AS AN AFFECT IN ADOLESCENCE

SAUL V. LEVINE

There are few words used as widely in the diverse literature on adolescence as "alienation"; but, as happens with most clichés, imprecision and variation in its use have blurred its meaning. Thus one has to know the context, the field of endeavor, the specific adolescents under discussion, and even the personal biases of the writer, before he can be certain of its intended connotation.

In our profession, alienation has been used to describe a wide range of states, from a normal and necessary factor in development (1) or a natural adolescent experience (2), to a result of early psychic trauma or a seriously impaired early mother-child relationship which interferes with later separation and individuation (3–6). Alienation has also been used to reflect a pathologic entity or syndrome (2, 4).

I use the word alienation in the sense of Seaman (7) and Keniston (8), and as I have seen it manifested in adolescents clinically and in research studies over the past decade. It includes the following facets:

*Isolation:* a sense of not belonging to the dominant group, culture, or society, not fitting in, lacking meaningful relationships, lacking feelings of solidarity, communal love, or support, and being alone.

*Meaninglessness:* a sense of lack of purpose or coherent meaning to one's life, a sense of futility, lack of a belief system, absence of a personal or social vision, or even the perception of one.

73

*Normlessness:* a sense of absence of universally acceptable norms of be-havior and values with which one is comfortable, confusion of expectations (from others) regarding values, attitudes, actions, and relationships, lack of stable traditions, and a sense of failure of predictability because of rapid change.

*Powerlessness:* a sense of having no influence or control, not only on the direction and activities of other individuals, institutions, or government, but even on the course of one's own life.

*Self-estrangement:* a sense of feeling withdrawn from oneself, of not knowing who one is or "should" be, and an unpleasant feeling of personal emptiness.

Clinically depressed, borderline, or even schizophrenic patients have some of these characteristics; in fact, they occur in many psychiatric disor-ders. But we should not label all who are disturbed as alienated, or what is far worse in my estimation, label as disturbed all who are alienated. Aliena-tion is not necessarily, and certainly not by definition, a clinical pathologic entity; it is a delineated affect. By "affect" is meant the "feeling-tone" accom-paniment of an idea, mental representation or symbol (9). Thus, alienation is an affective experience of some individuals whose disorders are diagnosed and treated by our profession, but it is also an experience shared by many young people who are *not* psychologically unstable and have *not* had trau-matic experiences early in life. Furthermore, and again like other affective experiences, alienation is a continuum both in degree and in kind: some persons are more intensely alienated than others; and one or more of its aspects (e.g., isolation or powerlessness) may predominate in the subject's feelings and preoccupations.

This view of alienation contains some elements included in Leighton's concept (10) of psychosocial disintegration, a reaction to rapid change in one's social system. Again, there is both a lack of norms and a sense of the futility of individual effort (powerlessness); there is also an absence of trust in leaders, or even an absence of leaders themselves. Social support net-works crumble, the future is bleak or unknown, and instability reigns. This sequence of events, like any other major crisis, can induce a wide variety of psychologic and psychiatric symptoms, ranging from severe anxiety to acute depression or even decompensation. And in many other instances, it results in the feelings described above, culminating in apathy and nihilism. Therefore, despite reactions to environmental or other stress in ways that do not conform to usual patterns of psychopathology, many persons mani-fest the hallmarks of alienation as an affect. This is exemplified in the fol-lowing case:

"Colin" was 17 years old when his father, a junior executive with an aircraft firm, was laid off after 27 years of steady employment. The family had to move to another town so that the father could find another job. Colin's behavior changed significantly, and his "new" fatalistic approach to life persisted longer than anyone expected (2 years). He told his parents that he wanted a more meaningful life than theirs, but he was pessimistic about accomplishing it. Both the change in Colin and the nature of his attitude and its persistence concerned his family. They and others were convinced that he needed psychiatric help, and a referral was made. Although Colin did not feel a psychiatrist could be helpful, he was willing to go for treatment.

To the psychiatrist, Colin expressed feelings of utter demoralization. The psychiatrist was told that Colin had always been a serious boy, concerned about others and sensitive to their needs, but according to all reports had appeared happy and outgoing, and had a positive sense of himself. His parents said that since the move he had become more serious, somewhat confused, and fatalistic. Colin, now 19 years old, stated that he felt there was little point to planning and striving for future goals, as he had no control whatsoever over his immediate or ultimate destiny. He didn't feel he had much in common with his peers, and didn't even feel comfortable within himself. He expressed feelings of low self-esteem and futility.

These feelings are not new: the literature of the ages is replete with examples of youth's alienation; and throughout recorded history the energy of alienation has been channeled into social movements like revolutions and wars. There are no exact statistics of the prevalence or incidence of alienation — neither the concept nor epidemiology has advanced that far — but some studies have shown that a significant proportion of our "normal" youth harbors these feelings to a varying extent (11, 12), and social-science and clinical studies have borne this out.

In fact, Colin's tnought processes were intact, without hallucinations or delusions, and his affect was appropriate to his expressed thought and mood. There were no vegetative, motor, or cognitive signs of clinical depression, and no evidence of a borderline psychotic process. The patient was not beset with anxiety, its derivatives or concomitants, and evidenced neither severe psychoneurotic nor characterologic psychopathology.

Nonetheless, this type of reaction to crisis is not universal: many people do not deteriorate or disintegrate; in fact, some grow via crises. But there are those who, like Colin, although not disturbed in a clinical or classical sense, react to crisis by feeling alienated and becoming highly vulnerable to the seductiveness of activities, individuals, or groups that promise to overcome their relatively painful affective state. In Colin's case, his problems were not resolved in psychotherapy, but were dramatically alleviated when he joined an inspirational group, an Anglican Youth Work group, which took an interest in him. He became more cheerful and more outgoing. He felt better about himself and others. Colin's family and friends noticed the transformation — they remarked on his new-found serious sense of purpose and his obvious commitment and contentment.

Our research studies and clinical work over the years with normal adolescents, draft dodgers in exile (13), drug-users (14), youngsters in communes (15) and with alternative life-styles (16), members of "fringe" religions (17) or unemployed (18), have revealed alienation as one common affective denominator that serves as a tremendous shaper of personal attitudes and behavior. The subjects, adolescents and young adults, had not been referred for diagnosis or therapy, nor had they been labeled as sick or disturbed; yet the extent of alienation they had evidenced before they pursued their respective courses of action was remarkable. Most of them had already, in attempts to combat their feelings of alienation, chosen paths that society largely deems destructive. And in many instances their alienation did indeed dissipate, as is illustrated later.

If one thinks of conditions which are ripe for a generation of alienation, the current one is ideal. It is encompassing a veritable explosion in knowledge, scientific discovery, and technologic advance, the most rapid change ever experienced in social values (e.g., sexual, family), and in the demise of the family (e.g., extended and even, lately, nuclear). These factors are intensified by economic instability and unpredictability about the near future, a soil obviously fertile for the development of alienation, at least as we have postulated it. Perhaps the term "environmental oppression" suggested by Frank (19) overstates contemporary social stresses and removes the concept of responsibility for one's actions, but there is no doubt of the accuracy of his description (20) of the "demoralization" that makes an individual alienated, vulnerable, susceptible to social groups, and even amenable to psychotherapy. Although psychotherapy was not successful in Colin's case, it may say something more about the specific modality used, rather than the process in general. Colin was not "disturbed" yet might have benefited from an active involving approach, concentrating on his obvious strengths. Paradoxically, the end-result of psychotherapy might have been the same, at least in principle, as occurred fortuitously. That is, he might have "decided" to join a socially active group after learning more about himself. But psychotherapy, even when exceedingly sensitive and well done, may not be able to "captivate" many young people, as in the case of Colin.

However, the causes and effects of alienation must not be generalized to all adolescents and young people. Offer and Sabshin (21) and others have shown that *Sturm und Drang* are not *sine qua non* of adolescence. Many adolescents are resilient, adaptive, and enthusiastic about their lives (21, 22), and some pass through this phase smoothly. We have found that the persons most prone to alienation are those who cannot adapt or cope, who have great difficulty dealing with transition states and crises. They feel the vicissitudes of life more painfully, and admit to feeling vulnerable and pessimistic.

We must likewise separate a sense of alienation during adolescence from psychopathologic disorders in adolescents. To apply a psychiatric label begs the question of the roots of alienation and is invalid. Furthermore, it is demeaning and destructive to large numbers of persons who are reacting to social stresses if we consider only intrapsychic etiology and the absence of autoplastic solutions.

Those who experience alienation derive no consolation from knowing that others feel similarly about themselves, their lives, and their society. In fact, alienation is but one possible answer to the existential questions posed in the course of defining one's identity (23) — "Who am I?" "Where am I going?" "How?" and "Why?" — questions that are not restricted to this age group. It seems to me that the narcissism of adolescence in itself is alienating, just as the narcissism of the "me generation" in recent times (24) is ultimately alienating and destructive. (In this regard, I am struck by the parallels of the letter I, in "identity-related issues," and the letter A, in "alienation-related feelings": Under the I of identity I would include impulse-control [sexual and aggressive], intellectual change [ability to abstract, hypotheticodeductive reasoning], industriousness, intimacy [sexual, romantic, friendly], independence/individuation and idealism/ideology: *all* the aspects of adolescent tasks can be related to the I; under the A of alienation one can list terms like apathy, Angst, anomie, ambiguity, anhedonia, anger, anxiety, antisocial, and affect.)

This dichotomy is not unique to youth: the self-involvement that our professions in part have been espousing, via self-awareness, self-actualization, and self-realization, leads ultimately to self-indulgence and selfishness; and when one is preoccupied with personal growth, getting "in touch" with oneself, and self-enhancement, others have to take second place. Narcissism does not encourage (or even allow) caring, altruism, and concern for and commitment to others; and intense, prolonged self-contemplation is fundamentally alienating. What makes this particularly significant for adolescents is that extreme alienation depletes the energy, social commitment, and ideology of this population segment that historically was at the forefront and the life-force of society. When their vitality is dissipated, society is endangered because, if those within their own social milieu cannot capture their imagination, there are alternative groups that most certainly can.

## BELIEF AND BELONGING

What we have termed "belief and belonging" (25) is a shorthand description of two of youth's powerful psychosocial needs that are an effective antidote and "vaccine" against alienation; we have found this in *all* of our studies and clinical work. One's belief system provides a coherent set of values, an outer-oriented ideology, a *raison d'être*, something intense to believe in. Belonging provides a sense of being part of a group of supportive like-minded persons, with shared aspirations, behavior, values, and emotions, and experiences of being accepted and cared for. A person who is feeling alienated — alone, demoralized, with low self-esteem — will be strongly attracted to any group that promises belief and belonging; his self-esteem will rise (26), and he will feel better, happier, and more vital. We may not like the group, agree with its tenets, or trust its motives, but it may be succeeding at doing something at which other potential support groups have failed. This may account for the recent and burgeoning success of all the group therapies, especially as promoted by the different parts of the Human Potential Movement. These groups use the principles of belief and belonging, although couched in other terms to a large extent.

This is well illustrated in the case of "Lenny," the son of a successful psychiatrist father and musician mother. Although not religious in an Orthodox sense, the family identified itself closely with Judaism. Lenny excelled scholasticaly, athletically, and socially, until his final year in high school, when his grades declined, he became sexually active and began experimenting with drugs. He got involved with a group of young people who disdained the educational system and used chemicals as a convenient way of escaping what they saw as an intolerable life style.

Lenny's behavior continued in the directions of self-destruction and self-absorption. He barely passed his final high school examinations, left the university during the first year, and continued to use drugs extensively. He was sent to see an experienced psychotherapist, who could make no inroads on his attitudes or behavior. Lenny felt miserable about his world, his friends, his behavior, and most of all himself, but could or would do nothing about it. Another psychotherapist tried, and was defeated by Lenny's lack of interest and cynicism. Lenny's personal habits deteriorated; he ate and slept poorly, was socially inactive, and was pessimistic about his future. He saw little point in middle-class pursuits. Those closest to Lenny began to give up on him, considering him a "loser" or ne'er-do-well.

While walking aimlessly downtown, Lenny was approached by two warmly expressive, enthusiastic members of the Unification Church (although they did not identify themselves correctly then), and accepted their invitation to a communal church dinner. Lenny was enthralled by that experience, and attended longer sessions in a rural retreat, becoming captivated and excited. He joined and remained a committed "Moonie." He stopped taking drugs immediately and permanently. Lenny liked his new friends, and felt closely akin to their values; he looked and felt better, and felt good about himself and his world.

Adolescents have always been susceptible to ideologies and purposeful social movements (27-29), but the climate has seldom been as conducive to this as it is today. Ironically, although we feel that belief and belonging are crucial needs and deterrents to alienation, it seems that they are becoming less apparent in contemporary society. Solidarity of the family, a major protection of youth against alienation (30, 31), is crumbling, and so is the sense of community and belonging that it engendered. Similarly, intense belief systems are less in evidence than ever before (28), as our society busies itself with material goals, competition, and self-absorption. Yet we complain when our impressionable youth gravitate to groups that fulfill these very needs (17). Like "Lenny," all of the young people we have studied experienced warmth with their group, a spiritual uplifting, and an awakening of a sense of purpose; and each got the feeling of being a worthwhile person. There are no absolute standards for what constitutes mental health (21, 32, 33), but there is little doubt that at least some of the criteria would be met by new groups that fulfill the traditional role of the family, and provide what is perceived as a warm association with a meaningful *raison d'être*. Certainly, a sense of purpose and personal security, heightened self-esteem, and significant communal experience are all in evidence. A checklist of psychiatric symptoms would show reduction in those related to depression and anxiety, and, unless the group itself espoused these behaviors, marked diminution in or absence of drug use and antisocial behavior. Whether flexibility and adaptability to change, and the ability to genuinely care for others, cope with inevitable stresses, even life's tragedies, and reason independently are similarly enhanced (or are hindered, as has been suggested) is not clear. However, the mental-health professions, whose nature some have likened to religion (34, 35), have not been able to reach many of these young people even when given the opportunity (36); and what youth perceives as a purposeless society has not been able to prevent their alienation.

Youth in small social systems based on intense ideology and group commitment (e.g., kibbutzim) possess more self-esteem and experience less alienation (37, 38) than their urban counterparts. Similarly, during times of outer-directed commitment—as during World War II, the civil rights marches in Selma, Alabama, the antiwar demonstrations in the late 1960s, and throughout the prolonged battle in Northern Ireland—there is a tremendous reduction in all of the indices of psychologic upheaval among youth (e.g., suicides, mental hospital admissions, and arrests). In these circumstances, alienation is less of a problem. Thus, unfortunately, destructive movements also can captivate youthful fervor, including belief and belonging, and reduce alienation.

By "needs," we are not speaking about the luxuries wanted by young persons or even the "metaneeds" that Maslow (39) postulated as necessary for self-actualization. A belief system and a sense of belonging are crucial psychosocial needs only one step from physiological needs, and are no less vital to human functioning, competence, adaptation, and development.

## SUMMARY AND DISCUSSION

Alienation will not be cured or eradicated, nor should it be. It is an affect we all experience from time to time, one that young people will always have to wrestle with. The salient question is whether it will become a dominant negative or positive force in a crucial period of a young person's life.

I have suggested that unless a social system—be it a family, group, institution, neighborhood, or society—can instill in its youth some degree of purpose and community, a substantial proportion of the adolescents, particularly those with low self-esteem and increased vulnerability (for whatever reason), inevitably will become society's problems. The statistics should concern us: more youth than ever before are engaging in antisocial behavior and vandalism, are fathering or having babies at a very early age, drinking alcohol or taking drugs, leaving home early, joining cults, dropping out of high school (40), or joining the ranks of the unemployed (18). They are engaging in these activities largely because of alienation and personal demoralization.

These are vulnerable youth—alienated, demoralized, with low self-esteem. Not all of these youngsters are candidates for psychotherapy: some need different kinds of social support; some could benefit from vocational, sexual, or educational counseling; others need various forms of rehabilitation, or even incarceration. But unless we attack the root causes of youthful identity diffusion, or look at *social* solutions, we shall only be plugging holes in the dikes. Keniston (8) has argued that our society lacks a vision of itself and of man that transcends technology. He feels that a society which is "worthy of commitment" is one that "harnesses our scientific inventiveness and industrial productivity to the promotion of human fulfillment."

This is not meant as a lament for a generation—the majority of our youth give us cause for enthusiasm. Furthermore, although alienation can be looked upon as an affect, it can also be a powerful motivating force for constructive outlets. In addition, it may provide us with an opportunity to re-evaluate where we are going and what we want as a society. It may give us the opportunity to instill in our young people, and ourselves, a sense of purpose which many of us have lost.

We—as mental-health professionals, as citizens, and as parents— should be searching for ways to harness that force, to "turn-on" our youth, to capture their inherent need for an ideology and group.

## REFERENCES

1. Settlage, C. F. (1970), Anomie, alienation, and adolescence: An editorial post-
   script. *J. Am. Acad. Child Psychiatry*, 9:278-281.
2. Berman, S. (1970), Alienation: an essential process of the psychology of adolescence. *J. Am. Acad. Child Psychiatry*, 9:233-250.
3. Blos, P. (1967), The second individuation process of adolescence. *Psychoanal.
   Study Child*, 22:162-186.
4. Cambor, C. G. (1973), Adolescent alienation syndrome. In: *Current Issues in Adolescent Psychiatry*, ed. J. C. Schoolar. New York: Brunner-Mazel, pp. 101- 117.
5. Freud, A. (1946), *The Ego and the Mechanisms of Defense*. New York: International
   Universities Press.
6. Williams, F. S. (1970), Alienation of youth as reflected in the hippie movement.
   *J. Am. Acad. Child Psychiatry*, 9:251-263.
7. Seaman, M. (1959), On the meaning of alienation. *Am. Soc. Review*, 24:783-791.
8. Keniston, K. (1965), *The Uncommitted: Alienated Youth in American Society*. New
   York: Delta.
9. Hinsie, L. E. & Campbell, R. J., Eds. (1970), *Psychiatric Dictionary*, 4th ed. New
   York: Oxford University Press.
10. Leighton, D. (1971), The empirical status of the integration-disintegration hy-
    pothesis. In: *Psychiatric Disorder and the Urban Environment*, ed. B. Kaplan.
    New York: Behavioral Publications, pp. 68-78.
11. Masterson, J. F. (1967), *The Psychiatric Dilemma of Adolescence*. Boston: Little,
    Brown.
12. Pasamanick, B., Roberts, D. W., Kemkau, P. M., & Krueger, D. B. (1959), A
    survey of mental disease in an urban population: prevalence by race and
    income. In: *Epidemiology of Mental Disorder*, ed. B. Pasamanick.
    Washington, D.C.: American Association for the Advancement of Sci-
    ence, Publ. No. 60, pp. 183- 201.
13. Levine, S. V. (1972), Draft dodgers: coping with stress, adapting to exile. *Am.
    J. Orthopsychiatry*, 42:431-439.
14. Levine, S. V., Lloyd, D. D., & Longdon, W. H. (1972), The speed user: social
    and psychological factors in amphetamine abuse. *Can. Psychiatr. Assoc. J.*,
    17:229-241.
15. Levine, S. V., Carr, R. P., & Horenblas, W. (1973), The urban commune:
    fact or fad, promise or pipedream? *Am. J. Orthopsychiatry*, 43:149-163.
16. Levine, S. V. (1976), Adolescents in alternative lifestyles. Presentation to the
    Meeting of the International Association for Learning Disabilities, Lon-
    don, Ontario, Nov., 1976.
17. Levine, S. V. (1978), Youth and religious cults: a societal and clinical dilemma.
    *Ann. Am. Soc. Adolesc. Psychiatry*, 6:75-89.
18. Levine, S. V. (in press), Psychological and social effects of youth unemploy-
    ment. In: *Children Today*, ed. Judith Reed. Proceedings, Annual Meeting,
    American Psychiatric Association, Chicago, Ill.: May, 1979. Washington,
    D.C.: U.S. Govt. Printing Office: Department of Health, Education &
    Welfare.
19. Frank, J. D. (1978), Self-centeredness vs. social action viz contemporary Amer-
    ican society. In: *Psychotherapy and the Human Predicament: A Psychosocial Ap-
    proach*, ed. P. E. Dietz. New York: Schocken, pp. 149-159.

20. Frank, J. D. (1978), Sources and functions of belief systems. In: *Psychotherapy and The Human Predicament: A Psychosocial Approach*, ed. P. E. Dietz. New York: Schocken, pp. 260–269.
21. Offer, D. & Sabshin, M. (1974), *Normality: Theoretical and Clinical Concepts of Mental Health*, 2nd ed. New York: Basic Books.
22. Murphy, A. E. & Toussieng, P. W. (1976), *Adolescent Coping*. New York: Grune & Stratton.
23. Erikson, E. H. (1968), *Identity, Youth, and Crisis*. New York: Norton.
24. Lasch, C. (1978), *The Culture of Narcissism*. New York: Norton.
25. Levine, S. V. (1979), Adolescence: believing and belonging. *Ann. Am. Soc. Adolesc. Psychiatry*, 7:41–53.
26. Rosenberg, M. (1979), *Conceiving the Self*. New York: Basic Books.
27. Adelson, J. (1975), The development of ideology in adolescence. In: *Adolescence in the Life Cycle: Psychological Change and Social Context*, ed. S. E. Dragastin & G. H. Elder, Jr. New York: Wiley, pp. 63–78.
28. Braungart, R. (1975), Youth and social movements. In: *Adolescence in the Life Cycle: Psychological Change and Social Context*, ed. S. E. Dragastin & G. H. Elder, Jr. New York: Wiley, pp. 255–289.
29. Toch, H. (1965), *The Social Psychology of Social Movements*. New York: Bobbs-Merrill.
30. Blum, R., et al. (1969), *Society and Drugs*. San Francisco: Jossey-Bass.
31. Keniston, K. (1965), *The Uncommitted: Alienated Youth in America*. New York: Harcourt Brace & World.
32. Frank, J. (1979), Mental health in a fragmented society: the shattered crystal ball. *Am. J. Orthopsychiatry*, 49:397–408.
33. Menninger, R. (1968), What troubles our troubled youth? *Ment. Hyg.*, 52:323–329.
34. Frank, J. D. (1977), Nature and functions of belief systems: humanism and transcendental religion. *Am. Psychol.*, 32:555–559.
35. Kiev, A. (1972), *Transcultural Psychiatry*. New York: Free Press.
36. Levine, S. V. (1979), Role of psychiatry in the phenomenon of cults. *Can. Psychiatr. Assoc. J.*, 24:593–603.
37. Bronfenbrenner, U. (1974), The origins of alienation. *Sci. Am.*, 231:53–61.
38. Spiro, M.E. & Spiro, A. G. (1975), *Children of the Kibbutz*, rev. ed. Cambridge, Mass.: Harvard University Press.
39. Maslow, A. (1967), Self actualization and beyond. In: *Challenges of Humanistic Psychology*, ed. J. F. T. Bugental. New York: McGraw-Hill, pp. 279–286.
40. Social Planning Council of Metropolitan Toronto (1978), Report: The Problem is Jobs...Not People. (Manuscript.)

# PART TWO

# CLINICAL SYNDROMES

INTRODUCTION

# PART TWO:
# CLINICAL SYNDROMES

## KLAUS K. MINDE

This section includes critical reviews of four clinical syndromes as they present in adolescence: attention deficit disorder, phobia, mood disturbances associated with physical illness, and borderline personality disorder.

Each author has not only been involved in outstanding research studies of his topic, but is also an expert clinician. This dual role of the researcher-clinician has allowed each contributor to present the reader with a broad vista, encompassing both the latest pertinent scientific data and its application in everyday practice.

The section begins with Paul Wender's paper which documents the persistence of attention deficit disorder (ADD) into adolescence. Wender initially discusses the advantages and disadvantages of various epidemiological methodologies used to study ADD; he concludes that only a prospective study can answer the question of the natural history of this disorder in adolescence. As such a study has not been done, Wender relies on studies which have re-examined various populations previously defined as hyperactive or showing other symptoms compatible with ADD. From these investigations, as well as from his own work, he concludes that a substantial number of adolescents continue to demonstrate such signs of ADD as impulsivity, lability of affect, and learning difficulties. He recommends providing such youngsters with educational remediation as well as drug treatment, and correctly emphasizes the great importance that a good personal relationship between the therapist and the adolescent has on the effectiveness of each therapeutic measure.

In the second paper, Lionel Hersov gives a detailed account of the history of the study of phobias as well as discussing their prevalence, incidence, possible etiologies and treatment in the adolescent population. He clearly documents the gaps in our knowledge, especially in regard to the epidemiology of phobias. We have only a very limited understanding of the natural history of phobias in this age group, and do not even have exact figures on its prevalence. Furthermore, there is still no strong evidence that any particular treatment method is superior to any other method or no treatment at all.

In discussing the management of phobic adolescents, Hersov stresses the need for a multimodal approach just as Wender before him. Hersov recommends that a detailed investigation of the phobia be undertaken before treatment is initiated. Treatment may include a combination of individual and family counseling, as well as psychotropic drugs. He exemplifies the need for such an approach in his thorough discussion of school refusal, the most common phobia of adolescence, which can be a symptom of hysterical, depressive, obsessive, or even schizophrenic disorders. In treating school refusal, parents and school personnel are also often utilized as parts of the treatment team.

The involvement and understanding of the life-space of the teenager in the diagnosis and treatment of mood disturbance in the physically ill adolescent is also the essential message of John Schowalter. In a comprehensive and sensitive treatise, he discusses the emotional impact of a variety of physical illnesses and other handicaps on the adolescent. Many of these illnesses, such as cystic fibrosis, were fatal disorders one or two decades ago, and even today carry an unknown long-term prognosis. Especially for teenagers, whose developmentally determined concerns are normally focused on future identity and adequacy, any serious physical illness will profoundly affect psychological well-being. Schowalter states that the likelihood of depression in the face of a physical illness is greater in those adolescents who have a premorbid history of mood swings. This in turn is often a reflection of the coping style of the adolescent's family and therefore, according to the author, is not primarily due to a genetic predisposition.

Schowalter also stresses the influence which medical and surgical interventions can have on the course of mood disorder in the physically ill adolescent. For example, the curtailment of physical activity following an operation or the side-effects of certain medications can cause depressive symptoms in adolescents; this is especially so since these youngsters, in contrast to younger children, have the cognitive ability to comprehend the meaning of their illness and its possible future consequences. Schowalter ends his paper by citing some measures which can prevent such depression. He points out that adequate pain relief allows these patients to feel more hopeful and in control; that contact with peers can bolster adaptive defenses; and that changes in ward routines to give adolescent patients the opportunity to express their views can alleviate the sick adolescent's concerns about helplessness and powerlessness.

The last paper of this section deals with disturbances of mood in the borderline adolescent. James Masterson, who has been associated for many years with attempts to understand and treat such patients, gives an excellent summary of his views. He states that the borderline syndrome is environmentally induced, and derives from a developmental arrest during the phase of individuation-separation. Masterson feels that during this developmental period the young child had been exposed to a primary caretaker who alternated between being emotionally available and being withdrawn. The child consequently experienced an "abandonment depression" against which the adolescent may defend himself with affects such as rage, panic, helplessness, depression, or guilt. Masterson states that it is these defensive aspects which the clinician initially encounters in these patients, and that treatment must aim at working through the defenses in order to confront the underlying abandonment depression.

While some of the concepts discussed by Masterson are highly complex, the author's style as well as his use of case vignettes serve to establish a link between theory and clinical work with this difficult group of adolescent patients.

Our knowledge of the clinical syndromes associated with mood disorders in adolescents has expanded significantly during the past 10 years; much of this advance can be directly attributed to the authors of these four papers.

CHAPTER SIX

# ATTENTION DEFICIT DISORDER IN ADOLESCENCE

## PAUL H. WENDER

Individuals who are diagnosed today as having attention deficit disorder (ADD) were formerly classified under the terms minimal brain dysfunction, minimal brain damage, and hyperkinetic-impulsive disorder. The new terminology, ADD, continues the identification and classification of young people with short attention span, impulsivity, motor abnormalities, interpersonal difficulties, altered emotionality, learning disabilities, and physical stigmata under this new rubric (1). Contrary to common belief among child psychiatrists attention deficit disorder *persists* into adolescence. This erroneous belief is surprising in view of the steady and increasing literature which has appeared since the 1960s asserting that "hyperactivity," "conduct disorders," and/or "dyslexia" may persist into adolescence and early adult life. I emphasize the word "persist" since no one has ever maintained that ADD arises *de novo* in adolescence; therefore its existence must logically reflect a continuation of a previously existing disorder.

I shall first review the evidence which suggests that ADD in childhood may continue into adolescence and adult life, then discuss the reasons why this fact may have been overlooked, and lastly examine the characteristics of the syndrome in the adolescent and differences in its optimal treatment from that of the preadolescent.

## METHODS OF STUDY

The ideal way to study the natural history of a disorder is to select an entire population, or a random sample of that population, and follow it longitudinally. The *only* large population survey of preadolescents has been conducted by Michael Rutter and his colleagues (2); but until this population is systematically rescreened, we are obliged to depend on a variety of *ad hoc* studies. Each of these can of course provide us with some information; however, for reasons of unintentional sampling bias, such information is invariably distorted.

In the absence of a population survey, the next best approach is to trace the fate of a cohort of individuals identified as having the disorder in question. This is a traditional technique in medicine, but is not easily generalizable to psychiatry. The reason for this is simple: the tradition began in medicine with disorders which were so severe that virtually everyone who had them came to medical attention (patients with penetrating head wounds, overwhelming infection, or neoplastic disease either died first or saw a physician); whereas such is not the case with psychiatry. (It is variously "guesstimated" that approximately one person in 50 suffering from a primary affective disorder reaches psychiatric attention.) Reasons for this phenomenon include an unavailability of facilities, lack of recognition of the disorder, and/or unwillingness to seek psychiatric care. Children who reach psychiatric clinics are likewise undoubtedly a small fraction of the population of psychiatrically disabled children; they may be assumed to be selected either because they are socially disturbing to others or have unusually psychologically minded parents.

Furthermore, given that the researcher wishes to do an anterospective study and lacks a time machine, he can merely identify a cohort of patients seen over a fixed period of time and wait ten years; but this method too is obviously flawed. Therefore, for the less than patient researcher, the standard technique is to go back to clinical records and attempt to select a cohort of individuals with the diagnosis in question. Since "hyperactivity" has been a popular diagnosis for only the last ten years, the supply of such "retrospective-anterospective" subjects is additionally limited. To complicate matters, the lack of operational criteria for psychiatric diagnoses in general, and "ADD" in particular, casts doubt about their validity.

The last alternative is to read through clinical records and attempt to identify children who would now be classified as having ADD. This too is difficult and bound to be inaccurate; important data often are not mentioned, and one is unable to separate questions not asked from those that were simply not recorded.

## EVIDENCE OF PERSISTENCE
## OF ATTENTION DEFICIT DISORDER

With all of these methodological *caveats* in mind, the following represents the available evidence that ADD persists into adolescence. The first retrospective strategy refers to the attempt to determine the current clinical picture of former patients who were likely to have been diagnosed as ADD, and to examine their present status and life histories. Using this technique, Morris, Escoll, and Wexler (3), O'Neal and Robins (4), and Menkes, Rowe, and Menkes (5) identified a group of such adults who had been treated as children and in adulthood showed a fairly high prevalence of serious psychopathology, including psychosis and antisocial personality. However, their findings, which are quite different from subsequent ones, are an example of the consequences of unconscious sample bias. Because of the epoch or the circumstances in which these children were treated (e.g., hospitals), they probably represented an unusually severely afflicted group. (For example, of the 14 children in the Menkes et al. study (5), 4 of the patients as adults were institutionalized psychotics, 2 were retarded and non-self-supporting, and of 8 who were self-supporting, 4 had been institutionalized for some time.)

More recent studies have documented the persistence of symptoms, but have found them to be much less severe. Weiss, Hechtman, Perlman, Hopkins, and Wener (6) have reported on 75 hyperactive and 44 matched control subjects, currently about 19 years old, who had been followed for 10 to 12 years. No operational clinical diagnoses were made, but the authors report that "only a small minority showed severe psychopathology...or had serious continued antisocial behavior." The patients were different in regard to "traits" as evidenced by the fact that "hyperactives" were more frequently characterized as "impulsive" and "immature-dependent" as compared to the control group. Cognitive evaluation of a subgroup of the same population, approximately 15 years of age, showed that the hyperactives performed significantly worse than the controls on measures of reading.

The same trends were documented in three anterospective studies conducted by Mendelson (7), Huessy (8), and Ackerman, Dykman, and Peters (9). These ADD children when followed up show varying admixtures of hyperactivity, distractibility, conduct disorders, and specific developmental disorders. Since most longitudinal studies fail to break children down into homogeneous subgroups, they have varying outcomes as the proportions of children with different subsyndromes vary. For example, severe reading retardation (which may occur independently although it is frequently associated with ADD) may have more serious developmental consequences than hyperactivity and distractibility per se. Rutter, Tizard, and Whitmore (2) found that a third of the children with specific reading difficulties showed antisocial problems, and a third of the antisocial children were seriously retarded in their reading. All one may conclude from the available anterospective studies is that variable numbers of "hyperactive" children continue to show symptoms of hyperactivity and distractibility, impulsivity, conduct disturbances, and learning difficulties through adolescence.

A second group of studies suggesting that ADD in childhood may persist into adult life, and presumably that it is present in adolescence between childhood and adult life, come from retrospective studies of adults with psychiatric disorders. Several studies have described ADD symptomatology in adult outpatients, and some have described its treatment responsiveness to stimulant medication and tricyclic antidepressants.(Mann and Greenspan [10], Rybak [11], Shelley and Riester [12], and Morrison [13]). Similarly, a number of studies of adult inpatients with "personality" or "character" disorders, mainly of an impulsive variety, have found that such individuals have an increased frequency of ADD symptoms in childhood and in adulthood, including soft neurological signs and abnormalities on neuropsychological tests (Hartocollis [14], Quitkin and Klein [15]).

The most direct technique of verifying the existence of ADD in adolescence is to identify adolescents with symptoms typical of childhood ADD, and attempt to validate the diagnosis through the use of other techniques such as the response to drug therapy. I know of only two such studies (16, 17). In the first, Safer and Allen (16) reported an open trial of stimulant medication in children whose "hyperactive" symptoms had been discovered and treated prior to adolescence and continued into adolescence, and in "hyperactive" children first diagnosed during adolescence. They found that the "hyperactive" adolescents manifested the same qualitative response as the younger children, and that the degree of appreciable improvemen: was approximately the same in both age groups (70%–90%). There was no tendency for the adolescents to abuse the medication and, indeed, one boy who tried to become "high" on Ritalin found he was unable to do so. Maletzky (17) conducted a placebo controlled trial of dextroamphetamine in 28 "delinquent" adolescents with prominent symptoms of hyperactivity, and found statistically significant and appreciable benefits. Obviously larger controlled studies are necessary.

Both of these studies are of particular interest in that they describe the "paradoxical" response of hyperactive adolescents to stimulant medication. It had generally been assumed that as ADD children reached adolescence and "outgrew" their symptoms, their "paradoxical" response to stimulant medication disappeared. It was believed that the "typical" ADD childhood response (calming, absence of euphoria, failure to develop tolerance) disappeared and that the typical adult response to psychostimulant medications (excitation, euphoria, and the rapid development of tolerance) would develop.

Because of our frequent clinical observation of the persistence of ADD symptoms into adult life, our group in Utah has completed two studies of presumptive ADD adults (18, 19), and is in the process of conducting a third. For these investigations we encouraged referrals and solicited symptomatic volunteers with the following diagnostic characteristics: persistence since childhood of hyperactivity and inattentiveness, together with current complaints of disorganization, impulsivity, affective lability, hot-temperedness, and poor stress tolerance. Individuals with any schizoid or borderline characteristics are excluded.

To further characterize these individuals, we have developed a number of rating scales which are currently being standardized. To provide one measure of validation for our presumptive diagnosis, we solicited questionnaire material from the patients' mothers describing them as they had been as children, and obtained similar data from socioeconomically matched mothers of normal adults. We used the Conners Abbreviated Rating Scale (20), a standard measure of childhood hyperactivity, which was standardized on the basis of concurrent teachers' judgments, not retrospective parents' judgments. (It is for that reason that we obtained a new normative sample.) Patients who meet our criteria have been described by their mothers as averaging in the 95th percentile of childhood hyperactivity as compared with the retrospective ratings of the mothers of normal adults. Additional data, consistent with the notion that our patients indeed suffer from the same disorder, is reflected in their psychological test performance. Both the men and women show impaired coordination; and the men show substantial deficits in spelling and arithmetic on standardized achievement tests.

In the last phase of our studies, we have entered these individuals in placebo controlled trials of psychostimulant drugs, pemoline and methylphenidate, and have found that they manifest a statistically significant improvement on psychostimulant medication. The nature of their drug responsiveness is similar to that seen in "hyperactive" children: they become calmer, do not become euphoric, and do not develop tolerance to the medication. In light of these findings and the prevalence of this syndrome in a number of outpatient populations, we conclude that the ADD syndrome in our patients could not have begun during adolescence, but persisted since childhood.

## PREVALENCE OF THE ADD SYNDROME IN ADOLESCENTS

Although relatively common in children, ADD is infrequently reported in adolescents. This probably reflects sampling bias. First, we can reasonably assume that only a small fraction of psychiatrically disturbed adolescents reach official psychiatric contact. Second, we can assume that those with major conduct and learning disorders, among whom we would expect to find a high concentration of ADD adolescents, are seen in other facilities, e.g., juvenile courts and technical or trade schools for non-retardates who perform poorly academically.

There are several studies conducted in a variety of settings indicating that "delinquent" children (predominantly boys) manifest a substantial degree of "learning disorders." This has generally been interpreted dynamically. It has been assumed that for psychological reasons such children have withdrawn their cathexes from academic activities, have strayed from the "straight-and-narrow," and have fallen further into a life of crime. It is very clear, however, that many dyslexics do not become delinquents; it is likewise very clear that dyslexia is frequently associated with hyperactivity and conduct disorders, and that children with these characteristics are at much greater risk for delinquency (Mendelson, Johnson, and Stewart [7], Huessy, unpublished observations). A systematic controlled study of children brought to juvenile court is needed (excluding those children brought in for what in the United States are called "status offenses," e.g., smoking in the bathroom, breaking curfew, and nonrepeated running away from home). Standardized investigation, involving rating scales, measures of attention, measures of coordination, and possibly experimental procedures, such as evoked potential, would be useful in determining what fraction of such children represent adolescents with ADD signs and symptoms which have persisted from childhood.

A third factor which tends to diminish the number of ADD adolescents we see is that adolescents, like children, are not generally self-referred for what in the old psychiatric literature are designated as "autoplastic" problems, those that are causing internal pain and suffering; rather, they come for "alloplastic" problems, those that are causing difficulties for others. Since the difficulties in question are generally antisocial, such children are more apt to appear in legal rather than psychiatric clinical settings.

In contrast, ADD adults are frequently self-referred, and we feel that they are a distinct subgroup of ADD adults; they are seen because they are hurting within themselves, and especially because they are suffering with a particular variant of mood disorder. The latter, sometimes diagnosed as "neurotic," often masks their typical ADD signs and symptoms.

## CLINICAL EXPERIENCE WITH ADD IN ADOLESCENCE

My clinical experience with ADD in adolescence derives from three sources: (a) children I have followed from preadolescence through adolescence whose symptoms persisted; (b) patients referred to me as adolescents and in whom I diagnosed ADD (even though the older literature denied them any right to possess this interesting syndrome); and (c) the many ADD adults seen in the course of our three studies. This last group was particularly helpful in my understanding the phenomenology of ADD in adolescence because these adults were self-referred, open and eager to communicate, and often, though certainly not always, more articulate than their younger fellow sufferers.

What have I seen with regard to signs and symptoms? Hyperactivity itself, as is frequently stated in the clinical literature, often diminishes in adolescence. Nonetheless, many of the adolescents and adults state that they have an internal feeling of restlessness, find it difficult to stay in one place, and must be up-and-about. Many, but not all, continue to fidget, foot and hand tap and wiggle.

In addition, attentional deficits continue to plague these people. Leaving school is a blessing to them because there are fewer formal demands. Many report that they cannot sit through a TV program or a movie, much less finish reading an article, and certainly never complete a book. In our controlled studies, one of the measures of drug efficacy which we had not anticipated is the rapidity with which patients fill out our entire questionnaires when they are receiving active medication. Many of them comment on this with pleased surprise, stating that they have never before been able to focus their attention without considerable difficulty. (An objective measure is simply that they complete the task sooner.) For those in school, concentration difficulties do not improve; they are as impaired in the 10th as in the 4th grade.

With regard to conduct disorders, their frequency is obviously related to such variables as the source of referral; these disorders are therefore ubiquitous in children referred from the juvenile court. In some children the symptoms become aggravated in adolescence, while among others they disappear. If they persist, their manifestations obviously change: rather than throwing spitballs, these adolescents are likely to be involved in more mature antisocial activities.

Impulsivity often persists. More intelligent children and those with intact parenting seem to develop better techniques for controlling it. The same holds true for disorganization, although often those who are most talented remain seriously disorganized. However, disorganization frequently shows a good response to medication; moreover, temper outbursts diminish with age, and one can often learn to contain them rather than express them.

Affective lability in ADD individuals is particularly interesting and unique. One of the most striking and most disturbing symptoms to our adult ADD patients is a form of mood disorder. This feature has never been specifically characterized, although it has previously been loosely designated as "neurotic depressive" or "affective lability." The ADD adults report this mood disorder as beginning in *childhood* and persisting thereafter, characterized by "ups and downs," lasting from hours to days. (Often a precipitant is noted but not always.) As the individual becomes older, the "ups" (which seem to be periods of excitement more than of hypomania) tend to diminish in frequency and duration. (The "downs" are not characterized by anhedonia as Klein has asserted [21], and which I agree is patho-gnomonic of biological depression and responsive to antidepressant medica-tion.) Both adolescents and adults can be "jollied out" of a depressive episode; if they go to an event they enjoy like a good party, movie, or football game, their symptoms remit. If, however, through a combination of bad judgment and general ineptitude, they dig themselves into a deep hole, their depressions may persist. In this sense their mood disorder is "reactive."

Another group of signs which frequently persist is that of learning dis-abilities. It is well recognized that in children with learning disabilities the absolute level of academic performance does increase with age. However, the discrepancy between the achieved and the predicted level increases fur-ther; therefore these children are apt to be academically further behind in high school than they were in elementary school. In addition, high school makes different educational demands from those in elementary school. Whereas earlier grades call for rote memory and regurgitation, high school performance demands the ability to organize, think through problems, and, to some extent, be creative. Since ADD adolescents have deficiencies in concentration and organizational ability, these learning difficulties may summate with the previously existing problems to make the academic aspects of high school especially noxious for them.

Many of the ADD adolescents, like ADD children, have an exagger-ated degree of social immaturity and imperceptiveness. Because of their lack of sensitivity, they lose friends and alienate people. As a result, they frequently complain of being friendless. And they are right; their sense of alienation is not neurotic, but a correct perception of how they are treated by others. They lack to an exaggerated degree what we all lack to some de-gree: the ability to perceive how our own behavior produces reactions in others. I term this the "Katzenjammer principle," basing this appellation on the popular U.S.A. cartoon series, the Katzenjammer Kids. This pair of mildly hyperactive, conduct-disordered preadolescents were always up to mischief and inevitably got their comeuppance in the end, both figuratively and literally. Their socializer, the Captain, always observed accurately that they "brought it on themselves."

## DIFFERENTIAL DIAGNOSIS

Every rigorous method should be used to distinguish between presumptive ADD and other disorders with which it may share some common features. The first among these, although not the most common, are beginning schizophrenias. Early schizophrenics frequently have social withdrawal, depression, and attentional deficits. To further complicate the matter, some (but not most) of these schizophrenic adolescents may have truly been "hy-peractive" in childhood. In general, the distinguishing feature of early schizophrenia consists of clear-cut symptoms (albeit mild in many cases) of the type termed "schizotypal" in DSM III (1), and referred to by us as "borderline schizophrenic" in our adoption studies of schizophrenia (22, 23).

Next is the distinction of ADD from affective disorders. Contrary to previous belief, primary affective disorders do occur in preadolescence; in preadolescent boys, they are often accompanied by conduct disturbances. In both preadolescence and adolescence, affective disorders are usually periodic, and attentional deficits and hyperactivity are generally absent between episodes. However, it should be noted that these two disorders, affective disorders and ADD, may coexist.

Lastly is the differentiation between ADD and "borderline" disorders — a term I use in the sense described in DSM III (1). In our studies of adults we expressly exclude individuals with these characteristics, whereas they are specifically sought out in adolescents who have ADD characteristics. There are several distinctive differences between the two disorders. Typical ADD adolescents may have anger, but it is short-lived; they do not brood or maintain anger over long periods of time; they do not have recurrent suicidal gestures; and they do not repetitively perform physically self-damaging, self-mutiliating acts.

It is essential to make these distinctions between ADD and schizophrenic, affective, and borderline disorders because each requires special methods of treatment, particularly different medications.

Psychometric tests may be helpful in completing the clinical evaluation. Those we find most useful (except for research) are standardized achievement and IQ tests to detect learning disabilities, and as an aid in prescribing remedial education when necessary. Neuropsychological tests and electroencephalography are indicated only if there are other reasons for suspecting the presence of neurological disease or seizure disorder.

## GENERAL MANAGEMENT

The therapeutic management of ADD in adolescents is similar to the management of ADD in children; the chief differences are in emphasis. These differences relate to four areas: (a) establishment of a therapeutic relationship with the adolescent; (b) special and/or remedial education; (c) management of medication; and (d) the use of psychotherapy.

### THE THERAPEUTIC RELATIONSHIP

The most important principle is the establishment of a working relationship with the patient. Younger children are usually taken to the child psychiatrist, and are indifferent or opposed to coming. Although their active participation usually facilitates treatment and makes it more likely that they will continue, some techniques of psychologic management used with younger children (e.g., behavior modification) require the child to play a relatively passive role; and medication is often given without the child's active involvement. However, these techniques and approaches work poorly, if at all, with older children. If therapy is needed into adolescence, the psychiatrist must shift to a more collaborative relationship. I find that the more actively involved the younger child, the smoother the course of therapy, and the more likely he is to continue in treatment (if required) as he becomes an adolescent. However, many preadolescent ADD children can be fairly well-managed without a topnotch therapeutic alliance. A passionate involvement in therapy is good, but acquiescence is often sufficient.

The adolescent patient with ADD is analogous to the adult with a personality disorder. His behavior is frequently more disturbing to others than to himself, and unless and until he can be helped to see how his own behavior "rebounds" on him (or is helped to recognize that aspects of his experience which he regards as intrinsic are products of his disorder), his active cooperation is difficult to obtain. The fact that he frequently has symptoms which cause him pain, such as moodiness, concentration difficulties, or hot temper, may serve as a starting point. Moreover, it is easier for the adolescent, as for the adult, to acknowledge his problems when they are attributed to biological differences rather than psychological "badness"; it is easier to accept disease than moral turpitude.

SPECIAL AND REMEDIAL EDUCATION

The same comments apply to the general management of specific developmental disorders and its implications for special and remedial education. "Specific developmental disorders" (a phrase legislated to be employed for a variety of cognitive deficits referred to as "dyslexia" in the past) are not unique to ADD, but are frequently associated with it. When these disorders persist into adolescence they are often the cause of school failure and literal or figurative withdrawal from school. Again, part of the management of the problem is educating the patient as to its nature. To the extent that the adolescent can be convinced that his specific academic deficit is due to the way his brain is wired and not due to either neurosis or retardation, his morale may be improved immensely. This is not always easy to do because learning disabilities have not been widely recognized until recently, and learning–disabled adolescents may have chronically been regarded as stupid and/or lazy. After the adolescent has received this message repeatedly for 8 to 10 years, it could be a sign of good mental health to accept it. Therefore, it is often difficult to convince him that the authority figures have been consistently wrong.

However, when the disorder is explained as a disease (e.g., "dyslexia"), the results can be striking. I particularly remember a 15-year-old girl whose chronic low self-esteem stemmed mainly from her academic problems. When informed that she was not "dumb," but only dyslexic, her mood brightened dramatically and she proceeded to share with her friends my evaluation of her situation; this further raised her self-esteem.

The next issue of management relates to the uses of special education. Unfortunately, there are no convincing data that such education appreciably improves the function of developmentally disordered children or adolescents; the best one can do is to institute an empirical trial.

Perhaps far more important is working around the child's disability. Blind people can get Ph.D.s, and there is no reason why "word blind" people should not. We are too apt to confuse the means with the end and forget that reading is a technique of gaining information, not an ultimate goal in itself. I have met several M.D.s and Ph.D.s with severe reading disabilities who mastered material through excellent auditory memories and through having material read to them both in college and graduate school. Many cannot spell, and if one becomes successful enough, one can hire a non-learning-disabled secretary. Arithmetic learning disability (mechanical, not conceptual) can be circumvented by the calculator, the spouse, or the accountant. I do not mean to minimize the difficulties such problems can cause, but rather to emphasize both that they may be irremediable despite the best efforts of "special educators," and that the difficulties need not interfere with success (including academic) if other cognitive functions are intact.

MANAGEMENT OF MEDICATION

The response to stimulant drugs in ADD adolescents is very similar to that in ADD children. (It may be the case that ADD children who outgrow their disorder also outgrow their therapeutic response to stimulant medication.) Thus stimulants, when effective, result in improved concentration, decreased physical activity, increased organizational ability, diminished moodiness, decreased temper outbursts, decreased impulsivity, and greater responsiveness to the wishes of others. A light-hearted psychodynamic point of view is that stimulant drugs chemically hypertrophy the patient's superego. This is illustrated by the case of a colleague's patient who stated that if she wanted to skip school and go surfing, she likewise had to skip her Ritalin or she would feel guilty. ADD adolescents show no euphoria in the ordinary dose range, nor the development of escalating tolerance as do abusers. As with younger children, methylphenidate and dextroamphetamine seem to be the most efficacious drugs and approximately equal in effect, although similarly, there are individual patient differences in responsiveness. The newest analeptic, pemoline (Cylert), clearly works with a small fraction of children, but an occasional adolescent may function best on it.

The problems with stimulant medication are not pharmacological; they are social. Methylphenidate is short-acting, and multiple daily doses must be taken; therefore, the patient must want to take the medication and desire its effects in order to be adequately medicated. On the other hand, dextroamphetamine comes in the form of long-acting capsules; a single dose per day is usually sufficient, and the decision to ingest it need not be made more frequently. The difficulty is that these drugs are clearly abusable by non-ADD adolescents, and there is cause for concern about the patients' not taking the pills themselves, and dispensing them to others. Pemoline is apparently considerably less abusable, but it is also appreciably more toxic. Although allergic or idiosyncratic reactions to methylphenidate and dextroamphetamine are extraordinarily rare, 1 per cent of individuals receiving pemoline develop marked elevation of liver enzymes; and, if treatment is continued, they may develop more serious hepatocellular damage. In view of the fact that the drug is less efficacious, and that liver function tests must be repeatedly obtained, pemoline's only benefit is that the ADD adolescent is less apt to give it to his friends.

I have found tricyclic antidepressants in ADD adolescents, as in ADD children, not very effective. The ADD adolescent, like the ADD child, is apt to get an immediate quasi-favorable response which lasts about 12 hours; it is characterized by some improvement in mood and decrease in motoric activity, but without an appreciable beneficial effect on concentration, impulsivity, or temper. Furthermore, tolerance usually develops within a few weeks, and increased doses provide no further benefit and usually give rise to irritability.

If the adolescent is compliant and does not have serious problems with acting out or up, the relatively short-acting stimulants are adequate. Giving abusable medication to impulsive individuals who consort with drug abusers is not comfortable either legally or ethically. What is therefore needed for the ADD adolescent, as for the ADD adult, is a long-acting, nonabusable, safe drug. Unfortunately, none is currently available.

PSYCHOTHERAPY

There are no hard empirical data to support the use of traditional psychotherapy, but it is my impression that some ADD adolescents can benefit from specific kinds of intervention. If a person has been chronically maladjusted, even if the maladjustment has a biological basis, reversing the physiological abnormality will not undo the distorted learning it engendered. In addition to the nonspecific benefits of a therapeutic relationship, many adolescents, like adults, can learn to work around their psychological differences and/or compensate for them and thereby adapt more effectively. Understanding one's weaknesses, realizing their effects on others, and learning to work with them can be very useful. Cognitive deficits may not be amenable to eradication, but in many cases can be circumvented with the use of psychotherapeutic techniques.

## CONCLUSIONS

We examined the thesis that attention deficit disorder (ADD) persists from childhood into adolescence and adulthood, and found that ADD in adolescence is far *more common* than is generally supposed. Its prevalence is underestimated because the ADD adolescent, particularly the adolescent from a lower socioeconomic class, is likely to be shunted into facilities outside the clinical setting, such as the training school or the trade school.

Many of the signs and symptoms of ADD in adolescence are very similar to those seen earlier in childhood. Yet some prominent and seemingly new ones, such as pronounced moodiness, may be either additive with normal adolescent changes or simply more evident because the adolescent is a better reporter of his subjective state.

As in younger children, traditional intervention techniques can be very useful in ADD adolescents. Medication can suppress many of the symptoms; educational maneuvers can minimize or circumvent areas of academic deficit, and psychological counseling and/or psychotherapy can further improve self-awareness and self-esteem.

I believe that intervention during adolescence may prevent significant adult problems, although it may need to be continued for many years. We are currently studying ADD adults whose symptoms have persisted to their late 20s and 30s, and anticipate that early and sustained intervention may prevent the development of later, learned social and psychological pathology.

## REFERENCES

1. American Psychiatric Association, Committee on Nomenclature. (1978), *Diagnostic and Statistical Manual of Mental Disorders*, 3rd ed. Washington, D.C.: American Psychiatric Association. Draft.
2. Rutter, M., Tizard, J., & Whitmore, K., Eds. (1970), *Education, Health, and Behavior: Psychological and Medical Study of Childhood Development.* London: Longman.
3. Morris, H. H., Jr., Escoll, P. J., & Wexler, R. (1956), Aggressive behavior disorders of childhood: a follow-up study. *Am. J. Psychiatry*, 112:991–997.
4. O'Neal, P. & Robins, L. N. (1958), The relation of childhood behavior problems to adult psychiatric status: a 30-year follow-up study of 150 subjects. *Am. J. Psychiatry*, 114:961–969.
5. Menkes, M. M., Rowe, J. S., & Menkes, J. H. (1967), A 25-year follow-up study on the hyperkinetic child with minimal brain dysfunction. *Pediatrics*, 39:393–399.
6. Weiss, G., Hechtman, L., Perlman, T., Hopkins, J., & Wener, A. (1979), Hy-

peractives as young adults: a controlled prospective ten-year follow-up of 75 children. *Arch. Gen. Psychiatry*, 36:675–681.

7. Mendelson, W., Johnson, N., & Stewart, M. A. (1971), Hyperactive children as teenagers: a follow-up study. *J. Nerv. Ment. Dis.*, 153:273–279.

8. Huessy, H. R., Metoyer, M., & Townsend, M. (1974), Eight- to 10-year follow-up of 84 children treated for behavioral disturbance in rural Vermont. *Acta Paedopsychiatr.*, 40:230–235.

9. Ackerman, P. T., Dykman, R. A., & Peters, J. E. (1977), Teenage status of hyperactive and nonhyperactive learning-disabled boys. *Am. J. Orthopsychiatry*, 47:577–596.

10. Mann, H. B. & Greenspan, S. I. (1976), The identification and treatment of adult brain dysfunction. *Am. J. Psychiatry*, 133:1013–1017.

11. Rybak, W. S. (1977), More adult brain dysfunction. *Am. J. Psychiatry*, 134:96–97.

12. Shelley, E. M. & Riester, A. (1972), Syndrome of minimal brain damage in young adults. *Dis. Nerv. Syst.*, 33:335–339.

13. Morrison, J. R. & Minkoff, K. (1975), Explosive personality as a sequel to the hyperactive child syndrome. *Compr. Psychiatry*, 16:343–348.

14. Hartocollis, P. (1968), The syndrome of minimal brain dysfunction in young adult patients. *Bull. Menninger Clin.*, 32:102–114.

15. Quitkin, F., & Klein, D. F. (1969), Two behavioral syndromes in young adults, related to possible minimal brain dysfunction. *J. Psychiatr. Res.*, 7:131–142.

16. Safer, D. J. & Allen, R. P. (1975), Stimulant drug treatment of hyperactive adolescents. *Dis. Nerv. Syst.*, 36:454–457.

17. Maletzky, B. M. (1974), d-Amphetamine and delinquency: hyperkinesis persisting? *Dis. Nerv. Syst.*, 35:543–547.

18. Wood, D. R., Reimherr, F. W., & Wender, P. H. (1976), Diagnosis and treatment of minimal brain dysfunction in adults. *Arch. Gen. Psychiatry*, 33(12):1453–1461.

19. Wender, P. H., Reimherr, F. W., & Wood, D. R. (1981), Attention deficit disorder ('minimal brain dysfunction') in adults. *Arch. Gen. Psychiatry*, 38:449–456.

20. Sprague, R. L., Cohen, M., & Werry, J. S. (1974), Normative data on the Conners teacher rating scale and abbreviated scale. University of Illinois: Children's Research Center. (Manuscript.)

21. Klein, D. F. (1974), Endogenomorphic depression: a conceptual and terminological revision. *Arch. Gen. Psychiatry*, 31:447–454.

22. Wender, P. H., Rosenthal, D., & Kety, S. S. (1968), A psychiatric assessment of the adoptive parents of schizophrenics. In: *The Transmission of Schizophrenia*, ed. D. Rosenthal & S. S. Kety. Oxford: Pergamon, pp. 235–250.

23. Kety, S. S., Rosenthal, D., Wender, P. H., & Schulsinger, F. (1968), The types and prevalence of mental illness in the biological and adoptive families of adopted schizophrenics. In: *The Transmission of Schizophrenia*, ed. D. Rosenthal & S. S. Kety. Oxford: Pergamon, pp. 345–362.

CHAPTER SEVEN

# PHOBIAS AND THEIR TREATMENT IN ADOLESCENCE

## Lionel Hersov

*We are so largely the playthings of Fate in our fears. To one, fear of the dark, to another of physical pain, to a third of public ridicule, to a fourth of poverty, to a fifth of loneliness —for all of us our own particular creature lurks in ambush.*
— Hugh Walpole, 1884–1941
*The Old Ladies.* New York, Daran, 1924, p. 149.

Although many might not agree that fears are determined by fate, but are related to unconscious conflicts, developmental factors, or learned experience, the above quotation brings out the differences in the fears that beset people during their lifecycle. A major concern here is with those disabling varieties of fear called phobias which occur during the period of development called adolescence. The *Oxford English Dictionary* defines adolescence as the growing-up period between childhood and maturity, usually extending over a period of some 10 years, including what is colloquially called the "teens" (i.e., the early and middle stages of adolescence).

An acceptable definition of a phobia is one proposed by Marks (1): "A special form of fear which is out of proportion to the demands of the situation, cannot be explained or reasoned away, is beyond voluntary control and leads to avoidance of the feared situation" (p. 3). Miller, Barrett, and Hampe (2) enlarged this definition, adding three features: persistence, maladaptiveness, and lack of specificity in relation to age and stage of development. The first two aspects are of clinical importance; the third is more contentious, because it refers to the difficult issues of the appropriateness of a fearful response to situations and stimuli at different ages. Bauer (3) has shown that the structure of children's fears reflects changes related to cognitive development as well as emotional and social development and experience.

The special quality of fear experienced by one who has a phobic disorder is hard to define. Phobia includes common behavioral manifestations and accompanying physiological changes, and these have been well described (1). However, it is the unreasonable or disproportionate quality of the fear response to what other persons would regard as benign or even ill-defined stimuli or experiences, that gives a phobia its unique quality. Phobic individuals usually recognize that their special fear is excessive and unrealistic, but they are unable to subdue it and are handicapped, or in severe instances disabled by it. Many phobic objects or situations are of everyday occurrence and not easily avoided, although some can give rise to such overwhelming anxiety that the patient goes to extreme lengths to avoid them.

The diversity of phobic objects and situations is reflected in the endless lists in some earlier texts, which Henry Maudsley criticized (4). This method of classification adds nothing to our understanding of their origin or psychological mechanisms; however, it has the merit of defining the object or situation more precisely, and is particularly useful for the planning of behavioral treatment of phobias.

Individual phobic symptoms have been described since the time of Hippocrates, but the first report of a syndrome of agoraphobia is credited to Westphal, in 1871 (5). He regarded it as separate from other psychiatric disorders in which delusional fears occur. In one and possibly another of his three male patients the symptoms had started in adolescence. G. Stanley Hall, writing in 1915 on *Diseases of Body and Mind* in adolescence, stated (5): "[Unquestionably] the insanity of doubt which Legrand du Saulle, Kovaleyski, Cowles and many have since studied under various names with its Grübelsucht, hyperscrupulosity, imperative and oft-repeated repetition of the commonest acts, misophobia, aikophobia, claustrophobia, agoraphc ia and all the scores of instinctual phobias, etc., is characteristic of the later stages of adolescence" (p. 291). More recently, Salzman (6), Adams (7), and Nagera (8) have described the relationship of phobias to obsessional neurosis as a phase in its natural history or intermingling with it in various degrees of severity. Half of the obsessive children reported by Adams (7) had phobic symptoms also; and, in Skoog's series (9), the older the children were when they became obsessive, the more likely they were to have phobias and compulsions. Evans and Acton (10) found phobic symptoms, sometimes quite disabling, in 24% of 329 adolescent inpatients in Edinburgh. They also found no significant relation to gender.

Phobic symptoms may occur in many adolescent conditions, such as depressive disorders, anxiety states, personality disorders, and even schizophrenia, often fluctuating with the degree of severity of the basic disorder. In these circumstances, treatment of the phobic symptom is part of the management of the major disorder. However, the present report is concerned with adolescents whose phobia is their main complaint or problem; in other words, the primary diagnosis is of a phobic state or disorder.

## PSYCHOLOGICAL MECHANISMS

The psychoanalytic concept of anxiety neurosis provided a new framework for the understanding of phobic disorders, supplanting notions of inherited or constitutional factors and psychotic disorders. Freud (11) divided the phobias into two groups according to the nature of the object feared: common ones (i.e., an exaggerated fear of all objects and situations feared to some extent by normal people) and specific phobias (i.e., objects and situations that do not inspire fear in normal people, like agoraphobia).

Anna Freud (12) has clearly affirmed the earlier distinction between "fear" (the attitude toward real dangers that threaten from external sources) and "anxiety" (the reaction to threats located within the mind, due to conflict between drives and internal opposing forces). In her view, fears, however strong, do not develop into phobias, whereas anxiety can. Anna Freud goes on to detail the mechanisms in the formation of a classical phobia in children who try to deal with various anxieties by profuse internal fantasy and many different defensive mechanisms. This precarious adjustment is easily upset by the so-called "intrusive event," an external happening that brings anxiety and panic to the surface: the child resorts to the defense of externalizing the source of danger, which is preceded by condensation of the fears and dangers into one encompassing symbol. The internal anxiety is exchanged for an imaginary external threat in the form of a symbol (e.g., animal, street, school); and as a supposed part of the external world, it is dealt with by avoidance. Anna Freud disagrees with the notion that phobic children not only avoid the phobic object, but also are compulsively drawn to it. Although this may occur sometimes, in her view school-phobic and agoraphobic children appear unaffected while left at home, as are animal-phobics when the dread animal is out of sight. This accords with clinical experience of the behavior of phobic adolescents; the explanation could well lie in reinforcement of avoidance behavior by the family as well as the blotting out of internal anxiety by defense mechanisms.

The psychoanalytic model of the development of phobias has held the stage for many years, but alternative formulations have been advanced recently. Some are modifications of the earlier views (13, 14), whereas others derive from learning theory (15, 16). The latter derivation assumes that phobias are learned via respondent conditioning or operant conditioning, or both (the two-factor theory [17]). However, neither model explains adequately how particular phobias develop and are maintained, why particular phobias predominate in certain clinical populations, or why agoraphobia and animal and social phobias are so common. The variety of explanations of the psychologic mechanisms in phobic disorders is well illustrated by later exegeses on Freud's "Little Hans" (18): this, the prototype of phobic resolution of internal psychic conflict, has been redefined by learning theorists (19), family therapists (20), and more recently, by Bowlby (21) in his concept of "anxious attachment."

## ADOLESCENTS' FEARS

Studies of adolescents' fears based on approximately eleven thousand 12- to 18-year-old children in Belfast were well summarized very recently by Bamber (22), who categorized his own findings in terms of the persistence of fears, and their increase or decrease through adolescence. The major groups in the first category were fears of physical harm, injury, illness, and disease, personal safety, and incapacity. A second category comprised fears related to social relations, social problems, and gossip, reprobation, and ridicule. Animal fears, and those of water, fire, and darkness, nightmares, and of aggression and aggressors, declined between 14 and 18 years of age. More fears were expressed by females than by males, particularly by those 16 to 18 years old. The difference between females and males was not significant. No hypothesis was put forward to account for these findings.

## PHOBIAS IN ADOLESCENCE: EPIDEMIOLOGY

It is difficult to discern from published studies the overall incidence of phobic disorders in adolescence because few reports separate nonhandicapping fears from handicapping phobias, and most include phobias under the general heading of neuroses or anxiety (23). Furthermore, studies that rely on parental information may be biased by the tendency for parents to underestimate the number of fears their children have (24).

In a systematic study of 325 subjects (who represented 0.5% of a population in Greater Burlington, Vermont), Agras, Sylvester, and Oliveau (25) estimated the prevalence of phobia at 77 per 1,000, but considered as disabling only 2.2 per 1,000 population. The incidence of common fears is high in childhood and, except for fears of death, illness, injury, separation, and crowds, falls off rapidly during adolescence and early adulthood. Phobias, however, appear to run a prolonged course and, for the most part, are mildly disabling. In their 5-year follow-up of 30 phobics identified in the above study, Agras, Chapin, Jackson, and Oliveau (26) found that the un-treated phobias tended to improve overall. The improvement rate showed a relationship to age, being significantly greatest for patients under 20 years of age: 4 had lost their symptoms entirely, and none of the other 6 evi-denced worsening of the phobia or their social functioning. The authors suggested that the steady decline in phobic avoidance was the result of the subjects' exposing themselves or being exposed by their parents to fear-arousing stimuli.

In the Isle of Wight surveys reported by Rutter, Tizard, and Whitmore (27), over 2,000 children aged 10–11 years were studied: 118 had a psychiatric disorder, and 16 of these had clinically significant and handicapping phobias. Specific situational phobias were most common and were of equal frequency in both sexes; specific animal phobias were only half as common and occur-red only in girls; and there were no cases of school refusal, handicapping social anxiety, or agoraphobia. In no case was phobia the only symptom, and it was the most severe symptom in very few. When the same population was restudied at 14–15 years of age (28), depression was much more common and school refusal was recorded for 15 children; in many cases these were part of a more widespread anxiety state or affective disorder.

Unfortunately, the published data give no individual prevalence fig-ures for school phobias or other specific ones. Rutter and his colleagues (27) remarked on the ready response of children's fears and phobias to sensible parental handling, which may account for the infrequent presentation of monosymptomatic phobias at child psychiatric clinics in the United King-dom. In Miller, Barrett, Hampe, and Noble's study (29), a factor analysis of parents' rating of their children's fears revealed three primary factors— physical injury, natural events, and social anxiety— constituting the major category of phobia. "Social" anxiety included anxiety about school, separa-tion, performance, social interactions, medical procedures, and traveling in a car or bus. It also included school phobia, although other data have sug-gested differences from the rest of the "social" anxieties. Follow-up of these children showed age to be a major prognostic variable: 96% of children under the age of 10 years, but only 45% of those aged 11 years or older were free of their phobia within 14 weeks.

From these few epidemiologic and clinical studies we can conclude only that the data on the prevalence and natural history of phobias in adoles-cence are much less substantial than those on fears and phobias in child-hood. The only exception is school phobia, which is dealt with subsequently.

## CLINICAL INCIDENCE

There have been relatively few clinical studies of age at onset and the pres-entation and prevalence of certain types of phobia. Marks and Gelder (30) recorded the age at onset of presenting phobias in adults receiving treatment at a psychiatric hospital. Specific animal and insect phobias, which were rare (3%) but the most clear-cut, usually started by the age of 5 years (mean age 4.4 years); and none started in adult life. Most occurred in females as a monosymptomatic phobia, with little generalization despite persistence over decades. By contrast, specific situational phobias (e.g., heights, darkness, travel, or thunderstorms) showed a wide age spread at onset, some developing before 5 years, but most in adult life (mean age 22.7 years). Social anxieties (shyness, blushing in public, public meals, meeting people, etc.) started mostly after puberty (mean age 18.9 years), possibly because adolescence is the age when increasing social demands are made on youngsters by their peer group. Agoraphobias appeared at any time from late childhood to middle life, but distribution was bimodal with peaks at late adolescence and around the age of 30 years; 75% occurred in women. The more diffuse varieties of agoraphobia merged into anxiety states, affective disorders, and obsessional disorders (30).

Clinical studies comparing populations of psychiatrically disturbed adolescents and control groups have yielded rather confusing data on the incidence of phobic disorders in adolescence. For example, Masterson (31) found phobic symptoms were more common in controls than in patients. He attributed this to the greater sensitivity of an interview schedule than of a clinical interview; review of the principal-symptom patterns by two clinicians reversed the finding. Haslam (32), who defined phobia as a morbid fear of some situation or object, found that monosymptomatic phobias were equally common in patient and control groups, and carried a good prognosis. The most common phobias appeared to be situational and social; some seemed to have followed a traumatic event, the resultant anxiety being focused on a specific situation that may have been coincident. Both Easson (33) and Hudgens (34) stated that a phobia in adolescence may be associated with another psychiatric disorder, such as anxiety state, affective disorder, or schizophrenia. Easson (33) linked separation anxieties during adolescent emancipation with the advent of phobic symptoms; the latter becomes more severe and pervasive as increased stress is experienced by an adolescent who has weak basic personality strength.

Miller, Barrett, Hampe, and Noble (35) emphasized the high frequency of school refusal in adolescence: among patients referred for treatment of phobic disorders, school phobia was the reason for referral of 69% of the adolescents, but only 1% of all patients. Their estimate in 1974 (2), that the ratio of professional papers on school to any other phobia was at least 25:1 shows the concern of parents and professionals. However, very recent studies show school phobia accounting for only about 5% of all psychiatric treatment referrals in childhood and adolescence (36) with a prevalence rate of approximately 1% (37). Similarly, a current review of the literature (15) revealed only 40 case studies of behavioral treatment of childhood fears (with school phobia the major fear in 86% of the cases), which accounted for only 6.8% (more girls than boys) of the caseload.

## TREATMENT

There have been few systematic studies of treatment methods and their outcome in specific phobias in adolescence, if we accept the diagnostic criteria outlined earlier. Most reports are of single case studies or, at best, small groups of patients; and studies comparing treatments are few. In many studies, particularly those in the behavioral literature, mildly fearful children and phobic parents have been grouped together, and generalized conclusions have been drawn. Although questionnaires of fear-survey schedules have elicited a great profusion of fears that affect children and adolescents, the range of phobias for which treatment is requested is comparatively small.

One of the few studies of different treatments was by Miller, Barrett, Hampe, and Noble (35), who compared the efficacy of reciprocal inhibition therapy and psychotherapy of phobic patients aged 6 to 15 years with untreated controls. Reciprocal inhibition included systematic desensitization within a broad range of methods derived from learning principles, such as restructuring contingency schedules that reinforced school avoidance. Psychotherapy focused on the child's "inner experience," hopes, aggressive and sexual fears, and dependent needs, as well as problems of daily living. The therapist encouraged the patients to examine and reorder their behavior and methods of coping, and the parents to remove secondary gratifications and reinforcements for avoidance behavior; in fact, the authors' descriptions indicated considerable overlap between the two methods of treatment.

Briefly, outcome analyses showed no overall difference between treated and untreated groups, or between reciprocal inhibition therapy and psychotherapy. However, in relationship to age, there was a better outcome with either method of treatment than with no treatment for children 10 years or younger. The authors (35) concluded: "The failure of either therapy to diminish phobia in children aged 11–15 years leads us to conclude that the first task is to discover an effective behavior change technique for this age group" (p. 276). They mentioned as factors influencing therapeutic strategies the child's size, increased social anxiety, the development of cognitive functions (formal operations), the waning influence of juvenile courts, and adults' intolerance of infantile behavior. In summing up, Miller and colleagues suggested that phobias in childhood and in adult life respond differently, and recommended the development of specific treatments for the various types of phobias.

At 2-year follow-up of 57 phobic children, most of whom were teenagers, Hampe, Noble, Miller, and Barrett (38) found freedom from symptoms or significant improvement in 80% (and persistence of severe phobia in only 7%). The good response to treatment had been maintained despite exposure of some families to stress that might have provoked phobic behavior. Age and time seemed important factors in recovery: phobias diminished rapidly in the group aged 6 to 10 years, reaching a low incidence at the end of treatment and remaining low at follow-up, but the reduction was less marked in the group aged 11 to 15 years. Only one of the children acquired a new symptom (obesity) over the 3-year period of the entire study, so there was little evidence of symptom-substitution. Indeed, as the primary target phobia diminished or disappeared, so did many associated deviant behaviors.

Berg and Fielding (39) randomly allocated to two treatment groups 32 school phobics (mean age 13 years) on a psychiatric inpatient unit for adolescents. Treatment was conducted on therapeutic community lines, without formal psychotherapy, but social therapists were given particular responsibility for individual patients, and all relevant staff and patients were included where possible in daily policy decisions. Treatment was continued for 3 months for one group and for 6 months for the other, and both groups were followed up at 6 months and 1 and 2 years after discharge. The results showed that length of stay made no difference to outcome in the boys, but that the longer stay was marginally more effective in girls.

There have been no adequate follow-up studies of the outcome of treatment of phobias in adolescence, apart from a very small number concerned with school phobia. Berg, Butler, and Hall (40) reviewed the outcome of 100 adolescents with school phobia treated on a psychiatric inpatient unit. A standard interview had been used throughout the years surveyed; it covered psychiatric symptoms and overall adjustment, and improvement was defined according to degree of incapacity due to symptoms and quality of social adjustment. The most severely ill group (17%) included five patients with agoraphobia, two each with severe depressive illness and severe schizoid personality traits, and one each with schizophrenic and severe obsessional disorder. The review revealed that many of the less severely ill adolescents retained their depressive features, anxiety symptoms, and obsessional traits to some degree after treatment. During the 4 years postdischarge, 10% remained ill, but those who had left school experienced fewer problems in going to work than they had in going to school, a finding which has been recently confirmed. (It is of interest in view of earlier studies relating school phobia to work phobia [42].)

Berg, Butler, and Hall (40) generally found that the outcome was worse in more intelligent children, and that school phobia carried an increased risk of psychiatric illness in later life: at follow-up, six patients were severe and persistent agoraphobics, and one-third of the sample had severe emotional disturbance and social impairment, which is in line with earlier findings (43, 44). Also, in two retrospective studies, approximately 10% (45) and 22% (46) of adult agoraphobics reported school refusal particularly in their adolescence. However, this recollection also occurs in adults with depressive illness, and one should bear in mind the weaknesses inherent in all adults' recollections of childhood experiences.

## RECOMMENDATIONS FOR CLINICAL TREATMENT

Although the psychologic treatments used to treat phobias in adolescents differ in terms of theory, techniques, and how the goals of treatment are defined, most now consist of active therapy in which the youngster is rapidly and firmly exposed to the object or situation he fears and avoids. Solely behavioral approaches are unsuitable, just as the classic psychotherapeutic approach cannot afford to omit the necessity for the patient to face the phobic situation in reality. Behavioral approaches are often coordinated with counseling, family approaches, and in some cases, psychotropic drugs, and the psychotherapist has to intervene more actively than is customary with traditional methods.

### SCHOOL REFUSAL/PHOBIA

The modern treatment of school phobia is a good example of the need for combined techniques. This phobia is the most common during adolescence, although social phobias and anxieties are prominent in many cases in association with school phobia, or as a separate problem with handicapping consequences. Monophobias such as those relating to blood, illnesses, injuries, dentists, and injections, are much less common.

I prefer the general term "school refusal," which includes instances of anticipatory anxiety and avoidance relating mainly to some aspect of school (school phobia), as well as cases due to fear of leaving home and separating from parents (separation anxiety). Although the latter also may be present, and must be taken into account in any treatment plan, clinical evidence does not support the hypothesis that general separation anxiety is the basic issue in all cases of school refusal/phobia.

School refusal is a syndrome of emotional disturbance that occurs in several psychiatric disorders, and appears at various ages and developmental stages in a child's school life. It is improbable that the etiology, psychopathology, and prognosis are uniform, or that one method of treatment will be appropriate for all patients (47). Each case is a unique clinical problem, even though the themes may often be common. Each patient requires systematic assessment and a clinical diagnosis in order to formulate a treatment program with the goal of early return to school. The clinician has to decide whether the avoidance of school can be designated as the main symptom and major behavior to be treated, or whether it is part of an obsessive, depressive or personality disorder, hysterical reaction, abnormal illness behavior, or schizophrenia. These decisions materially influence the choice of tactics and mixture of procedures in the treatment plan.

Complaints about the situation at school should be investigated systematically, whether they be about teachers, schoolmates, particular lessons, games and changing-rooms, violence and bullying, sexual talk, classroom size, change of teacher or school, or loss of a close friend or schoolmate. Such exploration may identify the phobic situation or object, or related situations that have led to loss of self-esteem, anxiety, panic, social isolation, withdrawal, and phobic avoidance; they will also reveal any situations the student enjoys or finds rewarding.

By the time they reach their "teens," most adolescents have acquired a measure of independence and self-reliance, and comfortable peer relationships outside their families. If the patient lacks these normal assets, and many school-refusers do, the treatment program must include training in social skills and help in learning how to sustain peer relationships.

Family factors are extremely important, especially their way of dealing with anxiety, anger, somatic complaints, stubbornness, dependency, passivity, illness, deaths, situational crises, and other stresses. The parents of an adolescent may no longer be able to exert sufficient authority or control, or provide the firm framework the youngster needs; this failure may relate to large generational gaps (a child of elderly parents), or to inconsistency in handling of the child over time or between parents. If the father has been absent physically or psychologically, this often requires special attention to return him to a more dominant and effective position within the family.

Although most treatments will occur on an outpatient basis, in certain instances there are advantages to inpatient or day-patient treatment. Less severely disturbed adolescents whose families are able to make independent decisions and exert their control can be helped to overcome phobic avoidance of school by attending as day patients. Initially they master their phobia by entry to the hospital school, and gradually generalize this gain to the ordinary school. Simultaneously, social relationships with other pupils (deterioration in these relationships is common) are re-established via membership of the hospital group. In other instances, where parents cannot exert control without using physical force, the home situation breaks down into "hysterical" behavior and self-recrimination: parents and youngster are locked in a struggle for dominance, and each failure to resolve the school avoidance leads to anger, anxiety, ambivalence, guilt-feelings, and increased anxieties over separation. In such circumstances, hospital admission means a planned separation, and provides a chance to help the youngster confront the feared situation on his own, with the support of therapists and nurses. Then, a program of gradual return to school from the hospital, with increasing time at home, can also be instituted (48).

Clinicians who are continually involved with the outpatient treatment of school refusal stress the need for active therapeutic methods whose major goal is the youngster's firm re-introduction to school as soon as possible. Rapid treatment with immediate return to school (49, 50) may be effective if the refusal is transient and the patient is referred within 2 to 3 days of onset. However, more gradual tactics are needed in the (usual) cases of poor attendance dating back to elementary school. In the first instance, the avoidance of school is clearly apparent and seems to be a simple response to a phobic stimulus, and to require a simple uniform treatment. Many of the case reports in the behavioral literature are simplified accounts of situation-specific avoidance behavior in young children. But in adolescence, the problem is more complex, requiring integration of various approaches to treatment by an experienced clinical team (51).

The main goal of treatment — return to school — must be made clear to the adolescent and his family from the outset, and some form of contract should be agreed to by all involved. My clinical team takes the view that all cases should be responded to as soon as possible within the limitations of clinic resources and the waiting list. After completing initial assessment and examination, we identify possible etiologic factors and try to anticipate the difficulties that might arise when the child starts back at school; these may be educational, social, or geographic factors. We consider carefully whether the youngster should attend a different school. However, although this course of action is requested by many parents, and suggested by many education and welfare personnel, it invariably fails because it does not attempt identification or resolution of the real issues. In many cases it is necessary to negotiate with the school authorities to change lessons, modify a timetable, or delete certain activities, and often the clinical psychologist is best placed to mediate.

We involve parents in the treatment plan from the outset, and help them take principal responsibility for the child's eventual attendance at school. If we remove the responsibility temporarily from them, it is because further failure would so reduce their confidence and authority as to render them incapable of exerting any authority at all, and we do so with the clear understanding that it will be handed back as soon as possible. This can be accomplished in a family with two healthy, concerned parents; but it is more difficult if one parent is handicapped by chronic illness, or where a single parent is trying to cope with a stubborn adolescent without the support of a spouse, family, or social network.

We use various combinations of treatment methods. Parents are regarded as active members of the team who need to understand the rationale of the approach: they take part in discussion, plan each stage, and are fully aware of the reasons behind each step. At the same time, social casework is provided for individual parents and to deal with family problems. We find that many youngsters who experience school refusal have been drawn into their parents' own depression or dependency needs and cannot make any move until they are freed of this burden. The parents may need a great deal of help to define reasons for their inability to relinquish attachment to their child, and to work toward allowing him more independence. Family sessions help to clarify issues with siblings who are brought into the treatment program where needed.

Most often, parents cannot make sense of the changed behavior and attitudes of their adolescent child, quite apart from the problem of school refusal. They misinterpret the sullenness, irritability, and anger that develop when school attendance is pressed, and cannot sense anxiety and panic behind the overt anger. Being unable to exert control and support their youngster because of the strength of their own feelings, they feel at a loss and may appear inadequate and hopeless. It is usually a relief to both parents if fathers are given sanction and support to take an active part, and at the same time are helped to resolve differences of opinion and action in handling the situation. Above all, parents must be helped to face up to the fact that allowing their youngster to remain at home reinforces the avoidance, and to appreciate that they may be fulfilling their own attachment needs by encouraging it. Some situations are so entrenched that progress is very slow, and the parents' resistances need continual attention and clarification.

Miller, Barrett, and Hampe (2) outlined major steps in establishing a treatment plan, as follows:

1. Establish a good, trusting relationship with the adolescent and his family.

2. Clarify the stimuli that give rise to anxiety and phobic avoidance.

These, we find, should be done without theoretical preconceptions, for the stimuli may be both in the school and at home. In particular, we discuss whether parental (usually maternal) threats of suicide, illness, or departure have been used to control the youngster and keep him at home.

3. Desensitize the adolescent to the feared situation.

We use imagination, relaxation, supportive psychotherapy with limited attempts at interpretation, cognitive rehearsal, and modeling, singly or in combination, as appropriate.

4. Expose the youngster to the stimulus gradually until he can remain in school on his own, and finally, can leave home for school without anxiety.

Medication may be needed sometimes, such as a morning dose of diazepam, since the anxiety is often at its height just before the child leaves home for school. We prefer a gradual, firm approach rather than sudden immersion in the full school day. One of the team may accompany the youngster to school initially; but this task is soon handed back to the parent, who continues until a companion is no longer needed. Close contact with the school is required during the phase of exposure, to negotiate increasing time in the classroom; and the teachers have to be prepared for the youngster's arrival after a long absence. Many adolescents dread the jibes of their schoolmates when they return; providing them with a reasonable "cover story," and rehearsing their response to such potential events gives them confidence to reenter with a coping repertoire of social skills. After the return we maintain close contact with family and school, so that we can intervene immediately if there are signs of faltering or an upsurge of anxiety. Constant vigilance is needed at this stage, at the beginning of a new term, and if the child becomes ill and must stay at home—times when the adolescents are particularly prone to anxiety and recurrence of the phobic avoidance.

Marks (52) stressed the importance of the strength of the patient's motivation to seek and complete treatment in behavioral psychotherapy. This applies particularly if the youngster's commitment to school and the family's valuation of school attendance are low. In some cases little can be done to alter these views, but strenuous attempts must be made before giving up. If family and patient value schooling and some rewarding experiences can be identified, social pressure to carry out a treatment program can help greatly to overcome initial objections.

OTHER SPECIFIC PHOBIAS

The reports of fears by Lapouse and Monk (24) and Miller, Barrett, and Hampe (2) contain no systematic data on specific phobias in adolescence, and most survey children only to the age of 12 years. Fears of blood were recorded by Lapouse and Monk (24) in 35% of children aged 6 to 12 years, more commonly in 6- to 8-year-olds, but by Miller, Barrett, and Hampe (2) in only about 2–3% of children aged 9 to 12 years. Thus it seems that handicapping blood phobias, especially in older children, are uncommon; therefore the following case history is of interest.

*Case 1*

"Alan," a 16-year-old, had a long-standing circumscribed blood phobia.

He had consulted the school psychologist because of concern that his phobic reaction to the sight or mention of blood would interfere with his becoming a motor mechanic. More immediately, as a condition for participation in a training program, he had enrolled in a first-aid course: he anticipated fainting if he saw blood at any time, thus ruining his chances; therefore he was referred for treatment. Inquiry revealed no problems with social adjustment, stability of mood, progress at school or family relationships. Alan was highly motivated to overcome his phobia: there was a strong family history of fainting at the sight of blood; both the patient's brother and an uncle had done so, but each had mastered the problem without treatment.

Alan had fainted on 20 occasions during science and biology classes, and became queasy and had to look away when blood or operation scenes appeared on television. He worried that, when a mechanic, he might see fellow mechanics injure themselves and would faint, which might endanger him and others.

Five 1-hour treatment sessions were given, which included an explanation of systematic desensitization, relaxation exercises, and the construction of a hierarchy of blood-associated scenes, followed by desensitization in imagination. The boy was subsequently shown a hypodermic syringe, handled it, and simulated giving an injection. Next he was shown a blood sample, watched it being drawn into a syringe, and did this himself. Then he watched while a doctor took blood from the therapist: this caused much tension and required strenuous attempts at relaxation. In the next session a sample of blood was drawn, although at the outset the boy had complained of feeling faint; he fainted, but recovered very rapidly. In the final session Alan went through the full procedure of having a blood sample taken; he became tense, but was able to relax; he did not faint.

When seen again, 2½ months later, the boy was much more confident about seeing blood on television, and stated that he now regarded the sight of blood as an everyday event and was not avoiding it.

*Comment*

Case 1 illustrates a highly specific phobia for which treatment with exposure and training in relaxation was highly effective. The history suggests that identification with or modeling on other family members may have played a part, rather than genetic factors. In Torgersen's study of twins (53), intraclass correlations for fears of mutilation, including fear of blood, was lowest in monozygotic twins and had a negative correlation in dizygotic ones.

MIXED PHOBIAS

Apart from agoraphobias and social, animal, and insect phobias,

phobias are said to be rare and usually monosymptomatic (1). The following case history of a young adolescent illustrates multiple changing fears and phobias related to stresses in the family.

## Case 2

"Brian," who was 13 years old, had long-standing fears of various objects and situations: as soon as his parents had dealt with one fear, another appeared. Current fears were of dogs, wasps and bees, flying, elevators, underground railways, and his own health. The parents had tried to deal with Brian's fears by encouraging him to approach the feared situation, but they had never pushed him or carried out a consistent plan. The boy could be distracted from his fears at times, but his response was unpredictable: his parents felt that Brian *wanted* to be regarded by his famly as a fearful child, to give him some status.

Brian was the middle child of three. He was viewed by his parents as less intelligent and successful than his siblings, but had no problems with school attendance, work, or peer relationships. He was healthy and generally happy at home, concerned about and helpful to other people, able to stand up for himself in a fight, and well-liked at school. Brian's parents were intellectual and artistic. His mother had had psychiatric treatment and was still under supervision; his father was competent and successful. The family appeared stable and financially secure, the only (important) concern being the mother's psychiatric illnesses and need for treatment.

Functional analysis revealed that the boy had two types of fears—one, the normal fears of prepuberty, which had persisted in an exaggerated form; and another, more severe variety, concerning injury, hospitalization and painful procedures (including anesthetics), and a very strong feeling of loss of control. On subsequent visits, careful inquiry narrowed the phobic symptoms to four main areas: visiting a dentist and having an anesthetic, traveling in elevators, being bitten by a dog, and flying. (The mother's only brother had been killed at age 22 in a flying accident.)

The treatment plan included sessions of training in relaxation to give Brian increasing control over his reactions before desensitization was attempted. An additional goal was to increase Brian's self-esteem. The parents were involved throughout the program, and able to reinforce their son with praise for any improvements in control of his fears and in his school work. Desensitization was based on a 20-item hierarchy for elevators, involving fear items such as their type and the absence or presence of other passengers. Actual exposure was to passenger elevators, first in nearby buildings and later on the London Underground, including travel in the train. After six sessions these fears had largely subsided, and a program was begun to desensitize Brian to visits to dentists. No work was carried out on the boy's fear of flying, but his sister was due to travel by air and he hoped he could learn from her experiences and overcome this on his own.

Toward the end of treatment, family tension came into the open, and it became clear that the boy was in the middle of warring factions. However, the parents were unwilling to deal with their problems via a family approach, and it remains to be seen whether the lessening of Brian's fears will be maintained.

*Comment*

Case 2 contrasts with the first in that there were multiple long-standing phobias, and family factors appeared to reinforce the persistence of the phobias, which kept changing. The absence of specificity makes the treatment more difficult and the prognosis correspondingly poorer.*

## CONCLUSIONS

School refusal/phobia is the most common type of phobic disorder in adolescence, followed in frequency by social phobias, agoraphobia, and miscellaneous ones such as blood, illness, and injury phobias. Phobic symptoms can also occur in association with other psychiatric disorders.

Many more outcome and prospective studies are required; however, the evidence thus far suggests a significant link between school refusal/ phobia in adolescence and psychiatric disorders and social impairment in later life.

The simple methods of treatment of situation-specific avoidance behavior that are useful in younger children and in many cases of circumscribed phobic disorders, are not effective against school refusal in adolescents. The latter requires an integrated approach including systematic assessment, clinical diagnosis, behavioral analysis, and family approaches, leading to definition of goals and the construction of a comprehensive treatment plan.

The multifarious nature of school refusal/phobia poses the following questions: What is the most effective combination of treatment procedures for the specified goals of treatment in particular adolescents and families? And how can the clinical team apply these most effectively, using various types of psychotherapeutic approaches?

## REFERENCES

1. Marks, I. M. (1969), *Fears and Phobias.* London: Heinemann Medical.
2. Miller, L. C., Barrett, C. L., & Hampe, E. (1974), Phobias of childhood in a

*I am grateful to my colleague, Dr. William Yule, clinical psychologist, who treated the two patients described here.

prescientific era. *Child Personality Psychopathol. Curr. Topics*, 1:89–134.

3. Bauer, D. H. (1976), An exploratory study of developmental changes in children's fears. *J. Child Psychol. Psychiatry*, 17:69–74.
4. Maudsley, H. (1895), *The Pathology of Mind: A Study of Its Distempers, Deformities, and Disorders*, 2nd ed. London: Macmillan.
5. Hall, G. S. (1916), *Adolescence: Its Psychology and Its Relations to Physiology, Anthropology, Sociology, Sex, Crime, Religion and Education*, Vol. 1. New York: Appleton.
6. Salzman, L. (1965), Obsessions and phobias. *Contemp. Psychoanal.*, 2:1–25.
7. Adams, P. L. (1973), *Obsessive Children: A Sociopsychiatric Study*. New York: Brunner/Mazel.
8. Nagera, H. (1976), *Obsessional Neuroses: Developmental Psychopathology*. New York: Aronson.
9. Skoog, G. (1965), Onset of anancastic conditions. *Acta Psychiatr. Scand.*, 41, suppl. 184.
10. Evans, J. & Acton, W. P. (1972), A psychiatric service for the disturbed adolescent. *Br. J. Psychiatry*, 120:429–432.
11. Freud, S. (1895), On the grounds for detaching a particular syndrome from neurasthenia under the description 'anxiety neurosis.' *Standard Edition*, 3:90–115. London, Hogarth Press, 1962.
12. Freud, A. (1977), Fears, anxieties, and phobic phenomena. *Psychoanal. Study Child*, 32:85–90.
13. Odier, C. (1956), *Anxiety and Magic Thinking*. New York: International Universities Press.
14. Rado, S. (1950), Emergency behavior, with an introduction to the dynamics of conscience. In: *Anxiety*, ed. P. Hoch & J. Zubin. New York: Grune & Stratton, pp. 150–175.
15. Graziano, A. M., DeGiovanni, I. S., & Garcia, K. S. (1979), Behavioral treatment of children's fears: a review. *Psychol. Bull.*, 86:804–830.
16. Rachman, S. (1968), *Phobias: Their Nature and Control*. Springfield, Ill.: Thomas.
17. Rachman, S. (1977), The conditioning theory of fear acquisition: a critical examination. *Behav. Res. Ther.*, 15:375–387.
18. Freud, S. (1909), Analysis of a phobia in a five-year-old boy. *Standard Edition*, 10:5–149. London: Hogarth Press, 1955.
19. Wolpe, J. & Rachman, S. (1960), Psychoanalytic "evidence." A critique based on Freud's case of Little Hans. *J. Nerv. Ment. Dis.*, 131:135–148.
20. Strean, H. S. (1967), A family therapist looks at "Little Hans." *Fam. Process*, 6:227–234.
21. Bowlby, J. (1975), *Attachment and Loss*, vol. 2. *Separation: Anxiety and Anger*. Harmondsworth, England: Penguin.
22. Bamber, J. H. (1979), *The Fears of Adolescents*. London: Academic Press.
23. Marks, I. (1970), Epidemiology of phobic disorders. *Br. J. Social Psychiatry*, 4:109–114.
24. Lapouse, R. & Monk, M. A. (1959), Fears and worries in a representative sample of children. *Am. J. Orthopsychiatry*, 29:803–818.
25. Agras, S., Sylvester, D., & Oliveau, D. C. (1969), The epidemiology of common fears and phobia. *Compr. Psychiatry*, 10:151–156.
26. Agras, W. S., Chapin, H. N., Jackson, M., & Oliveau, D. C. (1972), The na-

tural history of phobia. *Arch. Gen. Psychiatry*, 26:315-317.

27. Rutter, M., Tizard, J., & Whitmore, K., Eds. (1970), *Education, Health, and Behavior: Psychological and Medical Study of Childhood Development.* London: Longman.

28. Rutter, M., Graham, P., Chadwick, O. F. D., & Yule, W. (1976), Adolescent turmoil: fact or fiction? *J. Child Psychol. Psychiatry*, 17:35-56.

29. Miller, L. C., Barrett, C. L., Hampe, E., & Noble, H. (1972), Factor structure of childhood fears. *J. Consult. Clin. Psychol.*, 39:264-268.

30. Marks, I. M. & Gelder, M. G. (1966), Different ages of onset in varieties of phobia. *Am. J. Psychiatry*, 123:218-221.

31. Masterson, J. F., Jr. (1967), *The Psychiatric Dilemma of Adolescence.* Boston: Little, Brown.

32. Haslam, M. T. (1975), *Psychiatric Illness in Adolescence.* London: Butterworths.

33. Easson, W. M. (1969), *The Severely Disturbed Adolescent: Inpatient, Residential, and Hospital Treatment.* New York: International Universities Press.

34. Hudgens, R. W. (1974), *Psychiatric Disorders in Adolescents.* Baltimore: Williams & Wilkins.

35. Miller, L. C., Barrett, C. L., Hampe, E., & Noble, H. (1972), Comparison of reciprocal inhibition, psychotherapy, and waiting list control for phobic children. *J. Abnorm. Psychol.*, 79:269-279.

36. Hersov, L. & Berg, I., Eds. (1980), *"Out of School": Modern Perspectives in School Refusal and Truancy.* London: Wiley.

37. Berg, I. (1980), School refusal in early adolescence. In: *"Out of School": Modern Perspectives in School Refusal and Truancy,* ed. L. Hersov & I. Berg. London: Wiley.

38. Hampe, E., Noble, H., Miller, L. C., & Barrett, C. L. (1973), Phobic children one and two years posttreatment. *J. Abnorm. Psychol.*, 82:446-453.

39. Berg, I. & Fielding, D. (1978), An evaluation of hospital in-patient treatment in adolescent school phobia. *Br. J. Psychiatry*, 132:500-505.

40. Berg, I., Butler, A., & Hall, G. (1976), The outcome of adolescent school phobia. *Br. J. Psychiatry,* 128:80-85.

41. Baker, H. & Wills, U. (1979), School phobic children at work. *Br. J. Psychiatry*, 135:561-564.

42. Pittman, F. S., Langsley, D. G., & Deyoung, C. D. (1968), Work and school phobia: a family approach to treatment. *Am. J. Psychiatry*, 124:1535-1541.

43. Warren, W. (1965), A study of adolescent psychiatric in-patients and the outcome six or more years later. II. The follow-up study. *J. Child Psychol. Psychiatry*, 6:141-160.

44. Hodgman, C. H. & Braiman, A. (1965), "College phobia": school refusal in university students. *Am. J. Psychiatry*, 121:801-805.

45. Tyrer, P. & Tyrer, S. (1974), School refusal, truancy, and adult neurotic illness. *Psychol. Med.*, 4:416-421.

46. Berg, I., Marks, I., McGuire, R., & Lipsedge, M. (1974), School phobia and agoraphobia. *Psychol. Med.*, 4:428-434.

47. Hersov, L. (1977), School refusal. In: *Child Psychiatry: Modern Approaches,* ed. M. Rutter & L. Hersov. Oxford: Blackwell, pp. 455-486.

48. Hersov, L. (1980), Hospital in-patient and day-patient treatment of school refusal. In: *"Out of School": Modern Perspectives in School Refusal and Truancy,*

ed. L. Hersov & I. Berg. London: Wiley.

49. Kennedy, W. A. (1965), School phobia: rapid treatment of fifty cases. *J. Abnorm. Psychol.*, 70:285–289.

50. Kennedy, W. A. (1971), *Child Psychology*. Englewood Cliffs, N. J.: Prentice-Hall.

51. Yule, W., Hersov, L., & Treseder, J. (1980), Behavioral treatment of school refusal. In: *"Out of School": Modern Perspectives in School Refusal and Truancy*, ed. L. Hersov & I. Berg. London: Wiley.

52. Marks, I. M. (1976), The current status of behavioral psychotherapy: theory and practice. *Am. J. Psychiatry*, 133:253–261.

53. Torgersen, S. (1979), The nature and origin of common phobic fears. *Br. J. Psychiatry*, 134:343–351.

CHAPTER EIGHT

# MOOD DISTURBANCE
# AND PHYSICAL ILLNESS
# IN ADOLESCENCE

JOHN E. SCHOWALTER

There are a great many definitions of "mood." The one used here is that given in the *Diagnostic and Statistical Manual of Mental Disorders: III* of the Task Force on Nomenclature and Statistics of the American Psychiatric Association (1): "Mood refers to a prolonged emotion which colors the whole psychic life, and generally involves either depression or elation" (p. E 1). Although this definition limits discussion essentially to depression, it is important to remember that the term "mood" can represent a rich variety of feeling states. Indeed, because mood can also be thought of as a prolonged and prevailing emotional set, any emotion that is sustained can be considered a mood; Louis Linn has compiled an alphabetized list of 41 emotions from "anger" to "vengeful" (2).

## THE IMPACT OF ILLNESS AND
## LIMITATIONS OF PHYSICAL DEVELOPMENT

Apart from infancy, adolescence is the time of life when physical growth is most rapid. Although this upsurge in height and weight is usually gratifying, the speed of growth and the variation between individuals causes most ado-

Supported in part by a grant from The Office of Maternal and Child Health, Department of Health, Education, and Welfare; The Connecticut Department of Health; and grant MH 05442-30 from the Psychiatry Education Branch of the U.S. National Institute of Mental Health.

lescents to worry about whether they will grow normally. Thus, it is not surprising that most young persons who have had a chronic illness since childhood or who contract a serious or chronic physical condition during adolescence, fear, or even take it for granted, that their growth and development will be adversely affected. Therefore it is important that adolescents' physicians discuss this issue routinely with their patients, and not wait to be asked. The mental-health consultant or therapist also should explore the possibility that their patients fear failure or distortion of growth.

Many people consider their bodies to be billboards of themselves; a physical defect that shows on the outside is felt to reflect (or represent) some inadequacy or uncleanliness of mind or character. In her book *Illness as Metaphor* (3), Susan Sontag condemned the widespread assumption that people are sick because of what or who they are. There is no doubt that such beliefs are common, in both afflicted persons and judgment-makers. Calef (4) described a study by Winkler that well illustrates this: when he showed pictures of normal and handicapped children, and asked people to describe the children's personalities, the handicapped children were far more often described as vicious, suspicious, and hostile. The human tendency to "blame the victim" begins early. White, Elsom, and Prawat (5) studied the concept of death in children from kindergarten age through the fourth grade, using two versions of a story about an old woman who died; in half the stories the woman was portrayed as kind, and in the other half she was unkind. When questioned afterward, 22% of the children who had heard the story about the unkind woman attributed her physical problems and death to some unkind act she had committed.

Illnesses that may curtail or distort somatic growth in adolescence include hypopituitarism, hypothyroidism, malabsorption syndrome, renal failure, and cyanotic congenital heart disease. None of these is very common, but there are three conditions in childhood and/or adolescence affecting physical development that are relatively common: cystic fibrosis, diabetes, and anorexia nervosa. The first is discovered in childhood; the second may develop in childhood or adolescence; and the latter almost invariably begins during adolescence.

Cystic fibrosis is a fatal genetic disorder that severely retards physical and sexual growth and maturation. An even more powerful impact on mood, however, stems from the fact that most patients die during adolescence. When first described by Andersen, in 1938 (6), she stated that all affected children die by the second year of life, although some patients now live into their third and even fourth decades. Unfortunately, however, so much has been made of the fact that many patients who have cystic fibrosis die in their teens that some of them see arrival into adolescence as a death warrant, each birthday being a dreaded rather than a positively anticipated event. For these patients, resentment, anger, and fear combine with both mourning for development never gained, and anticipatory mourning for approaching death.

Diabetes also is a genetic disorder that causes a lag in growth and sexual development, but there is a modified growth spurt with the onset of puberty. This spurt is accompanied by a relatively rapid increase in insulin requirement. Discussion with patients in whom this event is anticipated can be very helpful, because a sudden increase in the need for insulin may depress a patient who assumes this is a sign of worsening disease rather than of burgeoning adulthood. Another problem for the diabetic adolescent is that keeping irregular hours and consuming large amounts of carbohydrates are typical for the age and, to a degree, necessary to his acceptance as normal by his peers. Such behavior, unfortunately, may raise havoc with control of the disease. Any attempt at strict control without the teenager's motivation is doomed, and usually triggers anger and depression in both physician and patient. Nonpunitive discussion of the patient's understandable wish to deny the illness, through refusing to do urine tests, omitting insulin, or eating irregularly, can help the patient acknowledge the self-destructive and dependency-producing results of such actions. It is also reassuring to make clear that both the wish and the ability to achieve better control of the disease usually develop toward the end of adolescence, when the exaggerated fear of being different subsides.

Diabetics have the further problem of daily self-administered injections. Because sexual and aggressive conflicts in regard to penetration are relatively common during adolescence, accompanying sadomasochistic fantasies and intrapsychic meanings can be very disturbing. On the other hand, to know that they keep themselves alive through personal control of a ritualistic action engenders an elated mood in some diabetic patients. For example, expressed dislike of injections is almost universal among our adolescent inpatients, the only exceptions being invariably the diabetics; and diabetics writing in our ward newspaper tend to chide fellow patients for complaining too much about injections and not realizing how positive and important they are (7).

Anorexia nervosa is a condition for which etiological theories and therapeutic approaches abound, but unquestionably its presence causes wasting. It has long been noted that most of these patients look sad, and of course, anorexia is common in depression. Cantwell and associates speculated that perhaps anorexia nervosa is an affective disorder (8), and there have been reports that tricyclic antidepressants are useful in its treatment (9, 10). An interesting aspect in this regard is the elated mood of some patients when they are triumphing in their wish to lose weight.

There is not, however, true anorexia in anorexia nervosa: nothing interests these patients more than food, and there is usually a powerful conflict between the wish to become thinner and the wish to gorge. Although some patients do seem depressed, this is more likely to become obvious when therapeutic measures are taken against the patient's wish or during an episode of bulimia. In fact, suicide seldom occurs during weight loss; it nearly always stems from guilt about binge-eating or a substantial weight gain. Carefully accumulated data of antidepressant therapy are too few for an authoritative statement, but my own experience and the remarks of colleagues lead me to believe that treatment of anorexia nervosa with tricyclic drugs is usually not successful in altering eating behaviors and in providing weight gain. There are, of course, some adolescents without anorexia nervosa who experience primary depression with profound weight loss and even, at times, amenorrhea, but these patients do not evidence the typical body-image distortion, the fear of fatness, and the belief that there is nothing wrong with them. For these patients, antidepressant therapy may well prove helpful.

## COMMON SOURCES OF MOOD DISORDER
## IN PHYSICALLY ILL ADOLESCENTS

Illness means losses for adolescents. Most common is the loss, at least in part, of who they thought they were, of their autonomy, and of their ability to function normally. Illness is often a blow to an adolescent's self-esteem (11); and low self-esteem, in turn, is a major determinant of whether psychosomatic symptoms will develop in an adolescent (12). A common dilemma for physicians is the need to determine how much a mood disturbance stems from an illness and how much it is an etiological factor. Although Goldberg and co-workers (13) recently showed that the group of depressed adults was no more likely than the control group to be admitted to a hospital because of physical problems, it is still true that many depressed adolescents have physical complaints.

Premorbid personality is usually a reliable predictor of whether a mood disorder will develop in a physically ill adolescent. If an adolescent was prone to depression before becoming ill, he is more likely to experience further mood disturbance, usually along previous lines. A patient's mood disorder is also affected by the mood style of his family: the parents' characteristic way of dealing with illness, and the family's typical use of sadness, despair, joy, or hope affect an adolescent's reaction to illness and his patterns of coping. Although the emphasis here is on the impact that parents and professionals have in preventing, worsening, and treating their patients' mood disturbances, the powerful effect of peers' comments must not be overlooked. It is easier for an adolescent to identify with peers; therefore, the immediate influence of peers on a patient's mood is sometimes equal to or greater than that of parents and professionals. It is well worthwhile to ask the adolescent what other patients have told him about surgery, side-effects of drugs, or overall prognosis; this is information that may need correction or merit reinforcement.

Illness takes its greatest toll when the disability affects the adolescent's strengths. For example, even a minor or temporary problem that disrupts reading ability can deeply depress an adolescent who reads for solace and self-esteem, and curtailment of physical activities is especially likely to trigger depression in athletic adolescents.

Feeling a loss of identity is readily aggravated by the dehumanization of sensory deprivation inherent in some treatments. Depression is especially common in adolescents who are in traction or full body casts, or are in isolation or receiving hemodialysis. The periods of despair that are common in adolescent paraplegics are coupled with fantasies of being held prisoner, and of punishment for real and imagined misdeeds (14). These same feelings may occur when constraints are part of an adolescent's treatment. However, although suicide is relatively common in robust male adults who suddenly become physically disabled (15), that depth of depression is uncommon in adolescents.

The adolescent's level of cognitive maturation influences the understanding that he can develop about an illness. Cognitive level probably best explains why reactive depressions are more common in this age group than in younger patients, but severe depressions and suicidal reactions are less common than in physically ill middle-aged or older persons. Compared with younger children, adolescents have a better sense of time and therefore are more likely to grasp the future significance of illness. However, adolescence brings an inherent sense of long-range optimism, an ingredient essential for continuity of the generations. Without a belief in their own eventual mastery, adolescents would not take up so willingly and enthusiastically the responsibilities of marriage and family or jobs at the bottom of the work force. I believe it is this same armor of optimism that protects physically disabled adolescents to a certain degree. But there is a negative aspect to this common adolescent belief that adulthood is bound to bring liberation and success. Many adolescents see childhood as a sort of indentured servitude, a necessary duty before one can attain the complete freedom believed to occur in adulthood. For the dying adolescent, all that servitude was for naught, and there is the special poignancy and despair of dying before liberation and fulfillment.

Although most adolescents look forward to adulthood, some become depressed by the emerging demands of adult responsibility and anticipated loss of dependency-gratification, and may use their illness to avoid further separation and individuation from the family. Adolescents with ulcerative colitis, asthma, or diabetes, through a show of mock independence, may not follow their therapeutic regimen; the result is the opposite of independence, a worsening of the disorder; this brings increased adult involvement, and perhaps the more complete care of hospitalization. Peterson, for example, found that adolescents who had a history of illness admitted to pretending to be ill more frequently than adolescents without such a history (16).

DEFENSIVE MANEUVERS

There is much written about "masked depressions" and "depressive equivalents" in childhood; essentially these are defensive maneuvers. Depressed adolescents are more likely than depressed children to have symptoms similar to those experienced by adults. These commonly include disturbances of sleep and/or guilt, and thoughts of death. Associated features may include sad appearance, withdrawal, anxiety, irritability, and fearfulness. However, it is not only young children who exhibit psychological maneuvers to avoid depression. Depressed physically ill adolescents often erect defenses such as increased activity (including counterphobic rushes into dangerous situations), and a tendency to be angry rather than sad; it is nearly always more comfortable to be active rather than passive, to be mad rather than sad. These defenses invariably tend to thwart caretakers' treatment plans, and may jeopardize the patient's recovery. In my experience, these actions usually represent defenses against depression, and only rarely are attempts at suicide by default; this is an important distinction, because it governs the urgency and type of treatment one should apply.

SHAME AND GUILT

The two other moods often associated with or substituted for depression are shame and guilt. Piers and Singer made a useful distinction between these two emotions (17), believing that guilt results from a superego transgression and is combined with fear of retribution, whereas shame results from not living up to one's ego ideal and is accompanied by fear of abandonment.

It is common for patients of all ages to feel that their affliction represents retribution. From discipline as children, we learn to associate doing wrong with being punished. In later life, whenever we feel punished we tend to assume that it is in response to an offense. If psychologically minded, one can nearly always dredge up a real or imagined psychological "cause." For a depressed patient it may not even be necessary to recall a transgression; this point was made very clear to me by a 17-year-old depressed boy who had ulcerative colitis: during psychotherapy he tried to couple the exacerbations of his colitis with expressions of anger toward others, links that I was not especially pushing for, but which his obsessive-compulsive quest for thoroughness demanded. He could not find any reasonable explanation for one rather severe episode of pain and diarrhea, and this led him to what he called "the Aunt Polly explanation." That year as a high-school junior he had read *Tom Sawyer*, and recalled an incident in which Tom had been unjustly punished by his aunt. Upon realizing her mistake, she said the punishment was still fair because Tom's behavior must have escaped notice many times when chastisement had been warranted. My patient concluded that his episode represented "a sort of catching up," an explanation that helped reinforce his sense of order, and made him feel expiated and less depressed.

As for shame, ill adolescents are probably more prone to this feeling than patients from other age groups. This is the time of life when attractiveness, strength, and energy are especially revered, and when one is to make final preparations for definitive sexual and vocational choices. Adolescent patients are likely to be unable, or fear they will be unable, to fulfill these ambitions. Because we live in a time of such rapid change, often there is also the fear of being left behind, abandoned, and unable ever to catch up. When shame leads to withdrawal from peers and regression back into the family, developmental drives are frustrated, and depression is likely to worsen.

## PREVENTION AND TREATMENT OF DEPRESSION

The first step in approaching any problem is to recognize it. People are notoriously poor at recognizing depression, for depression to a certain extent is contagious. Depressed patients often engender in those who are treating them feelings of helplessness, guilt, and anger. Compared with other affects and psychiatric diagnoses, depression is more likely to cause the staff pain and the feeling that they have not been sufficiently caring and therapeutic.

We are all aware that changes in mood are common in adolescence, and that physically ill adolescents are especially prone to depression. Recent studies have shown the extent of this. For example, in a study of almost 4,000 high-school students, 91% reported that they often or sometimes worry about their health (18); and another investigation showed that adolescents who had a history of chronic illness were twice as likely as controls to report not feeling as happy as their peers (16).

The question of prevention arises only when the problem of teenage depression is recognized. Prevention of physical illness represents the first and most general approach; when this cannot be accomplished, it should be remembered that patients with certain illnesses are most at risk for depression. These illnesses include infectious mononucleosis, ulcerative colitis, hepatitis, encephalitis, and a state of uremia. Patients with severe motor or sensory limitations, a history of depression, or from disorganized families, are also vulnerable. Physicians should therefore determine whether their patients are receiving medications that might trigger a depression (e.g., steroids, reserpine, levodopa, and methyldopa).

Reduction of anxiety generated by feelings of being a passive victim is a primary aim. It is crucial to keep patients informed about what is happening, what is to be done, and how they can help in the formulation and execution of therapeutic regimens. As mentioned above, to be active rather than passive in one's fate is a major weapon in combating the feelings of help-lessness and hopelessness so commonly linked with depression. Seligman found in severely burned children, that once hopelessness set in, death soon followed (19); and we learned that the greatest dissatisfactions experienced by less severely ill adolescent inpatients concerned insufficient information about their disorder, and not being involved enough in its treatment (20).

Reduction of pain is important: it allows patients to feel more hopeful and in control. Successful pharmacologic management of pain can help prevent secondary depression, especially in dying children (21).

Administrative structures, also, can help to keep patients from becom-ing overwhelmed. These include meetings of patients, and perhaps a ward newspaper; and venting one's anger about Fate, doctors, procedures, or food can help prevent the anger from being turned against oneself. Just as you never see "burn-out" in a fractious staff member, depression is rarer in patients who vent their frustration and anger. This was clearly illustrated by Seligman's identification of patients who, despite apparently overwhelm-ing adverse factors, survived because, as she put it, they were "too mean to die" (19).

Encouragement of peer interaction can be very important in prevent-ing depressions. Maintenance and stimulation of common interests can be enhanced through liberal visiting policies and group or "big brother/big sister" programs. In the latter, an adolescent who had adjusted well after a similar disorder or procedure acts as a mentor for the new patient.

A ward-policy change that made a difference in our unit was discontin-uing the danger list (22), a procedure in which critically ill patients were labeled by putting a red star on their chart and Kardex sheet. Aside from applying the stigma of "probably going to die," the practice ensured no serv-ice that could not be accomplished without the label. We also discontinued the policy of shutting all patients in their rooms behind closed doors when a patient died and was taken to the morgue. Comments by patients during the weekly meetings revealed that these actions to treat the seriously ill and dying with more respect and less secrecy had lifted their moods in general.

Both in terms of prevention and treatment, it is important to allow and foster adaptive defense mechanisms. Protest has already been mentioned. Intellectualization is another excellent one, because mastery tends to diminish anxiety which in turn lessens the likelihood or severity of depression. In fact, some patients become depressed primarily because of their anxiety, and the subsequent fear that it is a sign of their having mental *as well as* physical illness. The realization that anxiety is normal, and at low levels can be adaptive, is therapeutic for many patients (23).

Identification with the aggressor is another adaptive defense mechanism. This is not practiced solely by those patients who want to become nurses or doctors: *all* patients who feel they are treated negatively may tend to treat other patients and the staff similarly. As noted above in another context, the externalization of anger is a key defense against depression. This defense is hard on the staff, however, especially if taken personally, or if there is insufficient staff support. The realization by staff that a patient's anger and complaining are not necessarily personal, and can sometimes be therapeutic, is an important concept for both staff education and patient support.

Withdrawal can be a useful defense for some patients who are very ill. Although it is commonly a sign of depression and of giving up, in some patients it represents the husbanding of energy in an intense desire to survive.

Denial is still another defense that can be harmful or adaptive. Everyone uses some denial, but denial of facts prevents a patient from developing appropriate coping skills, and, in chronic illness or a long hospital stay, is usually maladaptive. However, there are data which suggest that denial can improve chances of survival from acute catastrophic illnesses (24).

Work with other members of the patient's circle can help prevent depression. A good relationship and communication with the patient's family are helpful, as patients seem more vulnerable to depression if they are under family stress at the time of admission or onset of illness. Furthermore, helping parents cope with their own needs is likely to help them provide support for their child.

Good staff morale is another obvious factor in prevention. When staff have an adequate support system, there is more consistency of care and less likelihood that staff and patient psychopathology will reinforce each other (25). In one study (26), most of the physicians who had changed opinions on emotional issues cited "clinical experience" as the cause of change, even when their approach had altered as much as 180° and when their previous approach also had been attributed to clinical experience. As it is unlikely that patients' behavior changes as much as the eyes of the beholder, it is crucial to educate the eyes of staff to see and to interpret their patients' emotions correctly.

As noted earlier, depressive feelings can be contagious. Depression tends to drive people away, and circular staff-patient reactions sometimes occur. In other words, staff often feel depressed when there are many depressed or dying patients on a ward. Staff who are demoralized can lower their patients' confidence, foster feelings of not being provided for, and encourage depression. The recent salutary move toward primary nursing provides patients and nurses with greater personal satisfaction; unfortunately, it seems also to increase the likelihood of staff burn-out. Primary nursing requires additional supervision because these strong relationships render a nurse more vulnerable when her patients are depressed, do poorly, or die.

The treatment of depression in physically ill adolescents includes continuation of the approaches mentioned as helpful for prevention. Psychotherapy is an important additional tool. Besides encouraging flexibility of adaptive coping mechanisms, psychotherapy often focuses on issues of failure, low self-esteem, changes in appearance, and ways to compensate for emotional, motor, or sensory losses. It can also elucidate problems in relationships with family members and staff, which often appear in the transference. Inclusion in group therapy with adolescents can be extremely helpful, especially if others have physical disabilities. Family therapy is indicated when family dysfunction or lack of support is a major component of the depression.

Antidepressant medication is usually not very effective, and is indicated chiefly in patients who cannot relate because of the depth of their depression. Amitriptyline (Elavil) inhibits serotonin uptake, but causes considerable anticholinergic side-effects. Desipramine (Norpramin; Pertofrane) and imipramine (Tofranil) inhibit norepinephrine uptake. When such therapy is indicated, we usually try amitriptyline first. For severe depression not responding to 150–200 mg. per day for 4 to 5 weeks, we may switch to a norepinephrine-uptake inhibitor; this is helpful in some cases. "Atypical" depressions that include hypochondriacal symptoms, which are uncommon in this age group, may respond to agents that inhibit monoamine oxidase. It is ironic that antidepressants are the most dangerous psychiatric drugs in terms of overdose and, therefore, usually contraindicated without close supervision in the treatment of adolescents who are suicidal. Weissman, Prusoff, Dimascio, Neu, Goklaney, and Klerman (27) have clearly demonstrated that pharmacotherapy is more likely to be efficacious when combined with psychotherapy.

## THE POSITIVE IMPACT OF MOOD

It is reassuring that relatively few physically ill adolescents become more than minimally depressed. Even though adolescence is a time when most adults are approached with doubt, adolescent patients often develop considerable hope, faith, and trust; this maintains optimism, and spurs motivation. Certainly, genetic makeup, personal experiences, family expectations, and peer support are important, but why some adolescents face adversity with hope whereas others give up is still an intriguing question. We do know, however, that the effect of positive moods on the body, especially the immunologic system, is as powerful as the impact of negative moods (28, 29). At the most basic level, deciding whether to take one's medicine or to accept a procedure or surgery is an example of the mind's ability to affect the body. The majority of adolescents cope well with their illnesses.

It seems important to remember that the mind, especially the unconscious mind, does not exclusively cause problems. More often, the mind and its moods are responsible for the adolescent's ability to accept help, to cope, and to learn to care for himself.

## SUMMARY

Physical illness has particularly severe effects on adolescents because of their need to feel autonomous and self-sufficient, the importance of strength and beauty, the usual vitality expressed by peers, and the special impact of debilitation or death occurring just before they finally reach maturity.

I have reviewed the typical impact of illness on the physical development of adolescents, discussed common causes of depression in physically ill adolescents, and presented useful approaches to its prevention and treatment. Although this paper focused on mood disturbance, the positive impact of mood on physical illness was emphasized as well.

## REFERENCES

1. American Psychiatric Association: Task Force on Nomenclature and Statistics (1977), *Diagnostic and Statistical Manual of Mental Disorders*, 3rd ed. (Draft.)
2. Linn, L. (1975), Clinical manifestations of psychiatric disorders. In: *Comprehensive Textbook of Psychiatry*, Vol. II, ed. A. M. Freedman, H. I. Kaplan, & B. J. Sadock. Baltimore: Williams & Wilkins.
3. Sontag, S. (1978), *Illness as Metaphor*. New York: Farrar, Straus & Giroux.
4. Calef, V. (1959), Panel Report: Psychological consequences of physical illness in childhood. *J. Am. Psychoanal. Assoc.*, 7:155-162.
5. White, E., Elsom, B., & Prawat, R. (1978), Children's conceptions of death. *Child Dev.*, 49:307-310.
6. Andersen, D. H. (1938), Cystic fibrosis of the pancreas and its relation to celiac disease; clinical and pathologic study. *Am. J. Dis. Child.*, 56:344-399.
7. Schowalter, J. E., & Lord, R. D. (1972), On the writings of adolescents in a general hospital ward. *Psychoanal. Study Child*, 27:181-200.
8. Cantwell, D. P., Sturzenberger, S., Burroughs, J., Salkin, B., & Green, J. K. (1977), Anorexia nervosa: an affective disorder? *Arch. Gen. Psychiatry*, 34: 1087-1093.
9. Needleman, H. L. & Waber, D. (1976), Amitriptyline therapy in patients with

anorexia nervosa. *Lancet*, 2:580.

10. Moore, D. C. (1977), Amitriptyline therapy in anorexia nervosa. *Am. J. Psychiatry*, 134:1303-1304.

11. Schowalter, J. E. (1977), Psychological reactions to physical illness and hospitalization in adolescence: a survey. *J. Am. Acad. Child Psychiatry*, 16:500-516.

12. Rosenberg, M. (1965), *Society and the Adolescent Self-Image*. Princeton, N. J.: Princeton University Press.

13. Goldberg, E. L., Comstock, G. W., & Hornstra, R. K. (1979), Depressed mood and subsequent physical illness. *Am. J. Psychiatry*, 136:530-534.

14. Geller, B. & Greydanus, D. E. (1979), Psychological management of acute paraplegia in adolescence. *Pediatrics*, 63:562-564.

15. Roth, M. & Kerr, T. A. (1970), Diagnosis of the reactive depressive illnesses. *Mod. Trends Psychol. Med.*, 2:165-199.

16. Peterson, E. T. (1972), The impact of adolescent illness on parental relationships. *J. Health Social Behav.*, 13:429-437.

17. Piers, G. & Singer, M. B. (1953), *Shame and Guilt: A Psychoanalytic and a Cultural Study*, reprint ed. New York: Norton, 1971.

18. Parcel, G. S., Nader, P. R., & Meyer, M. P. (1977), Adolescent health concerns, problems, and patterns of utilization in a triethnic urban population. *Pediatrics*, 60:157-164.

19. Seligman, R. (1974), A psychiatric classification system for burned children. *Am. J. Psychiatry*, 131:41-46.

20. Schowalter, J. E. & Anyan, W. R. (1973), Experience on an adolescent inpatient division. *Am. J. Dis. Child.*, 125:212-215.

21. Schowalter, J. E. (1973), Drugs, fatally ill children, and the pediatric staff. In: *Psychopharmacologic Agents for the Terminally Ill and Bereaved*, ed. I. K. Goldberg, S. Malitz, & A. Kutscher. New York: Columbia University Press, pp. 296-306.

22. Schowalter, J. E. (1974), Anticipatory grief and going on the "danger list." In: *Anticipatory Grief*, ed. B. Schoenberg, A. Carr, A. Kutscher, D. Peretz, & I. Goldberg. New York: Columbia University Press, pp. 187-192.

23. Janis, I. L. (1958), Emotional inoculation. In: *Psychoanalysis and the Social Sciences*, Vol. 5, ed. W. Muensterberger and S. Axelrad. New York: International Universities Press, pp. 119-154.

24. Weisman, A. D. (1972), *On Dying and Denying*. New York: Behavioral Publications.

25. Schowalter, J. E. (1971), The utilization of child psychiatry on a pediatric adolescent ward. *J. Am. Acad. Child Psychiatry*, 10:684-699.

26. Novack, D. H., Plumer, R., Smith, R. L., Ochitill, H., Morrow, G. R., & Bennett, J. M. (1979), Changes in physicians' attitudes toward telling the cancer patient. *JAMA*, 241:897-900.

27. Weissman, M. M., Prusoff, B. A., Dimascio, A., Neu, C., Goklaney, M., & Klerman, G. L. (1979), The efficacy of drugs and psychotherapy in the treatment of acute depressive episodes. *Am. J. Psychiatry*, 136:555-558.

28. Cousins, N. (1976), Anatomy of an illness (as perceived by the patient). *N. Engl. J. Med.*, 295:1458-1463.

29. Knight, R. B., Atkins, A., Eagle, C. J., Evans, N., Finkelstein, J. W., Fukushima, D., Katz, J., & Weiner, H. (1979), Psychological stress, ego defenses, and cortisol production in children hospitalized for elective surgery. *Psychosom. Med.*, 41:40-49.

# CHAPTER NINE

# ABANDONMENT DEPRESSION IN BORDERLINE ADOLESCENTS

## JAMES F. MASTERSON

Mood disturbance is a central feature of the psychopathology of borderline adolescents (and adults).* It is observed most often clinically as intense, labile depression and/or anger. Paradoxically, the patient may occasionally exhibit restriction or flattening of affect to the point of emotional emptiness.

The common occurrence of intense depression in these patients has led some observers to the thesis that the borderline syndrome is primarily an affective disorder akin to manic-depressive illness. Support for this notion has derived from comparisons of the frequency of depression in the family trees of borderline, manic-depressive, and schizophrenic patients, which found the number of depressed borderline families closer to manic-depressive than schizophrenic families. In my judgment, this point of view is mistaken, because the finding can as likely be due to developmental defects passed on environmentally as to genetic factors.

To understand the complex and multifaceted mood disturbance of the borderline, it is necessary to understand not only the quality of the patient's feeling state (i.e., how he experiences it), but also the conditions under which it occurs, and why these conditions produce it.

---

* The borderline syndrome as described in this chapter represents a specific psychopathological condition, a developmental arrest during the separation-individuation phase, which results in a fixation of both ego and superego development; it produces the specific intrapsychic structure of the borderline, i.e., the split ego and the split object–relations unit.

I have offered a developmental object-relations theory that the border-line syndrome represents a developmental arrest during the phase of separation-individuation related to the mother's alternating libidinal availability and withdrawal during the rapprochement subphase. The profound consequences of this arrest on the development of ego and intrapsychic structure, together with clinical manifestations and treatment have been reported elsewhere (1-11), and are not detailed here.

In this theory I use the term "abandonment depression" to unify the complex and varied, but crucial affective states of the borderline patient. The unifying features are the quality of the affective state of depression and its psychodynamics. The centrality of this underlying affective state, however, is often masked by the overt clinical picture; the latter, portraying the patient's defenses against the depression, can vary from externalized and acted-out rage, through phobic states, to inhibitory or internalized states such as anorexia nervosa. Not until these defenses have been worked through does the overriding importance of the abandonment depression become apparent.

Abandonment depression in borderline patients differs in several respects from the usual depression. First, it is not a single affect of depression but a complex of affects, including suicidal depression, homicidal rage, panic, guilt, passivity and helplessness, and emptiness. Second, the patient experiences the mother's withdrawal as the loss of part of himself and therefore experiences the depression as a loss of vital supplies.

Every patient will have all six affects. The degree to which one or more will predominate over the others depends greatly on the child's constitutional predisposition and the unique style of the mother's interaction. For example, mothers who use fear as a disciplinary technique shift the balance toward phobias; those who feature guilt shift it toward compulsive and inhibitory states; and mothers who feature domination and engulfment shift the balance toward compulsive states or acting-out behavior. I do not mean to imply here that the mother is the only contributor. The child contributes also, in terms of his basic genetic and constitutional capacities, i.e., some children are more fearful or more prone to inhibition or acting-out. Regardless of which clinical state is foremost, all of the patients have at the core of their affective state the abandonment depression with its assumption that, if they separate and individuate, they and their mother will die.

This state is so painful for the fixated, immature ego to tolerate that it must be defended against by the primitive defense mechanisms of splitting, clinging, acting-out, projection, projective identification, avoidance of individuative stimuli, and denial of separation. Consequently, what the clinician observes first is not the abandonment depression in its pure form, but some qualities of depression along with the patient's defenses. This has led some clinicians to deny the validity of the concept of abandonment depression, overlooking the fact that it does not appear in pure form until the defenses against it have been worked through in psychotherapy.

I will therefore consider, first, these components of the abandonment depression, and second, some of the types of defense that determine the clinical picture.

## THE SIX COMPONENTS
## OF THE ABANDONMENT DEPRESSION

### SUICIDAL DEPRESSION

The depression has qualities similar to that emotion described by Spitz (12) as anaclitic depression, i.e., feelings that spring from the loss or the threat of loss of part of the self or of supplies that the patient believes vital for survival. Many patients think of this in physical terms, as comparable to losing an arm or leg or of being deprived of vital substances such as oxygen, plasma, or blood. This aspect of the depression illustrates best how it differs in quality from the usual depression in adulthood, whose dynamics are predicated upon a sadistically cruel superego that persecutes the ego until it breaks it down.

The manner in which the depression emerges in therapy is itself a statement of its motivational power. In the first or testing phase of therapy, the patient may complain of boredom or a vague sense of numbness or depression, but his affect will appear quite bland and he will not seem to be suffering from a very intense feeling. This is a reflection of the fact that at this phase he is well defended against feelings of abandonment. As the defenses are successively interrupted, the depression becomes more intense, repressed memories emerge, and the patient's suffering becomes obvious. The patient intensifies his struggle to maintain his defenses; but, as the therapist confronts them, the patient gradually slides into the bottom of his depression—and there, almost always, lie suicidal despair and hopelessness. At this point, the patient is a genuine suicidal risk, and there is no longer any doubt in the observer's mind about the motivational power of the patient's depression.

One 16-year-old boy who was in an acute symptomatic state, unable to sleep, and with headaches, nausea, and diarrhea, was able to describe his feelings: "I'm going downhill. It scares me. I feel paranoid, I don't want to see anyone. When I go to class, I feel lonely, desolate, detached, alone on a brown place with no color, nobody around." He continued: "I feel like I'm dying. I feel powerless, sinking under 5,000 pounds of self-hate. I feel like a rotten tree with total despair inside. Hopeless, drained, no strength, I can't do it. Badly wounded, deeply hurt as though I'm being squashed, no way

out. My own emptiness frightens me. If hemlock was sitting here, I'd drink
it."

## HOMICIDAL RAGE

The intensity of the patient's anger and rage, and the rate of emergence
of these emotions in psychotherapy, parallel the depth of the depression.
The more depressed, the angrier the patient becomes. The content of the
rage at first is general, and very often projected upon contemporary situations. As memory of his feelings returns, the rage becomes more and more
focused on his relationship with his mother. Finally, at the bottom of the
trough, paralleling the suicidal despair, are homicidal fantasies and impulses directed at his mother. Thus the rage parallels and accompanies the
depression throughout the stages of psychotherapy.

## PANIC

A third component is the fear of being abandoned, which may be expressed as fear of being helpless, of supplies being cut off, of facing death,
or of being killed. Panic can dominate the clinical picture so strongly that it
conceals both the underlying depression and rage.

The degree to which fear is featured in the clinical picture seems to be
related to the degree to which the mother used the threat of abandonment
as a disciplinary technique. Many borderline adolescents were mesmerized
by the recent novel *The Godfather* (13). It is obvious that, being a best–seller,
this book must have appealed to many people without a borderline syndrome; nevertheless, the degree to which borderline patients were attracted
was very striking. The descriptions of the Mafia's use of terror and fear of
death to discipline and enforce compliance portrayed in concrete terms the
theme that had dominated these patients' early lives: if one complies, one
receives rewards; if one does not, one is actually killed. These patients live
in almost constant fear of abandonment, waiting for "the sword of Damo-
cles" to fall.

In the previously described case example, the threat of abandonment
apparently had been used as a disciplinary technique to inhibit self-assertion or expression of anger, and to enforce compliance. Therefore, as the
boy's depression and rage emerged in psychotherapy, the fear of being
abandoned for expressing these feelings rose simultaneously, sometimes
reaching panic proportions.

The role of intense fear leading to panic is suggested by another example, a female patient. As this girl's defenses were worked through, she became aware of her rage at her mother and expressed some of it in the interviews, albeit intellectually at first. The evening after she had expressed her
rage with full affect, she had a vivid nightmare in which she was pursued by

the Mafia, who wanted to kill her. This led to such feelings of panic that she was unable to sleep, and the next day she told me: "If I don't block out the feelings about my mother, I get depressed, self-deprecatory—I think everybody hates me and I hate myself. I have these ridiculous fantasies that nobody likes me. I'm even sure you think I'm a hopeless case and don't like me. I recognize that's ridiculous, but can't do anything about it."

Over a period of weeks, as the patient got closer and closer to talking about her rage at her mother, she became more panicky, and had repetitive nightmares of being attacked, tortured, and murdered.

GUILT

Guilt is a fourth affect behind the front line of the patient's defenses. This guilt, springing from introjection of the mother's attitude toward the patient, now becomes the patient's attitude toward himself. Because the mother greeted the expression of his self-assertion and his wish to separate and individuate with disapproval and withdrawal, the patient begins to feel guilty about the entire part of himself that seeks separation and individuation—that is, his own thoughts, wishes, feelings, and actions. Consequently, to avoid guilt feelings, he suppresses any moves in this direction and resorts to a chronic state of clinging and demanding, sabotaging his own autonomy. This aspect of guilt is seen most clearly in treatment after the environmental conflict with the mother has been more or less resolved; it is a time when an intense intrapsychic battle between the patient's wish to individuate and the guilt that this entails, comes to the fore.

PASSIVITY AND HELPLESSNESS

The mother withdraws her approval when the patient attempts to assert himself, viewing his self-assertion toward individuation as a threatened "loss of her child." Therefore, the patient associates the fear of abandonment with his own capacity for assertion. When faced with a conflict, he becomes overwhelmed with feelings of passivity and helplessness because the only tool that might give him mastery—self-assertion—brings with it fear of loss of his mother's love, i.e., abandonment.

EMPTINESS

The sense of void is best described as one of terrifying inner emptiness or numbness. It springs partly from introjection of the mother's negative attitudes (which leaves the patient devoid of positive supportive introjects), and partly from the failure of development of the self-representation.

DEFENSES AGAINST ABANDONMENT DEPRESSION

The styles of defense against abandonment depression determine the clinical picture. However, they are so varied that I have purposely minimized their contribution to an understanding of diagnosis in favor of defects in ego functions, i.e., reality perception, frustration tolerance, ego boundaries, impulse control, and the intrapsychic structure. Defects in these functions are the most enduring features of the disorder. These may manifest themselves in obsessive-compulsive and schizoid defenses; passive-aggressive, aggressive or hysterical acting-out; or heterosexual clinging.

## OBSESSIVE-COMPULSIVE AND SCHIZOID DEFENSES

"Bill," aged 15, was a model student. At about age 9 he had begun to experience outbursts of anger and aggressiveness at home, usually when his father (a successful theatrical producer) was away. His mother was permissive and indulgent, and Bill made excessive demands on her. Initially, Bill's tantrums were mild and infrequent, and did not involve destructive behavior. By age 11 or 12, however, the outbursts occurred more often, and Bill had begun to smash his own possessions, including a telescope he valued highly. (His parents replaced the objects.) Occasionally, if his father was at home when Bill had an outburst, the father would expel him from the house for the night, forcing him to sleep in the garage or at a friend's house.

Despite this history of acting-out, the patient's basic defenses were obsessive, schizoid, and paranoid. For example, his facial expression had the quality of a Greek mask, a superficial smile with almost no emotion underneath. The defense of intellectualization was manifested by his obsessive interest in science projects; his performance was excellent, but his meticulous attention to detail consumed endless hours. The schizoid quality of his character was illustrated by the fact that, although a good student with no behavior problems in school, he had no friends and acted as his class's clown to get attention. He also had fantasies of retreating to the North Pole, where he would have no contact with humans and could become like a machine; this was an endeavor in which he seemed to have almost succeeded. His idol was Mr. Spock of the television show *Star Trek*, because Mr. Spock was devoid of human feelings.

## PASSIVE-AGGRESSIVE ACTING-OUT

"Ben," a 16-year-old student in grade 10, had an early history of passive-aggressive response to conflict with his parents. Until age 2 he had clung to his mother, followed her around, and cried hysterically whenever she left him. His early development was reported to have been otherwise unremarkable. He had not evidenced separation anxiety when starting school, and was a good student until about the age of 7. Then, after being kept in bed at home for several months because of infectious hepatitis, he became an "underachiever."

By the summer of the ninth grade, at age 14, Ben had become depressed and apathetic and began experimenting with drugs. He used LSD, mescaline, and marijuana daily, claiming that these drugs did away with his "bad feelings" and allowed him to get closer to people.

Ben's course over the next 2 years was progressively downhill. Increasing passive-aggressive behavior resulted in his expulsion from several schools; and for several months before his hospital admission he had spent more than half the day in bed, getting up (to go out for his drugs) just before his parents returned from work.

### AGGRESSIVE ACTING-OUT

"Anne," who was 16 years old, had been adopted. She had suffered a cruel blow at the age of 10: the maid who had taken care of her died and her mother became ill, and the girl was left alone to care for her mother. Anne, always a problem, responded by acting worse. At home, she was rebellious, stayed up most of the night, and slept during the day; in school, she resented the teachers and dressed inappropriately.

As she entered her teens, Anne started to smoke marijuana, and at the age of 14 she was taken to see a psychiatrist. He considered her prognosis poor and recommended the girl's committal to a state hospital.

### HYSTERICAL ACTING-OUT

"Alice," who had been adopted, was 14 years old when she ran off to Greenwich Village. She had become bored and unhappy, and was doing poorly at school. (She was in grade 7.) In her new life she smoked "pot" every day, and said: "I feel free for the first time in my life, being taken care of by hippies." She adopted a pseudonym, Stefanie, which in contrast to her dull childish name, she thought symbolized a mature, well-liked, sexy, swinging, hippyish girl.

Her father's reaction was to break down and cry, saying: "Look what you have done to your mother and me. If you ever try that again, I'll stick a knife through your heart." The mother, on the other hand, calmly questioned Alice about her (still intact) virginity, accused her of being promiscuous, and took her to a gynecologist for a checkup.

### ANOREXIA NERVOSA

"Jean" was 16 years old. Her parents were divorced and her mother had anorexia nervosa. Already somewhat withdrawn in this unhappy situation, after her father's remarriage the girl became even more withdrawn, moody, and irritable. Then she threw herself into studying; in other words, she used obsessive study as a defense against her rage at being abandoned by both her sick mother and her remarried father. To make matters worse, soon after the father's remarriage, the brother to whom Jean was very close left home to spend all summer in camp. When Jean learned that her father was going to divorce his second wife, her defense broke down: she started a self-imposed diet, culminating in anorexia nervosa.

### HETEROSEXUAL CLINGING

"Martha" started at a new school when she was 14 years old, and there became increasingly unhappy and frustrated. She felt unable to communicate with her parents about her anxieties and missed her older sister, who had left for her freshman year at college. At first, Martha turned to her work to cope with her difficulties; but soon she began dating a 27-year-old man. She saw the man quite frequently, accompanying him to concerts and museums and visiting his apartment, and finally had an affair with him.

## WORKING THROUGH DEPRESSION

The extraordinary variety, tenacity, and dramatic intensity of these defense mechanisms may trap the unsuspecting into thinking they represent different disorders. However, careful working through of the defenses reveals the same underlying problem—abandonment depression. I shall illustrate with a brief report of the emergence of Anne's abandonment depression as her defenses were worked through.

By the seventh week of her hospital stay, Anne's behavior was no longer a primary issue, and the sessions began to move into the content of her abandonment depression. She was now tearful and frightened, and complained that her therapist made her feel worse. She began to have strong feelings which she had formerly avoided by withdrawing or using drugs. She complained: "You're making me feel worse. I feel there's a piece of glass between me and other people. I can't pay attention in school, everything seems different, nothing looks real. When I felt like this at home, my parents didn't know; and when I did something, they would ask me how could I ruin my little sister's life."

Moving further into her depression, she dramatically relived the scene when, also at the age of 10, she had come home from school and been told by her mother that her dog had been put to sleep and she shouldn't cry. Though she didn't cry then, now she wept unconsolably.

The tie to her mother was clearly expressed in a dream of running away from someone for fear of being smothered. Her first associations were trying to escape from her problems in the hospital, but then she said: "My mother haunts me, I can't get her out of my mind. Yes, just like in the dream. Oh, my God, I think it was my mother who was chasing me in that dream."

Anne then became resistant and stopped talking, saying it was much too painful and she couldn't take it any longer. Her behavior worsened; and when the therapist restrained her, her resistance broke down and the underlying homicidal rage burst forth. "You're just like her, I hate her. When she had the operation last summer, I hoped she'd die. And one day when she was 3 hours late because of the snow, I prayed that she had run into a tree. My God, how I really hate that bitch." After expressing these murderous fantasies, she began to talk more, and the acting-out stopped.

During the 14th week of therapy, Anne began to talk about her feeling that her parents had abandoned her, that they did not care for her. "When I talk about them, I don't get as angry as I used to; I get sad and upset. It's an awful feeling."

Her fear of loss of control was vividly expressed in two dreams. In one she was walking through the flames of a fire she had set in the center lounge of the unit; in another, she was driving at breakneck speed on an expressway when her therapist stopped her and told her to go and sit in a school bus. When her fear of abandonment was interpreted, her behavior improved. This improvement was further reinforced by help from her therapist in controlling her behavior and encouraging her to talk about these emotions in the sessions as a means of dealing with them.

In the trough of her depression, Anne confronted her feelings of utter hopelessness and despair. "I never felt they [the parents] really cared for me. If they did, they wouldn't have treated me the way they did. But I don't know if I'm worth caring about. If they don't love me, I don't care about myself, and then I do things to make them care for me even less."

This case sheds light on two questions posed earlier: What conditions impel the patient to experience the abandonment depression, and why? In brief, a separation in later life precipitates the condition by interrupting defenses the patient erected against his or her mother's withdrawal during the earlier separation-individuation phase of development. The breakthrough exposes the patient to the underlying abandonment depression.

## SUMMARY

Abandonment depression is a complex mood disturbance of central importance to the psychopathology of borderline adolescents. Therapists can be misled if they focus only on the defenses: they must work through those defenses to expose the underlying abandonment depression. As the characteristic feelings (depression, rage, panic, passivity and helplessness, emptiness and guilt) emerge, and are interpreted and discharged, their intensity attenuates. This enables the patient to alter his maladaptive defensive behavior and find new, more constructive means of coping.

## REFERENCES

1. Masterson, J. F. (1971), Diagnosis and treatment of the borderline syndrome in

adolescents. *Confront. Psychiatr. (Paris)*, no. 7, 125–155.

2. Masterson, J. F. (1972), *Treatment of the Borderline Adolescent: A Developmental Approach*. New York: Wiley-Interscience.

3. Masterson, J. F. (1974), Intensive psychotherapy of the adolescent with a borderline syndrome. In: *American Handbook of Psychiatry*, vol. 2 (Adolescence), 2nd ed., ed. G. Caplan. New York: Basic Books, pp. 250–263.

4. Masterson, J. F. (1975), The borderline adolescent. *Ann. Am. Soc. Adolesc. Psychiatry*, 2:240–268.

5. Masterson, J. F. (1975), The splitting defense mechanism of the borderline adolescent: developmental and clinical aspects. In: *Borderline States in Psychiatry*, ed. J. Mack. New York: Grune & Stratton, pp. 93–101.

6. Masterson, J. F. (1976), *Psychotherapy of the Borderline Adult: A Developmental Approach*. New York: Brunner/Mazel.

7. Masterson, J. F. & Rinsley, D. B. (1975), The borderline syndrome: the role of the mother in the genesis and psychic structure of the borderline personality. *Int. J. Psychoanal.*, 56:163–178.

8. Rinsley, D. B. (1965), Intensive psychiatric hospital treatment of adolescents: an object relations view. *Psychiatr. Q.*, 39:405–429.

9. Rinsley, D. B. (1968), Economic aspects of the object relations. *Int. J. Psychoanal.*, 49:38–48.

10. Rinsley, D. B. (1971), The adolescent inpatient: patterns of depersonification. *Psychiatr. Q.*, 45:3–22.

11. Rinsley, D. B. (1976), An object-relations view of borderline personality. Presentation to the International Meeting on Borderline Disorders, Topeka, Kansas, March 19–21. Topeka: Menninger Foundation and National Institute of Mental Health.

12. Spitz, R. A. (1945), Hospitalism: an inquiry into the genesis of psychiatric conditions in early childhood. *Psychoanal. Study Child*, 1:53–74.

13. Puzo, M. (1969), *The Godfather*. New York: Putnam's Sons.

# PART THREE

# DEPRESSION
# AND SUICIDE

INTRODUCTION

# PART THREE:
# DEPRESSION AND SUICIDE

## Quentin Rae-Grant

Adolescence is the prototypic analogue of transition. Its membership, defined less by age than by social designation, constitutes a driving force within societies where its existence is permitted. Adolescence, like divorce, used to be a prerogative of the affluent. In Europe the Grand Tour was reserved or available only to the families, more especially the males, of the most affluent sector of society. For most, the transition from the ignored status of childhood to the labeled status of adulthood occurred with no intervening transitional period, a condition that prevails today in less-developed countries. Thus, adolescence can at one level be regarded as a dispensable luxury, a sentiment that only half–facetiously bears echoes of harassed parents and slightly disgusted professionals. Parents have come to regard adolescence almost as a disease, luckily self-limiting, and only moderately contagious. The unifying factors are the dread of anticipation and the relief of ultimate safe navigation.

But adolescents have also provided a most articulate cutting edge for the shaping of society's future directions. Given the luxury, not the necessity, of marking time between childhood and adult status, collectively they combine caustic criticism of the past and cavalier contempt for the present with concerted concern for the future. They are the lightning rod for society's charges: the first in the streets to demonstrate, the first to espouse a new cause, the first to voice social problems, and the first to have their heads bashed in for their efforts. Adult society has no great love for an age group that so trenchantly attacks.

The degree to which this description is representative of adolescents as individuals is unknown. Until recently a well-thumbed aphorism held that adolescents who were not a noisy mixture of contradictions were psychiatrically sick or retarded. Adolescence, like no other period of life, has had imposed on it the yardstick of opposition to society, as a measure of the health of its individuals. Of course, as recent investigations have demonstrated, opposition may well be the attribute of only a vocal minority, not the majority of adolescents.

In general, neither adult nor pediatric psychiatrists are keen to work with the disturbed or disturbing adolescent. Adolescent pediatrics and psychiatry are still relatively underdeveloped professional areas. Perhaps, as Nissen points out, memories of adolescence are too close for comfort, and do not have the advantage of the rose-tinting of childhood remembrances. Also, perhaps, adult professionals may have difficulty dealing with the mourning and sadness encountered in adolescents as they relinquish their childhood, and the mourning by parents as they relinquish their children.

Adolescence has been compared by Anthony to the process of emigration and immigration. The excitement of leaving the old country and going to the adventures and opportunities of the new is counterbalanced by feelings of being a traitor to one's roots, and of drifting without an anchor. In the new country, comparisons at first are always with what previously was known: the customs and currency are translated into the old idioms, usually to the disadvantage of the immigrant host. For some, revisits to the old country, or even temporary return, are necessary preparation for the ultimate acceptance, use, and enjoyment of what the new country has to offer. Similarly, conflicts of loyalty characterize the adolescent as he ventures into the adult world, but periodically returns to charge his psychic batteries in the old and the familiar and within his family. The analogy is even closer if one recognizes that those who emigrate to get away from difficulties, problems, and disorders almost invariably find similar contentions in the new situation. Adolescence dredges up and replays the unfinished homework of childhood. Parents greet their child's adolescence, particularly its later stage, not only with concern, but also with vicarious excitement for their offspring, muted by a growing sense of the inevitable loss of "their child." This ambivalence crystallizes on the adolescent. It is not surprising that the adolescents most at risk are those with fewest family and societal supports.

The four papers of Part Three contain examples of the old and the new phases of North American psychiatry, and the middle and more stable grounds of European psychiatry. Anthony graphically illustrates how the two American positions regard each other. He puts the conflict in the past tense, but must know it continues. For a long time, theoretical debate centered on whether adolescents could become depressed and, if so, in what ways the depression would be expressed in pre-adult terms. One difficulty is that adolescents do not read theories — and, in any case, tend to be the creators of the next generation of replacement theories. The elegant, detailed, intuitive, and at times poetic, rendition of broad theoretical statements generalized from small numbers of intensely cared for individuals, seems rapidly to be giving way to the empirical collection of facts, and greater caution about generalized theory. Many clinicians try to maintain a balance between the two positions and avoid an either/or dichotomy, at the risk of accusations that range from lack of depth to the sin of heresy.

The new and exciting potential of psychopharmacologic agents is just beginning to enter the clinical practice of psychiatry for children and adolescents. They are particularly efficacious in the treatment of major psychosis but, because these medications are so potent, they also have serious and troublesome side-effects. The margin between clinical effect and adverse reaction is often small, and requires careful and specific monitoring. When drugs work they are indeed remarkable, and it is tempting to generalize from limited experience to overenthusiastic application. Regard for newly introduced medications, like others before them, will move through the cycle described by Laties and Weiss (1) as "panacea, poison, and pedestrian remedy." By themselves they are, as Wolpert clearly expresses, not the entire remedy for affective disorders. Continued attention will be required to understand contributory factors in an individual's experience that precipitate or prolong his disorder. One general caution, particularly cogent regarding the adminstration of drugs to children and adolescents, is that the effects of long-term administration are never known during the first wave of enthusiasm.

The problem of affective disorder is also examined from many angles, but uncertainties remain about the basic questions of what is meant and understood by depression in adolescents, as well as the definition of subgroups, and the place of depressive equivalents.

The concept of depression and affective disorder, particularly when one includes depressive equivalents, remains confusing, and leaves clinical judgment and preference as almost the only available guides. Most sobering, as reflected in the paper by Garfinkel and Golombek, is the continuing increase in the suicide rate. Despite improved treatment, more facilities, and multiple centers concentrating on prevention, depression continues to exact its toll not only of misery, but of mortality. The answers are not in, but the questions are being asked with a healthy savoring of fact, elbowing out of fashion the profundities of armchair experts.

Finally, with all this emphasis on pathology and illness, it is well to remember that adolescence is an adventure of great joy as well as great sadness, and of great hope as well as great despair. How and when to judge where the borderline lies between normality and psychopathology (which needs treatment) is the issue to which this section and its authors address themselves.

## REFERENCE

1. Laties, V. G. & Weiss, B. (1958), A critical review of the efficacy of meprobamate in the treatment of anxiety. *J. Chron. Dis.*, 7:500–519.

# CHAPTER TEN

# DEPRESSION IN ADOLESCENCE: A PSYCHODYNAMIC APPROACH TO NOSOLOGY

E. James Anthony

## A PREAMBLE TO THE CLASSIFICATORY PROCESS

Classification is both a scientific and a human activity, and the human aspect has a significant impact on the scientific one. As many as 30 nosologic systems of pediatric psychiatry have been produced over as many years, each with its own idiosyncratic point of view. In reviewing this state of affairs it was not difficult to reach the conclusions that taxonomy is not one man's business, and that every classification so far devised bears the unmistakable trademark of the classifier, whether biologic, psychodynamic, behavioral, or social (1). Furthermore, it seemed to me that over the years the classifying behavior of psychiatrists passed through stages of sophistication and elaboration somewhat akin to what Piaget and his colleague described in regard to the child (2). Thirty or more years ago psychiatric nosologists constructed independent "figural collections," from which have evolved systems that are more concise, coherent, and comprehensive, and that embody explicitly or implicitly some unifying principle or set of principles. It also appeared doubtful whether there would ever be an ecumenical diagnostic approach, for the simple reason that classifiers themselves were classifiable into diagnostic groups that in the main had little to do with one another and spoke different professional languages.

On the one side there were biologically oriented nosologists who, at one time, were fewer than their counterparts in adult psychiatry; at the oth-

151

er pole were the psychodynamically oriented, who worked within a developmental frame of reference with special attention to "internal" processes. In between were a growing number of nosologists who acknowledged the importance of constitutional, psychologic, dynamic, and social features, but still insisted on dealing almost exclusively with observable behavior as the most dependable of the classification criteria. Each group constructed its own classification because it found the classifications devised by antithetical groups unsatisfactory for its clinical or research work. It was also a sad but undeniable fact that the groups did not view one another with any kindness or understanding, and certainly did not regard their protagonists as the latter regarded themselves. For example, the biologically and behaviorally oriented were inclined to perceive themselves as scientific, objective, factual, and realistic; they, in turn, were seen by the others as restricted, compulsive, concrete, simple-minded, and shallow. The "internalists," on the other hand, saw themselves as dynamic, deep, imaginative, and complex, and were seen by the others as mystic, nebulous, unscientific, and subjective.

With such communication gaps built into the practice of nosology, it is not surprising that, even in the psychodynamic segment of the classification continuum, private and personal viewpoints continued to exist; however, these differences were often more semantic than real.

## CONSTRUCTION OF A PSYCHODYNAMIC NOSOLOGY

Consideration of the nosology of depression in adolescence within a psychodynamic context requires, first, a review of current concepts. Depressive affect and mood are now considered integral and ubiquitous parts of human existence (3), and, like the affects and moods of anxiety, potentially transformable by unfavorable human conditions into clinical depression. Either anxiety or depression may predominate as the presenting affect in certain circumstances and in certain individuals, but they frequently occur or recur together in primary or secondary form. The capacity to cope with these basic feelings as they impinge on daily existence has emerged as a measure of healthy mental functioning. In this respect, every phase of the human life-cycle — including adolescence — has its own constellation of depressogenic influences that challenge the individual's adaptability.

A complicating factor in constructing a psychodynamic nosology, as contrasted with biologic or behavioral nosologies, is the necessity to take into account the imponderables and intangibles of unconscious motivation. As the data for this cannot be culled from reliably administered questionnaires, it follows that a psychodynamic mode of diagnosis requires time for inner explorations and introspection; computer-banked diagnoses, which deal with tangible and surface aspects, unfortunately cannot be programmed to elicit such material. The motives associated with depression lie deeply buried along the lines of early development, and are interwoven in complicated ways with both the animate and inanimate developmental environment; access to this information necessitates delving into the past. Therefore, a protracted life history is an essential part of the process of diagnosis.

As the child is father to the adolescent, the latter inherits the dispositions and disorders belonging to the earlier period. Many of the disturbances that become apparent in adolescence are thus continued from infancy and childhood; therefore, nosologies for these different stages (and this is true into late adult life) overlap considerably. Even when childhood is relatively trouble-free, however, there is no guarantee that adolescence will run smoothly because the process of adolescence itself seems bound up with certain inherently problematic factors. Dynamically, adolescence is regarded as a time for mourning, when parental objects are gradually and painfully decathected. As with all cases of mourning, the reactions may be denied, postponed, or placed at a distance, so that no indications of loss are manifest; but clinical transformation into depression is always possible.

In theoretical psychodynamics, adolescence has been envisaged also as a time when so-called "primal" depressions, reserved or inferred from the child's behavior during the first five years, may occur. Thus the infantile "depressive position" (4), "depressive constellation" (5), basic depressive mood (6), "depressive-withdrawal" (7), and "depressive helplessness" (8) reappear in a curious admixture of adolescence on infantile formations. These theoretical considerations postulate that adolescents are at high risk for depressive disorders, a conclusion that in itself creates additional problems for the nosologist. Arieti and Bemporad (9) aptly stated: "The difficulty with this stage of development is that depression may be too ubiquitous. The normal mood swings of the adolescent may give the impression of an epidemic of depressive disorders occurring after puberty. The problem is in differentiating the truly depressed youngster from the normally moody adolescent who is showing transient episodes of dysphoric affect as an overreaction to relatively trivial disappointments" (p. 114).

The particular developmental tasks imposed on relatively immature psyches at this stage of life, the jettisoning of old ties and identifications, the forging of new identities for the future, and the struggle to live up to (often unrealistic) ideals are prone to generate stresses and strains to which the less resilient may succumb. Depression always appears to be lurking around the corner during adolescence.

## PROFILE OF DEPRESSION IN ADOLESCENCE

All of the best clinical descriptions in psychiatry seem to date from bygone days, when clinicians had little to depend upon but clinical acumen. An early description of depression in adolescence is that by Burton (10), in 1621, whose reference was chiefly to adolescent girls, but extended to mature virgins and nuns. According to this great anatomist of melancholy, depression in the adolescent female took the form of "troublesome sleep, horrible dreams, dejection of mind, much discontent, weary of all, yet will not, cannot tell where or what offends them though they be in great pain, agony and frequently complain, grieving, sighing, weeping, still without any manifest cause." Burton had no questionnaires or checklists to assist him, but all his recorded observations are remarkably sharp, and his encyclopedic survey of a nonclinical population (himself as a prototypical subject) includes every known symptom and sign in the contemporary repertoire of depression. He was aware of both the pleasurable and painful qualities of this affect, as well as its mysterious causes. During adolescence, he stated, one obtains the impression of "sadness emanating from nowhere."

Another good description was afforded by John Stuart Mill from personal experience; his detailed portrayal of severe unhappiness in adolescence demanded a separate diagnostic category of "analytic depression" (11), which is in sharp contrast to the anaclitic types. Mill thought his disorder stemmed from an undue analytic tendency that weakened and undermined his whole emotional life. It was, he said: "Favorable to clear-sightedness but a perpetual worm at the root of the feelings and, above all, fearfully undermines all desires and pleasures." Here we have the first suggestion in the literature that both cognitive and affective factors contribute to the genesis of affective disorders.

The most sensitive description of depression in an adolescent male has been furnished by Freud's well-known patient, the Wolf Man (12). As the description is retrospective, it is not surprising that it incorporates psychodynamic insights:

> After the death of Anna, with whom I had a very deep, personal, inner relationship... I fell into a state of deepest depression. The mental agony I now suffered would often increase to the intensity of physical pain... I could not interest myself in anything. Everything repelled me and thoughts of suicide went around in my mind the whole time.... I tried to fight this condition... but I was hardly able to listen to what was being said. My contacts with other people were reduced to a minimum.... My mental condition [was] so wretched... that I simply could not go on like this any longer.... I had fallen into such a state of melancholy after Anna's death that there seemed to be no sense or purpose in living, and nothing in the world worth living for [pp. 25–26].

This case reminds us of the association with loss, the painful nature of clinical depression, the conservation-withdrawal (7), persistent suicidal ideas and depressogenic family history. Elsewhere in the Wolf Man's story we learn that his mother was hypochondriacal and unavailable to him, that his father was manic-depressive, and that both his grandmother and sister suffered depression and committed suicide. Like other depressed adolescents, the Wolf Man complained despairingly of the meaninglessness of life, which also can be related to cognitive developments since childhood. Depressed children, even very intelligent ones, seem similarly unable to elaborate fully and systematically on their thoughts and feelings, the affects being either somatic or acted-out.

THE DEPRESSOGENIC SEQUENCE

In psychiatry as in the biologic sciences, a sound nosology rests on construction of a causal sequence; but in psychiatry the state of the art is such that clear delineation of etiology is difficult. Nevertheless, the construction of heuristic models is worthwhile to indicate possible connecting chains and stimulate further investigation. The pathway to clinical depression in the adolescent from its dim beginnings in infancy might occur as outlined in Table 1.

## ADOLESCENT DEPRESSION
## AND THE PSYCHODYNAMIC NOSOLOGIES

CLASSIFIED SYSTEMS

As might be expected, the psychodynamic classifications have much in common in addition to a shared vocabulary. There appears to be consensus on the following: that adolescents are more sensitive to loss because they are undergoing a process of loss; that their feelings of emptiness reflect the unperfected transitional period between decathexis and recathexis of objects; and that their depressions are reactivated primal ones or arise from *rapprochement* crises, that is, disturbances in the regulation of self-esteem, difficulties around autonomy and identity, persistent unsatisfied anaclitic needs, and from unresolved guilt originating from oedipal conflicts, disappointments, and frustrations.

I have described (11) the normal moodiness, "depressive equivalents," type-1 shame depression, type-2 guilt depression, and the more endogenous depressions observed in the children of manic-depressive and schizophrenic parents (Table 2).

Malmquist (13) has added three major areas to this nosology (Table 3). He focused on the important etiologic factor of loss, both current and past, and stressed the continuity into adolescence of certain childhood depressions, especially those associated with chronic illness or handicap, or masked by restlessness, somatic affects, and obesity. In addition, he emphasized the character depressions that make their initial appearance in adolescence,

## TABLE 1
## A PSYCHODYNAMIC MODEL
## OF THE DEPRESSOGENIC SEQUENCE

1. *Predisposing Factors*
   Constitutional vulnerability; excess orality; heightened narcissism; conserva-tion-withdrawal tendencies; primal depressions; oversensitive self-esteem.
2. *Precipitating Factors*
   Real or fantasied object-loss; frustration of instinct; disappointment; failure; narcissistic hurt.
3. *Perpetuating Factors*
   Inner disequilibrium; increased ambivalence; poor self-concept; diminished energy; anhedonia; loss of sexual interest.
4. *Defensive Mobilization*
   Hypomanic reactions; acting-out; increased dependency; phobic formation; angry withdrawal; obsessiveness.
5. *Increasing Symptom Formation*
   Moodiness; loneliness; boredom; hopelessness; helplessness; haplessness; un-worthiness; pessimism; loss of attention and concentration; guilt; shame.
6. *Breakdown*
   Developmental, reactive, neurotic, "masked," and endogenous depressive ill-nesses.
7. *Recovery Phase*
   Aggression turned back against object; lessening guilt, shame, and feeling of inferiority; increasing energy, sex drive, and self-esteem; renewed capacity for pleasure and happiness.

## TABLE 2
## CLASSIFICATION OF MOOD DISORDERS IN ADOLESCENTS
## (ADAPTED FROM ANTHONY[11])

1. Normal depression of adolescents
   — moodiness
2. "Depressive equivalents"
   — boredom, restlessness, nostalgia, stimulus-chasing, acting-out
3. Type-1 depression
   — cyclical development; crisis in self-esteem; narcissistic personality develop-ments; childhood onset (preoedipal roots); inadequate mothering; predomi-nance of shame and identity problems
4. Type-2 depression
   — noncyclical; masochistic trends; good–enough parenting; pubertal onset; predominance of guilt ("guilt-complex")
5. Borderline and psychotic depressions
   — especially in those at risk for (familial) manic-depressive and schizophrenic illness

## TABLE 3
## CLASSIFICATION OF DEPRESSION IN ADOLESCENTS
## (ADAPTED FROM MALMQUIST[13])

1. Mood lability as a developmental process.
2. Reaction to *current* loss.
3. Unresolved mourning for *current* loss.
4. *Past* losses being dealt with now by the ego.
5. Acting-out depressions.
6. Continuation of depression associated with chronic illness or handicap in childhood.
7. Continuation of latency depressions from loss or failure, "depressive equivalents" (somatization; hyperkinesis; overeating until obesity), and postponed grief reactions.
8. Character depressions (obsessional; anhedonic).
9. Psychotic depressive status (schizo-affective; manic-depressive).

## TABLE 4
## CLASSIFICATION OF DEPRESSION IN ADOLESCENTS
## (ADAPTED FROM FEINSTEIN[14])

1. Mourning reactions with degrees of nonresolution (denial, depressive shock, separation-individuation, rage toward lost object, reconstitution).
2. Normal depression of adolescents.
3. Depression with oedipal and latency fixations.
4. Depression with defective separation-individuation resolution.
5. Depression with anaclitic depression in childhood.

predominantly in obsessional or anhedonic forms. (In some cases of character disorder I have found depression alternating with masochism.)

As shown in Table 4, Feinstein (14) included mourning reactions, normal depressions, oedipal types of depression (analogous to those I classify as type-2), and a re-establishment form that develops from failure in the separation-individuation process (analagous to my type-1 category). He added a further category he labeled anaclitic, describing a depression continuing from childhood into adolescence. The general recognition of dependency as a critical factor in the onset of depression supports retention of this last category in the final accepted nomenclature.

Berman (15) (Table 5) constructed a nosology based on parent-adolescent transactions, matching each category of depression in the adolescent with a disorder or disturbance in the parent. It may be necessary to enlarge

TABLE 5

NOSOLOGICAL ASPECTS OF PARENT-ADOLESCENT
TRANSACTIONS IN DEPRESSION IN ADOLESCENCE
(ADAPTED FROM BERMAN[15])

| | Adolescent | Parent |
|---|---|---|
| 1. | Normal depressive moodiness | Normal parental empathy and sympathy |
| 2. | Grief reaction to current loss | Shared grief reaction |
| 3. | Mild transient depression relating to adolescence itself | Parental anxiety |
| 4. | Psychoneurotic depression; history of loss | Neurotogenic parent |
| 5. | Reactive depression; lowering of self-esteem | Depressogenic parents (disparaging, criticizing, humiliating) |
| 6. | Masked depression | Depressed, masochistic parents, generating feelings of rejection |
| 7. | Endogenous depression | Manic-depressive parent |

this important contribution to include the family of the depressed adolescent as a whole. Although individual links are not clear-cut, reactions in these adolescents (neurotic, reactive, masked, and endogenous depressions) seem to correlate with anxious, neurotogenic, disparaging, masochistic, and manic-depressive parents.

The epigenetic build-up of negative outcomes, through the sequence of psychosocial crises as described by Erikson (16), resembles a snowball effect by which the developing personality accumulates a heavy load of oppressive ingredients as it rolls toward adolescence (Table 6). However, this dynamic evolution does not account for the emergence of type-1 rather than type-2 depressions, which can only be adequately explained within the more comprehensive framework of psychosexual theory with its postulation of earlier and later fixation points to which the depressed individual regresses.

IMPORTANCE OF DISPOSITIONAL FACTORS FOR NOSOLOGY

Dispositional factors are not usually included within nosologic systems, even though they have the potential to illuminate diagnoses. Many of these factors, such as excessive orality, narcissism, or ambivalence, are little more than speculative, mysterious causal leaps. Schmale and Engel (7) made a better case for the thesis of predisposition, basing it on a developmental model which involved biologic, antecedent, adaptive feedback mech-

## TABLE 6
## AN EPIGENETIC BUILD-UP OF DEPRESSION
## (ADAPTED FROM ERIKSON[16])

| Stage | Gradual Accumulation of Negative Outcomes to Epigenetic Crisis |
|-------|----------------------------------------------------------------|
| 1 | Basic mistrust, lack of confidence, lack of hope, beginning pessimism. |
| 2 | Paranoid-projective orientation; shame and doubt; growth of dependency; low self-esteem. |
| 3 | Superego morality; guilt and sense of sinfulness; passivity and lack of initiative; beginning inhibition. |
| 4 | Inertia and inactivity; paralysis of action, helplessness; poor peer relations; feelings of inferiority. |
| 5 | Identity confusion and diffusion. |
| 6 | Isolated; unable to be close; hopeless. |

anisms that they referred to as "conservation-withdrawal." These mechanisms are a counterpart to the biologic arousal processes associated with the affect of anxiety. Their model also postulated a role for biochemical and genetic factors in augmenting or facilitating the individual's tolerance of helplessness and hopelessness. In addition, negative resolution of conflicts associated with these feelings can engender a predisposition to depressive neurosis or malformation of character. This model is a good example of the way in which modern psychodynamic theory is beginning to use empirical and experimental data from both biologic and psychoanalytic sources.

Primal depressions are thought to play a major role in predisposing the infant and child to depression in adolescence and adulthood (4-6, 8, 17-19). These primal experiences endow the developing child with a core of ambivalence, an unresolved depressive "position," a propensity to depressive-withdrawal, vulnerability to traumatic helplessness, a basically depressive mood, and preoedipal and oedipal experiences of disappointment, all of which conduce in their different ways to affective disorder. Given the relevant precipitating factors, a depressive illness results (Table 7). Disappointment makes an especially significant contribution not only to the predisposition to depression, but also to its precipitation during adolescence (18).

### THEORETICAL CONSIDERATIONS

The relatively immature psyche of the child and adolescent limits the application of classic psychoanalytic theory as propounded by Abraham (19) and by Freud (20), because this theory involves complex intrapsychic novas of both libidinal and aggressive drives. I consider Bibring's ego psy-

## TABLE 7
## DEPRESSION IN ADOLESCENCE: PREDISPOSING
## AND PRECIPITATING FACTORS
## DURING THE FIRST 5 YEARS OF LIFE

*Genetic Constitutional Factors*
Family history of affective disorder; excessive tendency to conservation-withdrawal; excessive orality; narcissism.

*Factors in Infancy*
Depressive constellation (Benedek[5]); depressive position (Klein[4]); depressive withdrawal (Engel[17]); traumatic helplessness (Bibring[8]); basic depressive mood (Mahler[6]); preoedipal disappointment (Jacobson[18]); oedipal disappointment (Abraham[19]); "primal parathymia" (Abraham[19]).

*Precipitating Factors in Adolescence*
Loss of parent by death or divorce; failure at school or work; menstruation; loss of love; failure with peers; loss of self-esteem.

chologic theory (8) as a better fit for what can be observed or inferred in depressed children and adolescents (21). Others have made use of the theory of an epigenetic ego coupled with regulation of self-esteem (18, 22), but Bibring's theory allows for the intercorrelation between psychosexual level, narcissistic aspiration, defensive need, the depressive reaction, and the nature of the central conflict (Table 8). The ego psychology cycle conceived by me (21) demonstrates how discrepancies between aspiration and achievement lead inevitably and cyclically to a sense of failure, lowering of self-esteem, feelings of helplessness, and depression, with *secondary* turning of aggression against the self, introjection of the ambivalently conceived object, and the use of depression to justify aggression (Table 9).

Arieti and Bemporad (9) have tried to link depression in adolescence, with its exaggerated urgencies, distortions, and impulsiveness, to the patient's failure to fulfill internalized parental ideals or to emancipate himself both internally and externally from the family. These authors prefer the framework of ego development devised by Loevinger (23), which links a particular type of dysphoria with a particular stage of ego development, a theory quite similar to Bibring's and to Piaget's "moral system." However, Loevinger does not differentiate between conformity to external rules, and conscientiousness with regard to internal rules in the context of shame and guilt; she appears to lump these together, which would impede differentiation of type-1 from type-2 depression in adolescence (11).

Arieti and Bemporad (9), like Beck (24) and myself, believe that the depression-prone individual has a distorted cognitive view of himself and others. According to them (9):

## TABLE 8
### AN EPIGENETIC EGO PSYCHOLOGY THEORY
### OF DEPRESSION (ADAPTED FROM BIBRING[8])

| | Psychosexual Level | | |
| | Oral | Anal | Phallic |
|---|---|---|---|
| *Narcissistic aspiration:* | To be loved To get supplies To be cared for | To be good To be loving To be clean | To be admired To be the center of attention To be strong and triumphant |
| *Defensive need:* | To be independent To be self-supporting | Not to be bad and defiant Not to be hostile Not to be dirty | To be modest To be inconspicuous To be submissive |
| *Depression follows discovery of:* | Not being loved Not being independent | Lack of control over impulses and objects Feeling of helplessness Guilt | Fear of being defeated Fear of being ridiculed Fear of retaliation |
| *Central conflict is over:* | Dependency needs | Controls | Competition |

## TABLE 9
### EGO PSYCHOLOGY CYCLE (ADAPTED FROM ANTHONY[21])

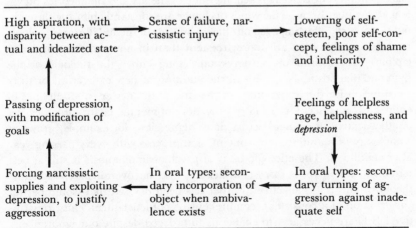

High aspiration, with disparity between actual and idealized state → Sense of failure, narcissistic injury → Lowering of self-esteem, poor self-concept, feelings of shame and inferiority

Passing of depression, with modification of goals

Feelings of helpless rage, helplessness, and *depression*

Forcing narcissistic supplies and exploiting depression, to justify aggression ← In oral types: secondary incorporation of object when ambivalence exists ← In oral types: secondary turning of aggression against inadequate self

The depressive has maintained a belief of the self and others that is typical of childhood...however, adult (and presumably adolescent) depression represents more than the resurgence of childhood cognitive beliefs. The individual continues to elaborate these encapsulated cognitions and to magnify their contents.... From this basic system of ideas...secondary cognitive structures are logically derived [pp. 476–477].

The adolescent, as understood by Piaget (25), enters a phase of thinking that is systematic, operational, and propositional. He therefore can evaluate his affects and their impact on others in terms of his new cognitive capacities, his newly developed ability to introspect, and his new potentiality for embroidering his affects and differentiating them in more subtle and varied forms. It is at this point that Beck's "cognitive triad" comes into being (24).

Adolescent patients, already predisposed to depression, may react to interpretations affecting their self-esteem with narcissistic mortification and transient depression. Thus, *iatrogenic* depressions often arise during prolonged analytically-oriented therapy and psychoanalysis. The depressions, however, usually respond to further interpretations of the mechanisms involved. During the transference neurosis, such patients also produce an outflow of depression, or reactivation of mourning postponed from childhood bereavement. Furthermore, they are prone to temporary depression with every break in treatment, with the anticipation of its termination, actual termination, and afterward. In a few cases the post-treatment depressions become more permanent, and require very careful therapy.

## CONCLUSIONS

Classifications of disorders reflect the state of the art and the theories prevalent at the time. Because the winds of change are constantly blowing throughout psychiatry, affecting even our basic concepts of mental illness, nosologic revisions in this area are more frequent than in any other medical discipline. Progressions or retrogressions along either the biologic or the dynamic diagnostic axis result in the addition of new categories, or their substitution for discarded ones. In the case of the newer subdisciplines of child and adolescent psychiatry, the developmental factor provides yet another source of change, across time; depression, for example, grows in complexity of manifestation, content, and process with every passing year after childhood. The etiologic basis of psychiatric diagnosis is still at best tenuous, and in most cases still lacking, and no overall psychodynamic theory of affect and affective disorder has been devised that would permit construction of a consistent, comprehensive nomenclature. Thus, descriptive labels are necessary, to enable us to proceed despite our ignorance.

Four views can be gleaned from the material presented, all still debatable. First, one may view depression as the twin affect to anxiety, ubiquitous and inherent to human existence. Second, there is a supposition that depression appearing in adolescence (as in adulthood) is a recapitulation of infantile depression, the earlier condition constituting a predisposition to the later one. Third, a more recent view suggests that cognition plays a vital role in the etiology, manifestation, course and prognosis, and treatment of depression. And fourth, it is postulated that there is an epigenetic build-up of depression which involves interplay between genetic-constitutional factors and environmental ones.

It must be emphasized that division into biologic and dynamic compartments creates an artifact, and contributes to the error that Whitehead referred to as a bifurcation of nature (26). Freud never relinquished his original leanings (27) toward a biological basis of depression; he predicted that, in the unlikely event the disorder would be completely understood, the ultimate explanation would be biological.

Many adolescents, especially gifted ones, are able to treat their own depressions. They use various ways (28), including self-psychotherapy, work projects, and self-medication; and in many persons who can call upon such internal sources, their depression in adolescence does not reach clinical proportions. Bertrand Russell, who grew up in a depressogenic family environment, recalled how as a teenager he often considered suicide. When he was 15, he wrote (29):

> There was a footpath leading across fields to New Southgate, and I used to go there alone to watch the sunset and to contemplate suicide. I did not, however, commit suicide, because I wished to know more of mathematics.

Here we have a striking example of the affect-cognition continuum that sometimes can turn the adolescent away from depression to creative productivity.

## REFERENCES

1. Anthony, E. J. (1967), Taxonomy is not one man's business. *Int. J. Psychiatry*, 3:173–178.
2. Inhelder, B. & Piaget, J. (1958), *The Growth of Logical Thinking from Childhood to Adolescence: An Essay on the Construction of Formal Operational Structures.* New York: Basic Books.
3. Anthony, E. J. & Benedek, T., Eds. (1975), *Depression and Human Existence.* Boston: Little, Brown.
4. Klein, M. (1940), Mourning and its relation to manic-depressive states. In: *Contributions to Psycho-analysis, 1921–1945.* London: Hogarth Press, 1948, pp. 311–338.
5. Benedek, T. F. (1956), Toward the biology of the depressive constellation. *J.*

*Am. Psychoanal. Assoc.*, 4:389–427.

6. Mahler, M. (1966), Notes on the development of basic moods: the depressive effect. In: *Psychoanalysis: A General Psychology*, ed. R. M. Loewenstein, L. M. Newman, M. Schur, & A. J. Solnit. New York: International Universities Press, pp. 152–168.

7. Schmale, A. H. & Engel, G. L. (1975), The role of conservation-withdrawal in depressive reactions. In: *Depression and Human Existence*, ed. E. J. Anthony & T. Benedek. Boston: Little, Brown, pp. 183–198.

8. Bibring, E. (1953), The mechanism of depression. In: *Affective Disorders — Psychoanalytic Contribution to Their Study*, ed. P. Greenacre. New York: International Universities Press, pp. 13–48.

9. Arieti, S. & Bemporad, J. (1978), *Severe and Mild Depression*. New York: Basic Books.

10. Burton, R. (1621), *The Anatomy of Melancholy*. New York: Tudor. Facsimile reprint, 1927.

11. Anthony, E. J. (1970), Two contrasting types of adolescent depression and their treatment. *J. Am. Psychoanal. Assoc.*, 18:841–859.

12. Wolf Man, The (1971), In: *The Wolf Man*, ed. M. Gardner. New York: Basic Books.

13. Malmquist, C. (1971), Depressions in childhood and adolescence. *New Engl. J. Med.*, 284:887–893, 955–961.

14. Feinstein, S. (1975), Adolescent depression. In: *Depression and Human Existence*, ed. E. J. Anthony & T. Benedek. Boston: Little, Brown, pp. 317–336.

15. Berman, S. (1979), The response of parents to adolescent depression. Presentation to the Annual Meeting of the American Academy of Child Psychiatry, Atlanta, Ga., Oct. 1979.

16. Erikson, E. H. (1968), *Identity, Youth, and Crisis*. New York: Norton.

17. Engel, G. L. (1962), Anxiety and depression withdrawal: the primary affects of unpleasure. *Int. J. Psychoanal.*, 43:89–97.

18. Jacobson, E. (1971), *Depression: Comparative Studies of Normal, Neurotic, and Psychotic Conditions*. New York: International Universities Press.

19. Abraham, K. (1911), Notes on the psychoanalytic treatment of manic-depressive insanity and allied conditions. In: *Selected Papers on Psychoanalysis*. London: Hogarth Press, 1927, pp. 137–156.

20. Freud, S. (1917), Mourning and melancholia. *Standard Edition*, 14:243–258. London: Hogarth Press, 1957.

21. Anthony, E. J. (1975), Childhood depression. In: *Depression and Human Existence*, ed. E. J. Anthony & T. Benedek. Boston: Little, Brown, pp. 231–277.

22. Sandler, J. & Joffe, W. G. (1965), Notes on childhood depression. *Int. J. Psychoanal.*, 46:88–96.

23. Loevinger, J. (1976), *Ego Development: Conceptions and Theories*. San Francisco: Jossey-Bass.

24, Beck, A. (1967), *Depression: Clinical, Experimental, and Theoretical Aspects*. New York: Hoeber-Harper, pp. 476–477.

25. Piaget, J. (1942), *Classes, Relations et Nombres*. Paris: Vrin.

26. Whitehead, A. N. (1938), *Modes of Thought, Part III: Nature and Life*. New York: Macmillan, pp. 173–232.

27. Freud, S. (1895), Extracts from the Fliess Papers. *Standard Edition,* 1:200–206.
    London: Hogarth Press, 1957.
28. Anthony, E. J. (1975), Self-therapy in adolescence. *Ann. Am. Soc. Adolesc. Psychiatry,* 3:6–24.
29. Russell, B. (1967), *The Autobiography of Bertrand Russell: The Early Years.* New
    York: Bantam.

# CHAPTER ELEVEN

# DEPRESSION IN ADOLESCENCE: CLINICAL FEATURES AND DEVELOPMENTAL ASPECTS

## Gerhardt Nissen

Depressive illnesses have always aroused far less public and scientific interest than other psychiatric disorders, even endogenous psychoses of the unipolar or bipolar type. It seems that depression, as well as mania, is a condition with which one can readily empathize, whereas the insane world of the schizophrenic is surrounded by walls that appear virtually impenetrable. To use an ornithologic metaphor, depression is to all of us as familiar and ordinary as sparrows and crows, whereas schizophrenia is an exotic bird—often highly colored, sometimes noisy and sometimes mute—that arouses curiosity and amazement wherever it goes.

Depressive syndromes do not constitute a well-defined clinical or nosologic entity. This is exemplified by the various forms in which they may present in middle-aged adults, who, when compared with adolescents, constitute a relatively homogeneous group. Even in these individuals, however, the diagnosis of depression is only a simple undertaking in typical cases; in most instances it is both difficult and uncertain. How much more diverse, therefore, is the presentation of affect in those who are going through adolescence—a most tempestuous phase.

No age group is immune to depressive syndromes; yet it is often said that some forms of depression, i.e., psychotic depression, do not occur in children. In adolescents, depression is accepted in principle as a possible diagnosis, but is often overlooked. Often this occurs because childhood is supposed to be a particularly carefree, happy period—a paradise on earth, and adults usually view this part of their own life through rose-colored spectacles that blot out all unpleasant experiences. However, most adults can remember depressed, sad, anxious, or retarded schoolmates or friends of their youth, one or more of whom tried, maybe successfully, to commit suicide. Some authors cite chiefly theoretical grounds in disputing the existence of depression in childhood, claiming that a child's ego is immature and incapable of fulfilling a repressive function. But they do not deny that depression can occur in feeble-minded or imbecile adults, and depression has even been induced experimentally in animals (1, 2). Others acknowledge that depressive syndromes can develop during the early years of life, but suggest that these should be termed differently. However, it would serve no useful purpose to introduce new terms to describe the varied affects of a particular disorder; this would only increase the linguistic confusion in psychiatry. Griesinger (3), who as far back as 1845 formulated the hypothesis that "Psychiatric disorders are disorders of the brain," drew a clear distinction between the endogenous, somatogenic, and psychogenic hurts responsible for behavioral disturbances in children. On the topic of depressive states in childhood, he stated: "The melancholic forms too, though decidedly less common, occur in childhood in all their variations."

The key to recognizing depression in adolescents does not lie simply in a good knowledge of depression in adults. Depressive illness in both age groups can be understood only if one considers it as a metamorphosis of depressive disorders in childhood, a metamorphosis brought about by a child's psychologic development into adolescence and adulthood. I shall thus begin by reviewing depressive disorders as they developmentally occur from childhood.

## DEPRESSIVE DISORDERS
## FROM CHILDHOOD TO ADOLESCENCE

The diagnosis of typical adult psychiatric disorders in children is made more difficult by the turbulent psychic development inherent in childhood. All attempts to divide normal psychic development into phases and stages are purely arbitrary because in many cases chronologic age does not correspond to developmental age. As far as the psyche is concerned, the difference between a healthy infant and a small child is greater than that between a healthy adult and a very old person. Moreover, psychic manifestations (such as depressive symptoms) are not only related to development and age, but also are dependent on intelligence. Thus there can be no depressive syndrome typical of the whole of childhood and adolescence.

I carried out a study designed to assess psychologic development in 105 children and adolescents who had moderate or severe depression (4). The subjects were selected from approximately 6,000 inpatients examined over several years; the depression had been present for at least 9–12 months in those of school age or adolescence. Upon follow-up 10 years later, 59 (57%) were still depressive, 9 (9%) had become schizophrenic, and 13 (12%) had other psychiatric disorders; in only 15 (14%) did the examination fail to yield any psychiatric findings of note (9 patients were not available at follow-up). Table 1 shows the relative frequency of "psychosomatic" versus "psychic" symptoms in these depressive children and adolescents according to their age group. Children in the youngest age group had chiefly psychosomatic symptoms; the only typical psychic features were inhibition of play and agitation. Some of the same symptoms and additional ones were evident in the group of young schoolchildren, the numbers of psychosomatic and psychic manifestations being roughly equal. By contrast, in the adolescents, psychic symptoms predominated, there being only one statistically significant psychosomatic symptom (headache). In short, a marked transition from predominantly psychosomatic symptoms to psychic ones occurred when one developmentally progressed from young childhood to adolescence.

The classic form of depression in adults in Western civilizations comprises chiefly psychic symptoms, such as feelings of guilt, self-accusation, and ideas of impoverishment; all of these are liable to be accompanied by retardation or agitation, diurnal fluctuation in mood, and psychosomatic manifestations. In adults, too, the severity of these symptoms is dependent on age (5). Cross-cultural research in psychiatry has revealed that the clinical features of depressive illness are influenced also by epochal (age cohort) and social factors. In the forms of depression found among intelligent adults in non-Western civilizations (e.g., some regions of Asia and Africa), psychosomatic symptoms predominate (6-10), although a shift toward a greater preponderance of psychic symptoms has been observed in the last 10 years (11).

It is particularly interesting that the components of the depressive syndromes in early to middle childhood are very similar to those in both mentally and educationally subnormal adults in Western civilizations (12) and depressive adults of normal intelligence in non-Western cultures. One can therefore formulate the hypothesis, albeit with caution, that depression marked mainly by psychosomatic symptoms, such as primary depression in early childhood, can be regarded as the "primordial" form of depression. In the light of this hypothesis, depression in adults appears to be a culture-dependent form of depressive illness; i.e., dependent upon the structure of the individual and collective conscience. In our civilization, ideas of duty, order, punctuality, and cleanliness are important; and their influence during the childhood and youth of depressed adults (13, 14) is becoming increasingly apparent.

## TABLE 1
## DEPRESSIVE SYMPTOMS IN CHILDREN AND ADOLESCENTS

| Children below School Age | Young Schoolchildren | Older Schoolchildren and Adolescents |
|---|---|---|
| *Psychic Symptoms* (listed in order of frequency) | | |
| Inhibition of play | Irritability | Brooding |
| Agitation | Insecurity | Suicidal impulses |
| | Inhibition of play | Feelings of inferiority |
| | Unsociability | Dejection |
| | Inhibition of learning | |
| *Psychosomatic Symptoms* (listed in order of frequency) | | |
| Paroxysms of crying and screaming | Enuresis (from 5th yr. of life onward) | Headache |
| Encopresis (from 3rd yr. of life onward) | Pavor nocturnus | |
| Sleep disorders | Genital manipulation | |
| Jactitation | Paroxysms of crying and screaming | |
| Appetite disorders | | |

The depressive youngster, whether child or young adolescent, whose conscience is still undeveloped or not fully developed, is not yet capable of waging the intrapsychic and often masochistic battles characteristic of the depressive adult. Depressive children either obediently and humbly follow their parents' and teachers' instructions, or argue aggressively with them, as if they represent an as yet undeveloped or only partly developed superego.

Depressive states and suicidal attempts are more common during adolescence than in childhood, but for various reasons they often pass unrecognized, i.e., in about 50% of cases (15). Many authors consider subdepressive states and hypomanic episodes a normal part of puberty. Although both brief and lengthy depressive mood disorders are noticed by many parents, they tend to regard them as indicating a need for educational measures rather than as psychopathological conditions. Diagnosis by a doctor is often hampered by the fact that many adolescents are very in-

hibited and unforthcoming, and whether healthy or suffering from a psychiatric disorder, tend to talk in "the dialect of adolescence," which encompasses both infantile and adult modes of expression. Many adolescents—
normal as well as depressed —identify themselves with the sociocritical and
revolutionary attitudes of their political idols; sensitive and receptive as
they are at this stage of their development, they are only too ready to
become involved in social or political problems. The language of most adolescents is so peppered with exaggerations and superlatives that it is often
difficult to differentiate between what they feel as individuals and what they
say as members of a group.

Adolescents of previous generations were relatively better adapted to
their environment because they regarded integration into society as their
ultimate goal. Although today's adolescents likewise must continually fight
to re-establish and consolidate their status in the twilight zone between
childhood and adulthood, they are dependent for a longer period than their
counterparts of yesteryear on the material and spiritual support of the family or State. They repeatedly respond with infantile modes of behavior, or
adult-type modes with which they have little experience and which are, as
yet, unintegrated. This and many other problems of individuation and
identification, particularly those relating to authority and sexuality, often
involve them in severe inner conflicts charged with anxiety, grief, and depression. Characteristically, during adolescence the individual begins critically to appraise values and persons in his environment that hitherto he accepted without question. Depending on its results, this appraisal can give
rise to personality-dependent developmental crises. The severe adolescent
crises of the past, e.g., embittered and seemingly insuperable father-son
confrontations, with the son demonstratively running away to sea, the army, or the Foreign Legion, are rare now because the hierarchical family
structure and the role of the father have changed.

The loss of loved objects induces a depressed mood characterized by
grief. In such situations grief is mobilized, appropriate, and understandable; it is in fact physiological, as long as it persists for only a limited period
and can be coped with adequately. (This process was referred to by Freud
as *Trauerarbeit*.) However, loss and conflicts of this type can trigger depressions that, when viewed objectively, appear insufficiently motivated. These
depressive syndromes for which there seems little or no objective explanation are quite common among adolescents. Although they usually disappear in time (unless they are of an endogenous phasic type), they do have
root causes which can be differentiated. In many cases the affected person is
predisposed to endogenous depression; but whether this predisposition will
lead to frank disease depends very much on developmental, psychologic,
and psychodynamic factors.

The clinical features of depression in adolescence are dictated by the adolescent's personality, his receptivity and ability to express himself, his emotionality, talents, and intelligence. The depressive state can be virtually asymptomatic or monosymptomatic, or may give rise to a wide range of psychic and somatic symptoms. According to Jaspers (16): "The way in which an emotional disorder presents itself in an individual reflects the grade of that person's psychic refinement." For example, a depressed adolescent who has difficulty learning may display a primitive and unreasonable fear of being poisoned, whereas a similarly depressed but highly intelligent adolescent may display an outlook on life which is complex and convincing. In both instances, the extent of the adolescent's bewilderment and confusion is explainable only in terms of his depression. After the depression has been overcome, the foundations of the depressive view of life may remain, but the individual no longer feels compelled to draw the same conclusions, e.g., contemplate suicide.

A co-worker and I examined 62 depressive adolescents (44 girls and 18 boys) (17) to assess the relative incidence of six depressive syndromes, descriptively differentiated. The three most common, in order of frequency, were as follows:

## Quietness and Resignation

The first depressive syndrome, "quietness and resignation," features symptoms such as grief, overadjustment, shyness, self-isolation, enuresis, nail-biting, unmotivated weeping, sporadic bouts of violent aggressiveness, and suicidal behavior. It characterizes withdrawn and quiet depressive adolescents who exhibit grief with which one cannot empathize, as well as dejection, boredom, and resignation. Such patients are very difficult to reach verbally. They have destroyed all their bridges to the outside world and, if not already paralyzed by feelings of hopelessness, sit waiting for some personal or collective disaster to wipe them out and thus spare them from taking personal decisions. Some of these adolescents display a "syndrome-shift" toward aggressive and suicidal behavior.

## Retardation and Loss of Drive

The second most frequent group, "retardation and loss of drive," features symptoms such as psychomotor sluggishness, apathy, insecurity, difficulty in learning, mutism, and passivity. It relates to adolescents who have little drive, lack motivation, and cannot think about the future. They are difficult to approach, laconic, apparently superficial, and lacking in emotional depth. They appear at ease with the world about them, but in fact are often in deep despair and incapable of critical introspection, and display little self-respect. They are monosyllabic or mute because they cannot describe their feelings. Any decision to change their circumstances costs them an enormous expenditure of energy, and every defeat they suffer serves to confirm, in their eyes, their inferiority to others. They are all too apt to let themselves be abused and exploited. Because of their lack of will-power, they are submissive and careless. Girls who suffer this type of depression are likely to allow themselves to become passive sexual objects, often simply to avoid losing a casual emotional contact.

## Agitation and Anxiety

The third group, "agitation and anxiety," features symptoms such as auto- and hetero-aggressiveness, insecurity, compulsive eating, unmotivated weeping, and suicidal behavior. It is typified by the aggressive, agitated adolescent: his delinquency represents a depressive equivalent, and is an attempt at self-consolation or self-cure or to find an alternative means of satisfying his needs. Acts of violence, as well as excessive drinking or drug-taking, in some instances are abortive experiments born of an impoverished or reduced dream activity and imaginative capacity. The same also applies to certain forms of promiscuity, e.g., the Don Juan-type behavior in boys that Kirkegaard (18) described, and nymphomania, its counterpart in girls. An unpredictable suicidal component is just as common in drug addicts as in adventurers, daredevil motorcyclists, and mercenaries. These depressive adolescents are less attached to life than others. They obey the "all-or-nothing" law, demanding either immediate fulfillment of their inner urges or oblivion.

The most common features in these three types of depressive syndromes are shown in Table 2. Comparison of these observations statistically showed suicidal behavior, rumination, and mood swings to be particularly characteristic of this age group. The high incidence of suicidal behavior is also partly due to the fact that adolescents in their first bout or phase of depression cannot appreciate the finite nature of their emotional trough: their depression seems endless, so they tend to seek definitive solutions. In contrast to depressive adults, ideas of impoverishment and sinfulness were seldom encountered; but feelings of inferiority were more common, engendered in particular by a sense of failure at school or at work, or when they compared themselves unfavorably to their parents.

### EXOGENOUS, ENDOGENOUS, AND REACTIVE DEPRESSION

Consideration of only the cross-sectional, phenomenological, or clinical features of a depressive syndrome rarely permits reliable nosological classification; this requires the addition of family history and in particular, findings derived from a developmental review. *Chronic* depression in children should often be construed as an *exogenous psycho-syndrome* due to brain damage in early life. These used to be classified as psychopathic or constitu-

## TABLE 2
## TARGET SYMPTOMS IN THREE DEPRESSIVE SYNDROMES
## IN ADOLESCENTS

| Rank Order of Symptoms | Symptoms |
|---|---|
| 1 | Sadness, brooding, boredom, suicidal behavior |
| 2 | Feelings of inferiority, dejection, social withdrawal |
| 3 | Emotional instability, refusal to attend school or work, obsessive-compulsive behavior |
| 4 | Headache, appetite disturbances, hypochondriasis |

tional depression. In adolescence, differentiation between *reactive* and *endogenous* depression is complicated by the fact that one is often dealing with first episodes; moreover, both are frequently triggered by psychic factors (19).

PHASIC-TYPE UNIPOLAR AND BIPOLAR PSYCHOSES

*Phasic-type unipolar and bipolar psychoses* are said to account for only 0.05–0.1% of affective psychoses in children and adolescents, but for 0.3–0.5% (20) to 3% (21) in the general population. However, almost without exception, statistics relating to the age at onset of manic-depressive diseases are based on retrospective information supplied by adult patients. Such information is of dubious value, for three reasons:

1. *The first phase of a depressive illness, especially if mild and short-lived, is seldom recognized.* Even Kraepelin (22) classified "Certain slight or very slight changes of mood, to some extent periodical, to some extent pathological which might still be consonant with the individual's predisposition" under the heading of periodic and circular disorders. According to this definition, psychogenic depression also could be confidently differentiated from affective psychoses only if it were extremely obvious. Thus the trend in psychiatry today is to refrain from such differentiations (23) in all instances where they cannot be made with absolute certainty.

2. *Manic-depressive adults are subject to illusions.* Autobiographical data frequently mislead physicians into wrongly interpreting as phasic many conflictual and depressive mood states commonly occurring during childhood and youth. There is a particular risk of faulty interpretation when an adult patient supplies information while suffering from a phasic mood disorder.

3. *The endogenous phases in question are atypical* and therefore not recognized at first. Follow-up studies reported between 1961 and 1973 (24-26) did not confirm the hypothesis that periodic behavioral disturbances in childhood can be regarded as equivalents of endogenous phasic disorders in childhood and adolescence. Even when endogenous phasic depression in a child or adolescent appears certain, the diagnosis often turns out to be wrong; for example, in none of 10 cases of "endogenous phasic psychosis" diagnosed in hospitalized children aged 6–16 years could this diagnosis be confirmed at follow-up 10 to 25 years later (4). However, these follow-up examinations yielded the surprising finding that the symptom "mood swings," observed initially in 19 of 105 patients, showed highly significant correlation with schizophrenia during adolescence and adulthood: schizophrenia was clinically confirmed in five of these patients, and personality development was extremely unfavorable in five others.

The following case summaries illustrate these findings.

*Case 1.* When first seen, this 17-year-old female was described as displaying "sweeping changes in mood." "At one time she would be morose, depressed, completely inhibited, uncommunicative, and monosyllabic, whereas at another she would be absurdly elated, pour water out of the window, be impudent and presumptuous, tear up paper, and turn the wireless full on." Eighteen years later, paranoid hallucinatory schizophrenia was diagnosed, and the patient was hospitalized for 6 years.

*Case 2.* A 16-year-old adolescent girl was said to be "as high as a kite one minute and down in the dumps the next." "At times, she was depressed and inhibited, disinterested, extremely slow, distrustful, withdrawn, and mute. She would then become insolent, impudent, and aggressive, and she would lie and steal. Lacking in self-assurance, she would weep quietly to herself. In addition to her phases of stealing, on two occasions when in a hyperthymic mood she set fire to things." Follow-up 25 years later revealed that she had had several bouts of a schizophrenic disorder. Three years previously, it had led to her admission to a psychiatric hospital, where she remained thereafter.

*Case 3.* Likewise, a 15-year-old hypochondriacal boy had been diagnosed as suffering from a manic-depressive disorder: "Abrupt changes in mood from exuberance to depression; wide fluctuations in mood; frequent depressive phases followed by manic exuberance and liveliness." Follow-up 18 years later revealed that the patient had completed training in commercial subjects. He was constantly under psychiatric care because of cardiac pain and headache, and displayed an obsessive-compulsive syndrome marked by obsessive washing and dressing rituals. It was impossible to differentiate the disturbance clearly from a schizophrenic disorder.

Dahl (25) reported similar findings in a study of 200 patients who, because of behavioral disorders, had been under inpatient observation by a pediatric psychiatrist 20 years earlier. In the interim, 30% had been admitted to various institutions. Manic-depressive psychosis was not diagnosed in any case, but schizophrenia was diagnosed in seven. Since one-third of the period in which affective psychoses usually become manifest had elapsed by the time of follow-up, it is safe to say that early symptoms of an endogenous phasic disorder had not been overlooked 20 years previously.

INFLUENCE OF THE CLASSIFICATION SYSTEM ON DIAGNOSIS

Just as the clinical features and content of a psychosis are dependent on epochal factors, so its nosology is influenced by the systems of nosologic classification prevailing at the time. It is well known, for example (20), that the frequency of diagnosis of manic-depressive psychosis almost doubled in the post-Kraepelin era. In the U.S.A., coincident with a trend to psycho-analytic research after 1935, this diagnosis decreased, whereas neurosis increased. In Germany, under the influence of Kurt Schneider, atypical pictures, transitional states, and mixed syndromes were long excluded from the manic-depressive group of disorders, resulting in a considerable diagnostic shift toward schizophrenia. Thus it is apparent that not only the content of a psychic disorder, but psychiatric knowledge is subject to phasic changes; or in the words of Popper (27): "Science is of an eternally temporary nature."

## SUMMARY

Depressive illness in children, even though its symptomatology may differ from that in adults, should be termed depression. The finding of depressive mood disorders in primates and severely retarded adults has demonstrated that the existence of ego or superego is not essential to the development of depression, but is simply a modifier of depressive features.

Depression is common among adolescents; however, it often tends to be regarded as an indication of need for educational measures rather than as psychopathology. Depressive adolescents express themselves in the same way as almost all other young people in this critical period of life; sub-depressive and hypomanic variations in mood are normal.

In all depressions, including endogenous phasic disorders, the content has a direct (even if distorted) connection with the patient's personal life story and with current social issues or "Zeitgeist" (28).

Depressive illnesses cannot be assigned to nosologic categories on the basis of clinical diagnoses alone: besides developmental, psychologic, and psychodynamic factors, family history and findings in longitudinal studies are of major importance.

Although they run an episodic course, illnesses marked by depression do not necessarily reflect an endogenous phasic disorder in childhood and youth. Rather, episodic depressive mood disturbances, especially if associated with fluctuations in mood, often represent initial stages or the first bout of schizophrenia.

Findings in follow-up studies indicate a highly unfavorable prognosis for persistent moderate and severe depression, psychotic and nonpsychotic, in childhood and adolescence. This conclusion demands intensive research into depressive syndromes of the young in the interests of preserving mental health, and preventing adult psychiatric disorders.

## REFERENCES

1. McKinney, W. T., Jr. (1976), Animal models of depression. In: *Depression: Behavioral, Biochemical, Diagnostic, and Treatment Concepts*, ed. D. M. Gallant & G. M. Simpson. New York: Spectrum, pp. 1–18.
2. Harlow, H. F. & Suomi, S. J. (1971), Social recovery by isolation-reared monkeys. *Proc. Nat. Acad. Sci. U.S.A.*, 68:1534–1538.
3. Griesinger, W. (1845), Die Pathologie und Therapie der Psychischen Krankheiten. Stuttgart: Krabbe.
4. Nissen, G. (1971), *Depressive Syndrome im Kindes- und Jugendalter.* Berlin-Heidelberg-New York: Springer.
5. Schwab, J. J., Holzer, C. E., & Warheit, G. J. (1973), Depressive symptomatology and age. *Psychosomatics*, 14:135–141.
6. Carothers, J. C. (1951), Frontal-lobe function and the African. *J. Ment. Sci.*, 97:12–48.
7. Rin, H. & Lin, T. Y. (1962), Mental illness among Formosan aborigines as compared with the Chinese in Taiwan. *J. Ment. Sci.*, 108:134–146.
8. Ammar, S. (1967), Médecine psychosomatique en Afrique. *Med. Hyg. (Genève)*, 25:142, 180.
9. Pfeiffer, W. M. (1969), Transkulturelle Aspekte der Depression. In: *Melancholie im Forschung, Klinik, und Behandlung*, ed. W. Schulte & W. Mende. Stuttgart: Thieme, pp. 93–99.
10. Rao, A. V. (1969), A study of depression as prevalent in South India. The University of Madras, April 1969. Dissertation (Psychiatry).
11. Prince, R. (1967), The changing picture of depressive syndromes in Africa. Is it fact or diagnostic fashion? *Can. J. Afr. Stud.*, 1:177–192.
12. Flugel, F. E. (1924), Das Bild der Melancholie bei intellektuell Minderwertigen. *Z. Ges. Neurol. Psychiatr.*, 92:634–643.
13. Kovacs, M. & Beck, A. T. (1977), An empirical-clinical approach toward a definition of childhood depression. In: *Depression in Childhood: Diagnosis, Treatment, and Conceptual Models*, ed. J. G. Schulterbrandt & A. Raskin. New York: Raven Press, pp. 1–25.
14. Tellenbach, H. (1978), *Melancholie.* Berlin: Springer.
15. Weiner, I. B. (1975), Depression in adolescence. In: *The Nature and Treatment of Depression*, ed. F. F. Flach & S. C. Draghi. New York: Wiley, pp. 99–117.
16. Jaspers, K. (1953), *Allgemeine Psychopathologie*, 6th ed. Berlin: Springer.
17. Nissen, G. (1975), Disguised depressions in children. *Acta Paedopsychiatr.*, 41: 235–242.

18. Kirkegaard, S. (1951), Entweder-oder, Bde. I-III. In: *Gesammelte Werke.* Dusseldorf: Diederichs-Verlag.

19. Kornhuber, H. (1955), Über Auslösung zyklothymer Depressionen durch seelische Erschütterungen. *Arch. Psychiatr. Nervenkr.*, 193:391–405.

20. Bellak, L., Pasquarelli, B., Parkes, E., Bellak, S. S., & Bravermann, S. (1952), *Manic-depressive Psychosis and Allied Conditions.* New York: Grune & Stratton.

21. Stenstedt, A. (1969), Die genetischen Grundlagen bei Depression. In: *Melancholie im Forschung, Klinik, und Behandlung,* ed. W. Schulte & W. Mende. Stuttgart: Thieme, pp. 10–16.

22. Kraepelin, E. (1923), *Psychiatrie: Ein Lehrbuch für Studierende und Ärzte,* v. 3. *Klinische Psychiatrie,* II: *Das Manisch-depressive Irresein.* Leipzig: Barth, pp. 1183–1395.

23. Perris, C. (1966), A study of bipolar (manic depressive) and unipolar recurrent depressive psychoses. *Acta Psychiatr. Scand.*, 42, suppl. 194.

24. Spiel, W. (1961), Die endogenen Psychosen des Kindes- und Jugendalters. Basle: Karger.

25. Dahl, V. (1971), A follow-up study of a child-psychiatric clientele, with special regard to manic-depressive psychosis. In: *Depressive States in Childhood and Adolescence,* ed. A. L. Annell. Stockholm: Almqvist & Wiksell. pp. 534–541.

26. Eggers, C. (1973), *Verlaufsweisen Kindlicher und Präpuberaler Schizophrenien.* Berlin: Springer.

27. Popper, K. R. Cited in Eccles, J. C. (1975), *Wahrheit und Wirklichkeit: Mensch und Wissenschaft.* Berlin: Springer.

28. Hegel, G. W. F. (1928), Vorlesung über die Geschichte der Philosophie. In: *Sämtliche Werke.* Stuttgart: Jubiläumsausgabe in 20 Bänden, neu herausgeben von H. Glockner.

# CHAPTER TWELVE

# THE TREATMENT OF MANIC-DEPRESSIVE ILLNESS IN ADOLESCENCE

## EDWARD A. WOLPERT

Cade's discovery in the late 1940s of the efficacy of lithium salts in the treatment of acute mania (1) ushered in a new period of treatment of manic-depressive illness. A symptom-complex destructive of careers and families, in many cases requiring months of hospitalization and at times electroshock therapy, became easily handled with a simple salt. The further discovery of the prophylactic use of lithium (2) led to the possibility of an illness-free life where previously the prognosis, although good for the individual episode, was poor for a lifetime because of the near certainty of recurrences.

As the numbers of manic patients treated with lithium increased, cardiovascular, renal, thyroid, and neurologic complications were noted and discussed (3). Gradually a new concept of the illness was developed, based on discoveries attendant upon elaboration of the new method of treatment.

Kraepelin (4), the great systematizer, originally described a number of affective disorders, all of which had a favorable prognosis, but noted that they were similar and at times interchangeable. In his final statement (5), he concluded that these are various manifestations of a single disease entity, manic-depressive illness. Such a concept was accepted by psychologically as well as biologically oriented psychiatrists. Indeed, the only significant writer who doubted its singular identity was Freud, who noted (6) two types of illness episodes, spontaneous and psychogenic. Abraham (7), who preceded Freud in studying manic-depressive illness, accepted Kraepelin's idea that all forms of affective disorder are one. But, unlike Kraepelin, who considered each episode of the illness as physiologically-based and the psychogenic factors purely fortuitous, Abraham regarded the psychogenic factors as causative.

In the third edition of the *Diagnostic and Statistical Manual* (8) compiled by the American Psychiatric Association, "manic-depressive illness" is replaced by the more general term "major affective disorder." The salient feature of the latter is a severe disturbance of affectivity which lasts for at least 2 weeks, and in most cases recurs throughout the patient's lifetime. Subvarieties of major affective disorder include major depression and bipolar illness; the latter is synonymous with the more specific "manic-depressive illness," which describes recurring manias and depressions.

Patients with bipolar illness are characterized by three alternating psychophysiological states—an activated state, a normal state, and a retarded state (9, 10). In the activated state, thoughts are speeded and have loosened, circumstantial, and bizarre associations; actions are increased; sexuality is expanded; sleep and dream times are decreased; and affect is expansive, elated, or euphoric. In extreme cases, thought fragments and physiologic variables are driven to a critical degree (i.e., manic excitement). In the retarded state, sleep and dream times are often increased, physiologic variables slowed, thought impoverished, affect depressed, and sexuality and action decreased. At times the activated or retarded state is precipitated by external events, or shifts of internal feeling states or ideas (i.e., psychogenic episodes); at other times no psychologic precipitant can be found (i.e., spontaneous episodes). In the latter case, prodromal symptom states (i.e., typical dreams or states of sensory panhyperarousal) (11) signal the appearance of a clinical episode.

These alternating psychophysiologic states strongly imply the waxing and waning of biologic functions, and have suggested to some observers a disorder of the biological clock (10, 12). As such, bipolar illness would fit well with Freud's definition of *actual* neurosis as the psychologic effects of sexual (physiological) hurts (13).

We recently summarized (14, 15) the evidence that bipolar depressive illness is basically a metabolic disorder in which the central fault is a periodic alternating surplus and lack of energy. In some patients these alternating energy states seem intrinsic, perhaps associated with menstrual or seasonal cycles; in others they seem precipitated by typical psychogenic factors. In many patients, both types of episodes occur. This alternation of energy state can coexist with other named symptomatic or character pathology, or may be found in otherwise normal individuals. The treatment of this illness is ideally both physiologic and psychologic: lithium to normalize the alternations of energy, and psychotherapy to remove psychogenic triggers that might override the lithium taken prophylactically (16).

Although many clinicians do not diagnose bipolar illness in adolescence, researchers who worked retrospectively with large groups of bipolar patients of all ages found that the first episode occurred earlier than 20 years of age in 20% (17, 18) to 33% (19) of their cases. Two independent studies of adolescents admitted to Renard Hospital at Washington University, St. Louis (20, 21) revealed that major affective illness accounted for about 35–40% of all such admissions. In Hudgens' study (21), 13 (12.7%) of 110 adolescent psychiatric inpatients had a bipolar disorder. Thus the clinical entity "bipolar illness" is seen in adolescence as well as inferred from histories of adult patients.

Studies of the outcome of lithium treatment in unselected manic-depressive patients, well summarized by Davis (22), indicate that prophylaxis with lithium carbonate is helpful in ameliorating the course of the illness and preventing recurrence. The findings are more pessimistic in studies of adolescent patients, however, both before lithium prophylaxis (23, 24) and after its introduction (21, 25). Only 10 (22.7%) of Landolt's 44 patients with bipolar illness (23) were well at follow-up at 5–25 years. Of Olsen's 28 patients (24), at an astounding mean follow-up of 25 years, 17 (61%) were symptomatic and disabled, 3 (11%) had committed suicide, and 8 (28%) had had recurrences, but were functional. Welner, Welner, and Fishman (25), who followed up 12 of Hudgens' bipolar patients (21), found an even more dismal course: 2 of the 10 who had been treated with lithium had committed suicide; all of the survivors were considered "socially disabled"; and all had a poor work history.

How can we understand the different results in these studies summarized by Davis (22) and in the follow-up work by Landolt (23), Olsen (24), and Welner et al. (25)? The major difference, of course, is that Davis' review summarized studies of populations of bipolar depressives of all ages whose illness had been identified at various ages, whereas the later studies were of populations whose illness had begun early and had been identified in adolescence. Also, none of the follow-up studies were very explicit concerning the therapist's approach between episodes, and this may be precisely where the success or failure of the overall treatment will be determined. The following representative case reports support this possibility.

## CASE REPORTS

*Case 1.* "Rita" was 18 years old when she requested a consultation in 1975 concerning her wish to discontinue lithium treatment. Her parents came to the consultation quite fearful and concerned. They stated that from 12 to 14 years of age Rita had experienced difficulty learning in school, insomnia, and low self-esteem, and for 6 months had undergone psychotherapy directed at her learning difficulty. Despite these problems, her parents said she was "a kindly, empathic, good-natured child" at that time. Previously she had been considered normal, with occasional periods of increased activity not thought to be unusual.

When Rita was 14 years old, her father learned he was to be transferred to Chicago in a year. Almost immediately the girl became "high," feeling she had many friends; and she started several projects, proclaiming her ability to do "many things." After about 2 weeks this mood ended abruptly, and Rita became "deeply depressed," lying in bed all day, refusing food and attendance at school. Because of her suicidal ideas her psychiatrist recommended admission to a hospital, but the parents rejected this; instead, they placed Rita under the care of another psychiatrist. After two visits the depression ended, and the girl appeared normal for several days; but after her third visit she became "vicious, high, aggressive all the time, using foul language, striking out, and wanting things immediately"; this time she was admitted to the hospital.

On admission, Rita was restless and kept calling out for her boyfriend, had accelerated and pressured speech, and increased motor activity. Associations were difficult to follow; flights of ideas, circumstantiality, and tangentiality were prominent (neologisms, blurring, and word-salads were absent). Her affect was expansive, self-satisfied, and confident. The girl denied suicidal thoughts, hallucinations, and delusions, but misidentified normal sounds as caused by her absent boyfriend. Orientation, memory, and intellectual function seemed normal, and no physical abnormality was detected. Blood urea nitrogen was 9 mg/dl, serum creatinine 0.6 mg/dl, blood glucose 90 mg/dl, and serum thyroxine was 10 mg/dl.

Treatment was started with chlorpromazine (600 mg/day), and from day 3 lithium carbonate (starting with 900 mg/day) was added. The girl remained quite active and for the first few days desired continuously to go home; at times she appeared quite suspicious, which seemed consistent with her hypomania. On day 4, Rita was feeling light-headed, so the chlorpromazine dosage was decreased. By day 6, her speech was less pressured and she had begun to socialize; haloperidol (Haldol) was begun and the dose of chlorpromazine was further decreased. Rita's mood changed markedly on day 10 (the seventh day of lithium treatment): she felt "normal," looked back at her previous "high" as quite unpleasant in many ways, and now began to feel "tired." On day 12, a rash appeared, accompanied by minimal pruritus; the chlorpromazine was discontinued. One day later, when the dosage of lithium carbonate was 1200 mg/day, the patient's serum lithium level was 0.82 mEq/liter.

Rita was discharged home on day 14, to be followed up in the Lithium Clinic. She was seen briefly at the Clinic monthly for 6 months, but the discharge plan for referral to a psychiatrist and for family therapy was not carried out. The girl discontinued visits to the Clinic, explaining: "They only checked my blood level. I didn't need them to tell me I was doing well and was stable." She continued to take lithium and to have her blood level checked by her pediatrician.

The family moved to Chicago in 1973. In 1975, because of her good progress in school and absence of "highs" and "lows," Rita decided to discontinue lithium. Her parents persuaded her, with some difficulty, to seek psychiatric consultation, during which time it became clear that the patient had made many strides forward. She was doing well intellectually, had many friends, seemed to be making reasonable plans for a vocation, and had apparently normal relationships with boys. Her only conflict with her parents concerned lithium usage. On that one point she was adamant; she did not need it! She knew that some experts advocated prophylaxis only after three manias, and felt that her having had only one justified her decision.

The patient readily consented to thyroid and kidney studies, which showed no abnormality. In discussion with Rita and her family, I recommended continuing prophylaxis; but the girl refused, saying she would recognize the onset of symptoms, and would avert the illness by reinstituting lithium if needed.

Two years later, with no obvious precipitant and at a time when Rita appeared to be doing well, a second mania developed — so fast that the girl could not recognize its presence until she made multiple errors in judgment, and was arrested for driving above 80 miles per hour. Since then, Rita has taken lithium prophylactically and is undergoing psychotherapy.

*Case 2.* "Jean," then 14 years old, was taken by police to a general hospital in another city after being found wandering aimlessly through the streets, disheveled and talking incoherently. Amphetamines were found in her pockets, but toxicologic blood and urine screens were negative. Her behavior in the emergency room was described as delusional; her thoughts were loose and tangential, with flights of ideas; and bizarre movements of her extremities were considered autisms. She tried to unclothe and assault the nurses.

Jean's parents came from their home, several hundred miles away, and accompanied her when she was transferred to a nearby psychiatric hospital a few days later. There a history was obtained of acute confusion and depression, progressively worsening in the previous 2 weeks. The girl was described as attractive and well-dressed, exhibiting increased psychomotor activity, rapid speech, bizarre and loosened associations, and flattened affect. She said she might have a nervous condition but sometimes thought she was pretending. She described herself as "completely depressed." "I wanted to commit suicide 2 days ago. I was looking at the window thinking it would be nice to fall and fall." In association she added: "I was thinking how pretty that color is (referring to the red of her fingernail polish), and how if someone had an accident, and was injured, they could be put back together." She thought the interviewer's entry into the waiting room was a hallucination. "I was thinking of what ashes would do if they got together and decided to march against someone else." Although her sensorium was clear, her comprehension, intellectual functioning, insight, and judgment were grossly impaired.

The differential diagnosis was acute schizophrenic episode, manic-depressive illness of the manic type, or drug intoxication by amphetamines or other drugs.

Jean's history was remarkable for the absence of gross traumas. She was the second of three girls born to apparently happily married parents, and her relationships to siblings and parents were not unusual. Childhood was said to be normal, but she had sucked her thumb until age 6. She was described as gregarious with girls, shy with boys, and behaving responsibly in relation to others, to school, and to belongings. Some vague depressions were noted, but no history of clear-cut "high" spells could be elicited. There was no family history of mental illness. Physical findings and results of routine laboratory blood tests were normal.

Jean was treated for 100 days with antipsychotic medication, first with perphenazine (Trilafon), later replaced by haloperidol; group and individual therapy was added. Improvement was slight, so lithium carbonate was started (2400 mg/day); on the seventh day the blood level of lithium was 0.8 mEq/liter, and remission of the mania was clinically apparent.

A maintenance dose of lithium carbonate, 300 mg tid, was established, and Jean returned home and to school and started psychotherapy three times a week. After three years of psychotherapy, Jean seemed outgoing without being forward; her shyness had disappeared; and she enjoyed a varied social life and worked productively at school. The intensive psychotherapy was terminated smoothly, and the girl handled well the necessary change of therapist when she entered a college in another city. She still takes 900 mg lithium daily and has experienced no more gross incidents.

## DISCUSSION

Case 1 demonstrates some of the difficulties in recognizing and treating bipolar depressive illness. A psychiatrist accustomed to adult patients would have recognized this 14-year-old girl's presenting symptoms (insomnia, low self-esteem, inability to study) as typical of depression, but the original therapist was not attuned to such a diagnosis in adolescence and could direct treatment only at the problem-complex "learning difficulties" present since age 12. Earlier hints of periodic hyperactivity were too vague to warrant a diagnosis, and the therapist was not alert to the possibilities they might signal. The development of mania made the diagnosis clear, and the patient was admitted to a psychiatric hospital where a psychiatrist instituted treatment with lithium carbonate: this both terminated the mania and apparently prevented recurrences of both manias and depressions for three years. However, the therapy failed ultimately because of failure to attend to the patient's psychologic state; although referral to a lithium clinic after discharge was accomplished, referral for individual and family therapy was not.

By the time I saw the patient she resisted both the continued use of lithium and psychotherapy; therefore prophylaxis was discontinued until a recurrence of gross illness forced the issue. It is of note that her second mania began two years after the girl stopped taking lithium.

Unless the patient has some physical illness contraindicating use of this agent, we recommend lithium prophylaxis for all who have experienced a clear-cut mania. We consider that the possible psychologic, social, or economic damage that could accrue from a further manic episode greatly exceeds possible lithium-induced physical damage. Some patients who unilaterally stop lithium experience a mania almost immediately; in other cases, as in this one, latency lasts much longer. Had Rita been treated psychologically after her first hospital stay, her resistance to taking lithium, apparently an issue in her age-appropriate struggle for autonomy, might have been controllable, and hence the second hospitalization avoided.

Case 2 illustrates that early bipolar depressive illness may be confused with schizophrenic or a drug-induced state. Once the correct diagnosis is made, the acute episode controlled, and lithium prophylaxis begun, psychotherapy becomes possible and conflicts can be controlled, removing a psychogenic trigger of affective disorders. In this case, unlike Case 1, psychotherapy was considered essential in addition to physiologic monitoring of the lithium treatment. Such a dual approach is more likely to resolve conflicts and strengthen the ego. Thus in Jean's case, treatment was "successful," whether measured by socioeconomic or scholastic criteria, or by absence of affective recurrence requiring readmission to a hospital.

## SUMMARY

Manic-depressive illness, viewed as an *actual* neurosis in Freud's sense of the term, is highly amenable to treatment in adolescents as well as in adults. It is critical to recognize that treatment of only the physiologic aspect of the illness is insufficient. In addition, psychologic conflicts must be resolved, so that psychic triggers of the affective episodes are removed.

It remains to be seen whether long-term follow-up studies of bipolar depressive patients will yield a pessimistic prognosis (as in Case 1) or optimistic results (as in Case 2). Because bipolar illness is a function of both physiology and psychology (15), success in treating such patients demands equally careful consideration of both aspects, and flexibility in the treatment plan devised for each individual patient.

## REFERENCES

1. Cade, J. J. F. (1949), Lithium salts in the treatment of psychotic excitement. *Med. J. Aust.*, 2:349–352.
2. Hartigan, G. P. (1963), The use of lithium salts in affective disorders. *Br. J. Psychiatry*, 109:810–814.
3. Johnson, F. N. & Johnson, S., Eds. (1978), Lithium in Medical Practice; Proceedings of the First British Lithium Congress, University of Lancaster, 1977. Baltimore: University Park Press.
4. Kraepelin, E. (1904), *Lectures on Clinical Psychiatry*. London: Baillière, Tindall, & Cox.
5. Kraepelin, E. (1921), *Manic Depressive Insanity and Paranoia*. Edinburgh: Livingstone.
6. Freud, S. (1921), Group psychology and the analysis of the ego. *Standard Edition*, 18:67–143. London, Hogarth Press, 1955.
7. Abraham, K. (1927), Notes on the psychoanalytical investigation and treatment of manic depressive insanity and allied conditions. In: *Selected Papers of Karl Abraham*, Reprint ed. London: Hogarth Press, 1968, pp. 137–156.
8. *Diagnostic and Statistical Manual of Mental Disorders*, Third Edition (DSM III) (1980), Washington, D.C.: American Psychiatric Association.
9. Wolpert, E. A. (1975), Manic depressive illness as an actual neurosis. In: *Depression and Human Existence*, ed. E. J. Anthony & T. Benedek. Boston: Little, Brown, pp. 199–221.
10. Bunney, W. E. (moderator) (1977), The switch process in manic-depressive psychosis. *Ann. Intern. Med.*, 87:319–335.
11. Wolpert, E. A. (1977), Nontoxic hyperlithemia in impending mania. *Am. J. Psychiatry*, 134:580–582.
12. Jovanovic, U. J. (1977), Chronobiologic aspects of psychiatry. *Waking & Sleeping*, 1:335–341.
13. Freud, S. (1917), Introductory lectures on psychoanalysis. General theory of the neuroses: the common neurotic state. *Standard Edition*, 16:378–391. London: Hogarth Press, 1963.
14. Wolpert, E. A. (1979), Manic depressive illness: the relation of biology to psychology. In: *Biological Psychiatry Today*, ed. J. Obiols, C. Ballus, E. Gonzalez-Monclus, & J. Pujol. Amsterdam: Elsevier, part A, pp. 530–534.
15. Wolpert, E. A. (1980), Major affective disorders. In: *Comprehensive Textbook of Psychiatry*, Vol. 3, ed. A. Freedman, H. Kaplan, & B. Sadock. Baltimore: Williams & Wilkins, pp. 1319–1331.
16. Wolpert, E. A., Wolpert, G. Y., Holinger, P. C., & Preodor, D. (1979), A follow-up study of lithium carbonate treatment of manic depressive illness. In: *Biological Psychiatry Today*, ed. J. Obiols, C. Ballus, E. Gonzalez-Monclus, & J. Pujol. Amsterdam: Elsevier, part B, pp. 1111–1116.
17. Wertham, F. I. (1929), A group of benign chronic psychoses: prolonged manic

excitements: with statistical study of age, duration, and frequency, in 2000 manic attacks. *Am. J. Psychiatry,* 9:17–78.

18. Preodor, D. & Wolpert, E. A. (1979), Manic-depressive illness in adolescence. *J. Youth Adolesc.,* 8:111–130.

19. Winokur, G., Clayton, P. J., & Reich, T. (1969), *Manic Depressive Illness,* St. Louis: Mosby.

20. King, L. J. & Pittman, G. D. (1970), A six-year follow-up study of 65 adolescent patients. *Arch. Gen. Psychiatry,* 22:230–236.

21. Hudgens, R. W. (1974), *Psychiatric Disorders in Adolescents.* Baltimore: Williams & Wilkins.

22. Davis, J. M. (1976), Overview: maintenance therapy in psychiatry. II. Affective disorders. *Am. J. Psychiatry,* 133:1–13.

23. Landolt, A. B. (1957), Follow-up studies on circular manic-depressive reactions occurring in the young. *Bull. N.Y. Acad. Med.,* 33:65–73.

24. Olsen, T. (1961), Follow-up study of manic depressive patients whose first attack occurred before the age of 13. *Acta Psychiatr. Scand.,* 37, suppl. 162, pp. 45–51.

25. Welner, A., Welner, Z., & Fishman, R. (1979), Psychiatric adolescent inpatients: Eight- to ten-year follow-up. *Arch. Gen. Psychiatry,* 36:698–700.

CHAPTER THIRTEEN

# SUICIDAL BEHAVIOR
# IN ADOLESCENCE

BARRY D. GARFINKEL and HARVEY GOLOMBEK

## INTRODUCTION

Social attitudes to self-inflicted injury vary in different cultures, and at least in our Western society, have changed over the years (1). Early Christian societies characterized suicide as a sin. Saint Augustine, for example, saw a need for moral strictures to prevent self-destruction by overzealous converts as a demonstration of their new-found faith in an afterlife. As the State increasingly shared with the Church the responsibility for the control of human behavior, suicide became a criminal offense; it was viewed as robbing the State of the individual's contribution to society. Subsequently came the belief that suicide was invariably a symptom of mental illness, and most recently, that it represents an interaction of biological, psychological, and situational influences. Current psychiatric opinion does not view suicide as a sin or a crime (in Canada, suicide was struck from the Criminal Code in 1973), nor pathognomonic of any form of mental illness.

The increase in reported rates of suicide has led to intensified study of its causes. However, the study of self-destruction by youth has been

This article is based on a paper delivered by Dr. Barry Garfinkel at the Hincks Symposium, November 2, 1979.

The authors wish to acknowledge the Ministry of Community and Social Services of the Government of Ontario and The Hospital for Sick Children, Toronto, Ontario, for providing financial assistance for research in the area of suicide by children.

hindered by biased, limited attitudes, particularly the inability to acknowledge that young people can experience depression to a degree that results in
suicidal preoccupation and behavior.

Several theoretical and methodological approaches to the study of
suicide emerged in the last century. In the mid-1800s Esquirol reviewed
case history material (2) in an attempt to isolate factors associated with suicidal behavior, whereas Durkheim, 50 years later, chose to examine suicide
demographically (3). The latter excluded psychological factors and stressed
sociological ones; this approach was contrary to that expressed by Zilboorg
(4), an early psychoanalytic theorist who had stressed the major contribution of childhood experiences to suicidal behavior, such as identification
with an absent father. Similarly, Hendin's (5) study of transcultural developmental patterns suggested that child-rearing practices, which differentiated
Swedish, Danish, and Norwegian children, determined their later suicidal
behavior.

Each of these approaches examined only part of the subject; furthermore, their limited observations were understood within the context of
existing theoretical models. For example, the study of psychological factors
alone neglects major social, environmental, and situational aspects that
contribute to crises and depression. On the other hand, a purely
sociological perspective emphasizes social structure, cultural styles, and
important situational events, but ignores psychopathology.

Later investigators have sought to integrate the various perspectives in
an attempt to link social, cultural, and environmental factors to significant
intrapsychic ones. Halbwachs (6) has been the most successful in relating
sociological population statistics to individual psychological functioning.
This union allows not only a clear description of the characteristics of suicidal individuals, but also a ranking of relevant antecedent events. It must be
borne in mind, however, that even the broadest approach yields incomplete
data: for cultural and social reasons, record-keeping of suicides is subject to
large errors of omission.

Self-destructive behavior in adolescents has emerged as a multifarious
problem ranging from suicidal communication to completed suicide. Several investigators have reported a ratio of eight attempts to every completed
suicide by persons under the age of 25 (7, 8), although Weissman (9) "conservatively estimated" the rate to be 30–40 to 1; Jacobziner suggested there
were as many as 50 attempts to every suicide (10), then revised this to 100
to 1 (11). Many unsuccessful attempts are motivated by intentions equal
to those that result in death: the attempter wishes to die, but makes the
attempt in a nonlethal fashion; or because of fortuitous circumstances, his

self-destructive act does not end in death. Thus the observation that some persons survive and some die from suicidal acts obscures the underlying aim of all attempters, which is to die from the self-inflicted injury. It follows, therefore, that attempted suicide is different from suicidal gestures, where self-inflicted injury is primarily an attempt at communication, and does not represent a conscious wish to die.

PRESENT STUDIES

In an attempt to characterize adolescents at risk for suicidal behavior, the records of young persons who had committed suicide or survived the act were studied. Completed suicide was studied demographically in a province-wide youthful population; attempted suicide was investigated through individual medical records in an urban pediatric hospital.

The aims of the investigations were to delineate a set of descriptor variables of young people at risk for completed and attempted suicide, and to define a typical pattern of life experiences that led to the act.

*Completed Suicide*

Study of information given at coroners' inquests and in police and necropsy reports obtained from the provincial Registrar General and Statistics Canada revealed 1554 suicides by 10 to 24 year olds in Ontario during January 1971 through August 1978 (12). This figure exceeds by more than 10% the official statistics for this age group during that period.

Since the number of official suicides is obviously lower than the researched number, and only those cases in which suicide was unquestionable were included, the findings presented here reflect a conservative statement of the actual problem.

*Attempted Suicide*

Review of all available emergency-room charts for young people treated between January 1, 1970 and January 31, 1977, at The Hospital for Sick Children, Toronto, for injuries deliberately self-inflicted, showed a total of 605 suicide attempts by 505 persons between the ages of 6.0 and 20.9 years (13). The attempters were matched with 505 nonsuicidal (control) subjects for age, sex, and time of visit to the emergency department (within 10 visits of that by a suicidal patient); and the data of both groups of subjects were analyzed from as many aspects as possible.

As not all of the emergency-room records were complete or available, these data also are a conservative reflection of the suicide attempts presented.

## COMPLETED SUICIDE IN ONTARIO

FEATURES OF THE SUICIDAL ACT

*Rate*

This investigation revealed 42% more suicides in 1977 than in 1971; and even when adjustment is made for a 9% population increase, the figure is still as high as 32%. On the average, each week more than five young people committed suicide in Ontario in 1977. As suicide is attempted at least 30 to 50 times more often than it is completed (9, 14), the five completed suicides probably represent at least 150 to 250 youthful suicide attempts each week. (There were about 2,366,300 10- to 24-year-olds in this province in 1977).

The suicide rate increased 124% for 15- to 19-year-olds, and 132% for 20- to 24-year-olds between 1961 and 1975 in the U.S.A. (14); and suicide among those under 25 years of age is known to have increased world-wide over the past decade. This increase in self-inflicted injury among youth has coincided with an increasingly greater incidence of breakdown of traditional life in the family and society (15).

There was also a seasonal fluctuation in the rate — highest in the fall and winter months, and lowest in spring and summer. It appeared to divide the year in half, September through February having a 25–40% higher rate than March through August. (However, the rate peaked dramatically in June to a one-third increase over May; in July it dropped to the previous level.)

Clearly, depressive mood and self-destructive behavior in youth increased during the colder months, possibly reflecting limitations of physical activity and social contacts in harsher weather. The marked increase in June was identified in all occupations and subgroups, and could not be attributed solely to students' experiencing tension during final examinations or conflict over leaving school; rather, it may partly reflect the abrupt cutoff of many cultural pursuits and community events that occur in Canada toward the end of May. Seasonal variation did not relate to independent variables such as sex, area of residence, occupation, or method of suicide.

These findings concurred with the longtime recognition that suicide does not occur at a uniform rate throughout the year, showing seasonal fluctuations that Sanborn, Casey, and Niswander (16) have attributed to changes in barometric pressure (a variable that was not studied). A review of suicides over 20 years in the U.S.A. as a whole (14) revealed a peak period in April and May and, during the 1970s, a second peak in autumn. A 1971 report of suicides in upstate New York (17) similarly identified high

rates in May and October. The Ontario findings best concur with Eastwood and Peacocke's (18) demonstration of a trend to higher frequencies in
early autumn and early to mid-spring for *all* age groups in Ontario.

METHOD OF SUICIDE

Table 1 shows the frequency of use of various methods of suicide.
It demonstrates that firearms were the predominant choice for 10- to 24-
year-olds.

Overall, firearms are the major means of self-destruction in North
America, and their use is increasing (1, 14, 19, 20). In Philadelphia (19)
and Los Angeles (1), during the 1960s the recorded rates of their use for all
ages were 28% and 44%, and in 1975 (14) firearms and explosives accounted
for 55% of suicides nationwide; ingestion of drugs or poison was the next
most common method (13.8%) (14). Holinger (20) reported methods of
suicide used by age group 10–14, 15–19, and 20–24 years. In the two older
groups, firearms were used in 55% of cases, hanging was the second most
common method (16% and 19%), and drug overdose accounted for about
14%. In his youngest group, firearms accounted for about 47% of suicides,
hanging for 45%, and ingestion of poisons for 5%; thus, hanging was more
than twice as common than in the older groups. By contrast to the above
studies, the very close restriction of firearms in Britain is reflected in Shaffer's (21) report: 43% of the children had died from gas inhalation, 17% by
hanging, and 13% from drugs; only three had used firearms.

The Ontario study showed the choice of suicidal method was also influenced by the person's sex. Gun use was 12 times, and hanging 7 times,

TABLE 1

METHODS OF SUICIDE RECORDED IN 1554 CASES
IN ONTARIO DURING JANUARY 1970 TO AUGUST 1978

| Method | Percent |
| --- | --- |
| Gun | 40% |
| Hanging | 20% |
| Drugs | 18% |
| Inhaling carbon monoxide | 7% |
| Jumping from a high place | 7% |
| Jumping in front of a moving vehicle | 4% |
| Drowning | 2% |

more common for boys than for girls, whereas the male:female ratio for
jumping to one's death was only 2:1. Drug overdose was equal for both
sexes. These findings concur with Liberakis and Hoenig (22), who reported
that firearms were used 10 times more often by males than females nationwide in Canada, and 20 times more often in Newfoundland; and Holinger's
(20) report that the male:female ratio for ingestion of a harmful substance
was about 1:1 for all adolescents.

In addition, the Ontario study demonstrated a changing trend in the
choice of suicidal method, especially in the use of more violent means by females since 1975. (The percentage of male violent suicides remained constant.) This may reflect the departure by women from their traditional role
in society toward a more equal status since the mid-1970s (which could
have influenced choice of method without increasing suicide frequency).

By relating choice of method to geographic location, it was found that
firearms accounted for 60% of the rural but only one-third of the urban suicides, whereas drugs were used in 23% of the urban suicides, but only 10%
of the rural ones. The use of firearms also showed regional variation: they
were used in 60% of the suicides in northeastern and northwestern Ontario
(predominantly rural areas), but only 32% in the southeastern and south-
western (chiefly urban) regions. The disproportionately greater use of firearms in rural communities, where guns are more available, and the more
prevalent use of prescribed drugs for overdoses in urban communities, con-
note accessibility in the choice of suicidal method. Similarly, more suicides
by jumping occurred in cities, where there are subways, higher bridges, tall
buildings, and a greater density of moving vehicles. Carbon monoxide poisoning was more common in rural areas which may reflect easier access to
motor vehicles as well as less likelihood that someone will come by. Clearly,
availability and access as well as common usage or observation of a method,
determined at least partly the means by which young people inflicted self-
injury. Confirmation of the influence of geography on choice of method
was found in Myers and Neal (23), who reported urban/rural differences
similar to our own; and in a study of the Yukon (24) which reported a disproportionately high incidence of drowning.

The young person's occupation also influenced the choice of method:
52% of the housewives took an overdose of drugs (and only 13% used firearms); almost equal numbers of government employees took a drug overdose (35%) or used a gun (31%); whereas the most common method used
by laborers and unemployed students was firearms (49% and 38%, respec-
tively).

*Age*

Sixty percent of the suicides were young adults, about one-third were 16 to 19 years of age, and only 7% were in the 10–15 year age group. A logarithmic curve of the number of suicides plotted against age revealed a rapid increase from 15 to 17 years, less rapid from then until a peak at mean age 20, and a plateau from 20 to 24 years.

*Gender*

Sex-type differences were found: the male:female ratio overall was 4:1.

A notable finding was the increasing trend since 1975 for girls to use more violent suicidal methods: violent self-inflicted injury was the cause of death in about 15–20% of all female suicides during 1971–1974 and increased to 35–54% during 1975–1977. This diminishing influence of sex on method, as noted earlier, may reflect changes in sexual and social attitudes.

Two reviews of suicide in the U.S.A. have shown a greater increase in the suicide rate for males than for females (14, 20). The rate rose more than 200% among males and about 128% among females aged 10 to 24 years from 1955 to 1975 (14), and the male:female ratio increased from about 3.5:1 in 1961 to 4.2:1 in 1975 for the age group 15 to 19 years (20). Thus, while the frequency of suicide was rising alarmingly for both sexes, the rate of increase among males was further widening the male:female ratio. Correlation of the ratio with other factors like age and geographic location showed additional differences. The largest differentials appeared among children under 15 years of age (21) and the smallest for those aged 20 to 29 years (7). Geographically, there was a 2:1 ratio in an urban population of 15- to 24-year-olds, but 9:1 among a rural population aged 11 to 19 years (25).

Seventy percent of the suicides occurred in familiar surroundings, at home (e.g., farms, apartment houses), or at the place of work. (The remainder occurred in locations corresponding to the method used, e.g., many hangings occurred in jails.) About twice as many suicides occurred in urban areas (67%) as in towns, villages, and farming communities (33%). This may simply have been an artifact of the greater proportion of youth living in cities in Ontario; i.e., the "sheer numbers involved" (14).

There were regional differences, also, in the rates of suicide. (Ontario comprises five major regions— three, mainly urban, in the southern sector, which contains the greatest proportion of the adolescent population; and two, mainly rural, in the north.) During the 8½ years of the study, the rates were relatively low in the southern regions, and high in the northern ones. More recently, however, the incidence has remained relatively constant for the three southern regions, but has fluctuated considerably in the northern ones (in both, there was a decrease from 1975 to 1976, but a marked increase in 1977). In addition, the five provincial regions are subdivided into counties. Similar to the above findings, counties in the southern regions had rates as low as 3 per 100,000, whereas counties in the primarily rural north had incidences ranging from 12 to as high as 40.

Dizmang, Watson, May, and Bopp's (1961–1968) study of American Indians on a reservation (26) recorded a prevalence of 98 suicides per 100,000; over half were by persons under the age of 25. These investigators showed that significant family disorganization or breakdown, resulting in increased rates of divorce, desertion, arrest, and multiple caretaking, differentiated the Indians who committed suicide from those who did not attempt it. Our findings indicated a higher rate of completed suicide in rural northern regions, in particular the counties with a large Canadian Indian population, the majority of whom live on reservations. The rates in these counties were two to four times the provincial average, and social disorganization, family dysfunction, and cultural and economic stresses appeared more common than in counties with smaller Indian populations.

By contrast with Ontario's regional rates, in the less-populous more-isolated province of Newfoundland the rate of youthful suicide during 1969–1971 was about one-tenth of Canada's national average (22). This low rate despite Newfoundland's severe economic problems again suggests that the greater incidence of suicide in rural Ontario is primarily related to family breakdown and social disorganization in a social environment that limits the opportunity for a troubled young person to find support from stable adults when crises arise.

*Occupation*

One-third of the subjects were students, and one-third were employed as laborers. Only 11% were unemployed, a figure well below both the provincial and national averages for this age group. The remaining one-quarter were employed as sales, business, or clerical personnel, housewives, civil servants, peace officers, or in social service. In general, therefore, these young people were pursuing an education, active in the work force, or establishing a household or family.

Previous studies, also, have shown that most adolescent suicides were employed or students at the time of death (27) (which contrasts with the finding that most adult suicides are unemployed or non-students). Two 10-year studies in Britain, 20 years apart, in fact indicated that university students are at highest risk: In 1959 Rook (28) noted the suicide rate at Oxford and Cambridge was 4 to 5 times the national average for a comparable age group, and in 1978 Hawton, Crowle, Simkin, and Bancroft (29) reported that suicides at Oxford were 2 to 5 times the national average for 15- to 24-year-olds.

ANTECEDENT CONDITIONS

Physical illnesses and/or character disorders were noted in only 3-5% of the cases. This contrasts with the reports by several other groups of investigators (7, 23, 30) of a high frequency (30-40%) of physical illness preceding suicide. (Furthermore, unlike Weinberg's finding [31] of physical illness as a major causal factor of suicide in males more than females, there was no sex-related trend in our incidence.)

Significant psychiatric conditions were noted at the time of the inquest or necropsy in 25% of the cases. Most often recorded was a combination of depression and previous suicidal behavior, and in 19% (5% of all cases) a schizophrenic condition had required hospitalization and treatment with major tranquilizers. These findings accord with other reports (21, 23, 32, 33) of a high frequency of psychiatric illness in those who commit suicide. In Shaffer's sample of young children (21), about 30% were receiving or awaiting psychiatric care at the time of death; Balser and Masterson (32) reported that 62% of their adolescent subjects had had symptoms of schizophrenia; and Myers and Neal (23) reported depressive illness in 45%, but schizophrenia in only 13% of their cases. These different rates probably relate to the age of the groups studied; Eastwood and Peacocke (33) demonstrated two significant clusters of psychiatric conditions: mood disorders characterized older suicides, and schizophrenia and personality disorders the younger ones.

Only 19% (5% of total) of our subjects for whom antecedent conditions were recorded had used intoxicants just before or as the method of suicide. This coincides with a case-study of ten adolescent suicides (25); but others have reported a high frequency of alcoholic intoxication at the time of suicide (24).

COMMENTARY

Youthful suicide in Ontario was most often associated with depressive illness and previous suicide attempts. As late adolescence is the period when affective disorders and schizophrenia commonly emerge, the association of these major psychiatric illnesses with suicide is not surprising. In addition, there was a virtual absence of notable medical illness at the time of death.

Pursuit of school and vocational achievement by these young people stands in marked contrast to a sudden and debilitating psychiatric illness that inteferes with the utilization of external help and the tolerance for out-side stress. A preceding state of intoxication was less often recorded, indi-cating that, unlike adults, few adolescents need to disinhibit themselves with intoxicants to carry out the self-destructive action.

## ATTEMPTED SUICIDE PRESENTING AT A
## PEDIATRIC HOSPITAL IN TORONTO

### FEATURES OF THE SUICIDAL ATTEMPTS

*Rate*

Six hundred five suicidal attempts in 505 patients were studied during the period of investigation. One hundred seventy-six (37%) patients had made more than one attempt. Other investigators (34) have reported repe-tition rates between 8% and 60%.

Kreitman (35) in 1976 noted a 10% increase in the rate of suicide at-tempts among 15- to 24-year-olds, and Wexler and co-workers (36) demon-strated a continuous global rise in the rate of suicide attempts particularly among the young. One-fifth of young people in a nonpsychiatric population manifested suicidal gestures, attempts at suicide, or serious suicidal ideas (37); and about 8% of the children in a child-guidance clinic displayed serious suicidal behavior (38).

The present data revealed distinct periods of increased frequency of suicidal attempts in relation to season. October through April were the peak months of admission for attempted suicide, twice the rate for May through September. As May and June had low frequencies, it appears that the rate did not relate to the stress of final examinations and leaving school. Several other authors, also, have reported seasonal fluctuation in the rate of suicide attempts by adolescents not unlike that for completed suicide. How-ever, studies in two countries in the northern hemisphere (Sweden and the U.S.A.) have revealed differing variation, and one group in Los Angeles (7) noted no such variation. In Sweden (8), the rate peaked in November and was lowest in June and July; in the U.S.A., one study (10) showed the frequency highest in spring and lowest in autumn, whereas another (39) reported a low rate in spring and peaks of twice that incidence in both summer and autumn.

Variation was also found in the rate in relation to time of day, about 25% of attempts occurring between noon and 6 p.m. and 50% during the evening. This accords with other reports (8, 40), that two out of every three attempts take place between 3 p.m. and midnight (40), and that the majority occur between early afternoon and 12 p.m. (8). It seems that, in contrast to adults, relatively few adolescents attempt suicide in the early morning.

## Method of Suicide Attempt

Eighty-eight percent of all attempts were made with a drug overdose. The next most common method was laceration (8%), then hanging (2%), and jumping (1.5%). About 20 persons (4%) used two or more methods. The medications most commonly used were household analgesics (37%) acetylsalicylic acid, acetaminophen, and combination tablets), benzodiazepines (24%), and barbiturates (19%). Phenothiazines, solvents, or inhalants and street drugs were each used by about 5%. Although the drugs may have caused many medical emergencies, serious life-threatening effects were noted in only 8% of cases.

Several studies have shown that a majority of adolescents attempt suicide by drug overdose (39-43): between 50% and 87% had taken an overdose of medication; the remaining attempts were by hanging, inhaling gas, jumping, or laceration.

## Risk and Rescue Factors

Two assessments of severity of the 605 attempts were made. Initial ratings on a three-point scale (low, moderate, or severe) indicated that about 8% had involved a high degree of danger. Re-rating on Weisman's risk/rescue scale (44) indicated that 90% of the attempts were of low to moderate risk, and had a moderate to high likelihood of rescue. It also identified a distinct group of attempters (1 in every 10) whose act was of moderate to high risk with a low to moderate likelihood of rescue, a group that represents the bridge between those who complete suicide and those whose attempts do not end in death. Barter, Swaback, and Todd (45) reported similarly that 87% of the attempts by adolescents were of low to moderate lethality; but others have reported higher rates of severity of the attempts, 19% "severe" (10) and 29% "seriously life-threatening" (7).

Attempters were less likely than controls to have parents nearby at the time of their injury; and only 43% of them (but nearly 70% of the controls) were accompanied to the hospital by their parents. The suicidal child was six times more likely to be accompanied by a professional, such as a social worker, child-care worker, or other mental-health worker, and seven times more likely to be accompanied by police. Thus, in general, during a time of crisis and major need, fewer of the attempters' parents were available to provide assistance.

Jacobziner (10) reported that the mother was in the home at the time of the attempt by nearly 29% of his adolescent patients, and Lukianowicz (38) also found others were present in many cases.

## Management

It had been anticipated that self-inflicted injury could be handled

quickly, but overall the index patients required more extensive and prolonged treatment than the control group; fewer than 50% (but 80% of the
controls) were discharged within 8 hours. Furthermore, over 60% of the
attempters (but only 20% of controls) were admitted to the hospital, and
their average stay exceeded that of the controls; attempters were twice as
likely to be kept in the hospital for 3 days or more. About 20% of the suicidal patients were sent home after medical treatment but were referred for
outpatient psychiatric assessment, and only 17% were not advised to receive further medical or psychiatric care. Approximately 50% of those who
were admitted were referred for further investigation.

Thus, in general, the suicide attempts were handled as more severe,
demanding medical emergencies than the acute problems of controls. Since
the attempters were much more likely to be admitted to the hospital, this
typically resulted in referral and investigation. Even if the patient was sent
home after emergency treatment, there was a greater than 20% chance that
he or she would be referred to a psychiatric service.

Other cited figures have been relatively lower than ours: in a study by
Mattson, Seese, and Hawkins (46), 44% were admitted to a hospital; the
remainder were referred for outpatient assessment and management, but
only 60% complied; Toolan (47), in the U.S.A., reported that 39% of his
sample of adolescents were referred to a psychiatric hospital for observation
or treatment; and Bergstrand and Otto (8), in Sweden, stated that of 69%
assessed psychiatrically, about one-third were referred for outpatient or
residential psychiatric treatment.

DEMOGRAPHIC CHARACTERISTICS

*Age*

The mean age at the time of the attempt was 15 years. Approximately
two-fifths of the attempters were in the 15 to 16.9 years age group, boys
more commonly in the younger age group and girls in the older group.

Recent findings indicate that the peak age of suicide attempts is
between 20 and 25 years; and Weissman (9) concluded from a review of the
international literature that persons under 30 years of age constitute 50%
of all attempters.

*Gender*

There were 381 female (75%) and 124 male attempters. This female:
male ratio of 3:1 is in line with other studies of suicide attempts in adolescence: 4:1 in Sweden (8), 3:1 in New York City (10), and 2:1 in Scotland
(41).

The findings that more girls attempt suicide, but more boys complete it differentiates adolescent suicides and attempters; i.e., their gender appears to influence the lethality of self-destructive acts.

## Religion

Lukianowicz (38) considered religious affiliation insignificant in relation to suicide attempts by young people, an opinion concurred with by Mattson and co-workers (46). The latter added that Catholic affiliation, which severely condemns suicide, does not significantly diminish suicidal behavior; in fact, Toolan (47) found the highest rate of suicide among Catholics, which included a large group of Puerto Ricans. White (48) noted a similar trend toward a higher incidence of attempts among Roman Catholic adolescents in Birmingham, England; and Schneer and Kay (49) reported a high frequency of suicide among Catholics and Jews.

The Hospital for Sick Children in Toronto services a large downtown area whose population is largely Roman Catholic. In the suicidal group, however, Protestants were overrepresented (53%, versus 44% in the control group), and there were fewer Roman Catholics (40%) and Jews (3%) than among the controls (46% and 6%). These differences are statistically significant (p < 0.05). Thus, in Toronto, the family's religion appeared to influence the rate of suicide attempts. This finding may relate partly to the greater number of subjects here than in the other investigations, and the hospital's proximity to many close-knit communities largely composed of first- and second-generation immigrants from southern Europe who have maintained close religious observance.

### ANTECEDENT CONDITIONS

Ninety-four percent of the attempters had experienced psychosocial problems, chiefly difficulty at school and family conflict. Table 2 presents a comparison of antecedent conditions between suicide attempters and the control group.

## Medical Illness

Physical illness was documented in control patients (43%) less often than suicidal ones (54%) (p < 0.01). Neurological symptoms (mostly nonspecific headaches) were more frequent among attempters, whereas minor trauma and orthopedic problems were more common in controls. The index group also had almost three times the control rate of pregnancy and of gynecological conditions such as infections, and almost twice the control rate of gastrointestinal complaints. Organic illness has been considered an etiologic factor in some suicide attempts by adolescents (50), and 6% of one group stated that concern over a physical illness was the precipitating

TABLE 2
ANTECEDENT CONDITIONS OF SUICIDE ATTEMPTERS

| Antecedent Condition | Attempters | Controls | $p$ |
|---|---|---|---|
| Prior street drug use | 37.2% | 5.5% | $<0.05$ |
| Current psychiatric symptoms | 68.2% | 16% | $<0.01$ |
| Previous psychiatric symptoms | 82% | 50% | $<0.001$ |
| Previous therapy or counseling | 63% | 18% | $<0.001$ |
| Physical illness | 54% | 43% | $<0.01$ |
| Family suicide | 8% | 1% | $<0.01$ |
| Family psychiatric illness | 52% | 16% | $<0.01$ |
| Family medical illness | 52% | 45% | $<0.05$ |
| Father unemployment | 14% | 7% | $<0.01$ |
| Mother outside employment | 50% | 36% | |
| Parental separation or death | 53% | 16% | $<0.001$ |

cause of the attempt (48). In another study (51), 86% of the adolescent attempters had physical complaints for which no specific organic diagnosis had been made, and about half had specified "psychosomatic" illness. A greater prevalence of somatic complaints, in particular gastrointestinal symptoms, has been recorded for male suicide attempters than for matched psychiatric controls (52).

*Psychiatric Illness*

A significantly greater number of current psychiatric symptoms were identified in those who had attempted suicide (68%) than in the control group (16%) ($p < 0.01$). More than half of the attempters had affective symptoms, and many had more than one psychiatric symptom; hostility or aggression was observed in 40%, and specific reactions to situational disturbances were noted in one-third. In contrast to findings of completed suicide, few attempters showed symptoms of schizophrenia or drug abuse.

About two-thirds of those who attempted suicide, but only 18% of the controls, had previous legal, psychiatric, or social-service involvement ($p < 0.001$): 38% had received professional help within 2 years of their attempt, approximately 50% had attended an outpatient psychiatric clinic; 21% had been psychiatric inpatients, 15% had had trouble with the law, 14% were wards of the Children's Aid Society, and a few were being helped by a physician, school guidance counselor, or social agency. Clearly, the attempters were experiencing diverse psychosocial problems.

The great majority (82%) of the suicidal, and 50% of the control patients had a longstanding history of psychiatric symptoms ($p < 0.001$). The attempter group was differentiated by a marked prevalence of chronic complaints such as sadness, isolation, withdrawal, aggression, and histrionic and neurotic symptoms, whereas a greater percentage of the control group had psychophysiological symptoms. This has been confirmed by other studies which suggest that psychiatric problems are common in suicidal adolescents, and in many cases noted before the attempt. For example, depression has been reported in 35–80% of cases; and it has been conservatively estimated that depressive states precede 40–45% of suicide attempts (11, 39, 52, 53). In addition, psychometric testing of a group of suicidal adolescents indicated minimal brain dysfunction in 60% (39).

SCHOLASTIC ACHIEVEMENT AND PROBLEMS

More than half of the attempter group were experiencing failure at school or were dropouts. However, when the severity of the attempt was rated on a three-point scale, "severe" correlated with success at school, and "minor" and "moderate" attempts were significantly associated with failure at school. This corroborates the completed suicide study in which suicides were more commonly associated with industrious and productive individuals.

Difficulties at school accounted for 38% of current problems and 35% of chronic ones. Other common recent difficulties included conflict with parents, with family rules in general, and with boy- or girlfriends. Longstanding problems also most often related to school or with family, friends, or police; other factors were abuse of alcohol or drugs, living away from home, and residence in a group- or foster-home. Delinquency and parental divorce or separation were noted in some cases.

Other investigators also have identified scholastic problems, including truancy in 4 of 10 adolescent attempters (38). Repeated studies 10 years apart (53) showed poor adjustment and performance at school, but truancy and defiance predominated in the later study. Examination of school records of one group of adolescent attempters (39) revealed exceptionally poor performance by 75%; 19% had failed one or more grades, and 35% had left school early or were chronic truants. However, other studies have yielded contradictory findings: a comparison with matched psychiatric controls showed no difference in relation to scholastic performance alone except for children who had made more than one attempt (54); and 36% of the adolescents studied by Teicher (55) were not enrolled in school at the time of the attempt, and few had left school because of poor marks.

*Precipitating Events*

Conflict had precipitated the attempt in about 75% of cases, which helps to explain why the psychiatric symptoms most frequently noted on admission were sadness and hostility, often in response to a crisis. Conflicts were most often with parents, although more pervasive family discord and conflicts with a boyfriend or girlfriend were also recorded. If frequencies are combined for all problems relating to family, parents, and siblings, about 70% of precipitating events were within the family. School-related problems were identified as precipitating events in 11% and problems with the law in 8%. In 4% of cases the event was the attempted suicide of a friend, a finding that offers limited support to the theory of "psychic contagion," i.e., that a vulnerable adolescent, becoming aware of another person's suicide, is directed to self-injury.

In 3%, the major precipitating event was abuse or severe neglect by parents. Thus, one repercussion of child-abuse may be a greater likelihood of self-inflicted injury and disregard for one's own safety.

Many authors agree that the most common precipitants of suicide attempts by adolescents are conflicts with parents, breakup and loss of a heterosexual relationship, sexual conflicts, problems at school, and pregnancy (8, 45, 46). Nonspecific family conflicts were reported in 38% of attempters (40), whereas an investigation of suicidal adolescent girls (56) identified a more chronic pattern of parental rejection exacerbated by a specific conflict, such as rejection by a boyfriend immediately before the attempt. In approximately two-thirds of the adolescent attempters studied by Barter, Swaback, and Todd (45), the precipitating event was the actual or threatened loss of a highly emotional relationship; in many cases a significant heterosexual relationship had led to conflict with parents, culminating in crisis.

Others have reported problems at school as the direct precipitating factor in 5–8% of cases (57). On re-examining a subgroup of children for whom such problems appeared to have motivated the attempt, Otto (57) reported that nearly 47% cited poor academic performance, 13% described problems with teachers and/or schoolmates, and 11% stated a wish to leave school.

FAMILY CHARACTERISTICS

*Family Discord and Breakdown*

The attempters had experienced three times the control rate of parental separation or death (p < 0.001) and almost twice the control rate of parental divorce. Approximately 50% of their fathers (but only 14% of the controls' fathers) were absent. In most single-parent families the mother was raising the child; and the mothers of over half of the attempters worked outside the home. These findings describe a breakdown of the family unit primarily as a result of the father's absence.

Most of the children separated from both parents were living in group-homes; the rate of placement of attempters was about 8 times higher than among the control group. This high rate of suicidal attempts in group-homes may reflect several factors: the frequent referral of suicidal or depressed children to group-homes; the tendency for these homes to receive the community's most severely disturbed children, increasing the likelihood of their providing suicidal models (psychic contagion); the staff's difficulty in dealing with severely disturbed children; and group-home procedures which often require that all who attempt suicide be taken immediately to a pediatric hospital emergency service for treatment and assessment.

Dorpat, Jackson, and Ripley (58) described an increased prevalence of disorganization of the families of suicidal adolescents. They identified broken homes in about 64% of cases, most commonly because of divorce; and death of a parent was often noted, having occurred in about 40% of cases when the child was between 12 and 17 years of age. Other studies have yielded similar findings: Barter, Swaback, and Todd (45) reported that more than 50% of the suicidal adolescents had lost one or both parents, most commonly through divorce, and in Ackerly's study of preadolescent attempters (59), about one-third had experienced separation, divorce, or death of parents. In five other studies (39-41, 45, 48) during the 1960s and 1970s, between 25% and 88% of suicidal youngsters were not in contact with one or both parents (39, 41, 45); and a 50% rate of family breakdown resulted from separation, divorce, and death (40, 48). In still another study (11), the fathers of 12% of the attempters had died, a loss that Cantor (60) considers has greater impact on suicide attempts by first-born adolescent girls.

Such findings suggest that the absence of a parent in itself may predispose a child to attempt suicide. In contrast, however, death of a parent did not significantly differentiate suicidal from nonsuicidal individuals in other studies (54, 61). Crook and Raskin (61) stated that parents' marital discord and conflicts before breakdown of the family related more significantly to the attempt. Similarly, although a comparison of suicidal adolescents and matched psychiatric patients (54) showed a significantly higher incidence of conflict and threatened loss of parents among suicidal families, there was no difference in the overall incidence of actual loss of a parent. (However, significantly more of the suicidal patients had lost a parent before age 12.)

Connell (34) considered family disorganization the norm for suicidal adolescents. He found that one-third of attempters' parents were divorced or separated, and about half had severe marital problems. By contrast, Schneer, Perlstein, and Brozovsky (53) claimed that neither broken homes nor absence of the father significantly differentiated suicidal adolescents from controls.

*Parents' Employment Status*

Unemployment of fathers of the youthful attempters (14%) was twice the control rate (7%) (p < 0.01); and 50% of the attempters' mothers were employed outside the home compared to 36% of controls (p < 0.01). This may indicate the mothers' need to seek employment as a result of the fathers' chronic unemployment, or because they are the sole breadwinners in single-parent families.

These findings confirm that families experience stress created by both a father's unemployment and a working mother's absence from the home, and concur with reports that family stress (30, 58) resulting from economic problems (10, 20, 62) is a factor in suicide attempts by adolescents. A father preoccupied with financial worries and concerned about his self-esteem may be less able to respond to crises and sadness in his children's lives. Similarly, a mother's involvement in work and interests outside the home may diminish her attentiveness and availability to her troubled child when the need arises.

*Medical Illness in the Family*

Medical problems were recorded for nearly half of the attempters' families and over 40% of control families: the difference in rate was more obvious among fathers (20% vs 13%) than among mothers (27% vs 20%). Illness of siblings was of equal frequency in both groups.

The types of illnesses differentiated the two groups of fathers, but not the mothers. Compared with controls, more index fathers had cardiovascular disease or diabetes, twice as many had gastrointestinal illnesses or organic brain syndromes (including epilepsy), and five times as many had orthopedic disease. Thus, the attempters' fathers had a greater prevalence (p < 0.05) of chronic and debilitating illnesses, whereas the control fathers had predominantly acute and less-debilitating conditions, such as allergy, respiratory illness, and nonspecific neurologic problems.

Although the medical history of relatives of suicidal adolescents has seldom been studied, our findings confirm the impression that these families probably suffer an increased incidence of physical problems. Physical illness in the family may trouble an adolescent in two ways: concerns about the illnesses may directly disturb him; and parents chronically preoccupied with their own ill health may be less responsive to their child's need for help in coping with difficulties and stresses.

*Mental Illness in the Family*

Psychiatric illness was identified in 52% of the index families but only 16% of controls, a difference that is highly significant (p < 0.001). The rate was 20% higher than for control fathers and mothers, and 10% higher than for control siblings.

For all members of the index families (fathers, mothers, and siblings), the most common recorded problem was alcoholism or substance abuse. About 60% of the fathers with psychiatric symptoms were alcoholics, and about 7% were noted to have neurotic, schizoid, and aggressive symptoms, but there were few suicidal and affective symptoms. Alcoholism or substance abuse constituted one-third of all psychiatric disturbances recorded for index mothers. Of the mothers with psychiatric symptoms, about 18% were described as neurotic, almost 12% had affective symptoms, and 6.5% displayed aggressive or schizoid features. Notably, alcoholism or abuse of other substances constituted one-quarter of the mental illness recorded for siblings. Similarly, Bergstrand and Otto (8) reported alcoholism in 15% of parents of adolescent attempters, and other emotional disorders in 28%; and two other studies (39, 51) recorded alcoholism in one or both parents in approximately one-third of cases.

The high rate of mental illness in the families of those who attempt suicide in youth suggests a causal relationship. The attempt may be a reaction to psychological disturbance, particularly alcoholism or other substance abuse by the parents, or other members of the family. Young people experiencing the turbulent period of adolescence may have difficulty coping with the stress of psychiatric illness of an immediate family member. Suicide attempts may also be the adolescent expression of the common genetic vulnerability of the family that is expressed in other family members as alcoholism and drug abuse. Certainly the relative absence of psychiatric illness in our control group links suicidal behavior in youth with forms of psychiatric illness in other family members.

*Family History of Suicidal Behavior*

The recorded rate of suicide or attempted suicide was more than seven times higher for index (8.3%) than for control (1.1%) families (p < 0.01). Suicide had been committed by eight immediate and three other members of the attempters' families, but none was recorded for the controls' families. Attempts had been made by 25 immediate members of index families, but only four in the control group, and by one more distant family member in each group.

The current literature supports the view that certain families are disposed to suicide (37, 63). As many as 44% of those who make the attempt have a family history of suicide (51); and Jacobs (27) found a high incidence of suicidal behavior in the relatives and friends of attempters, but no attempts in the families of his control group. This tendency for suicide to cluster in families suggests that family factors, whether genetic or environmental, influence adolescent suicidal behavior. The occurrence of both suicide and attempted suicide within index families supports the hypothesis that they are part of a continuum of self-destruction across generational lines.

COMMENTARY

Typically, the suicidal young person was experiencing many serious and pervasive situational conflicts, and lacked adult support and guidance in his or her efforts to cope with them. The picture that emerged was one of chronic family discord characterized by major problems such as divorce, separation, and alcoholism, in many cases coupled with a family history of suicidal behavior. Within a continuum of psychological and social assaults on the individual, the attempt at suicide appeared to constitute the most recent manifestation of many painful life experiences.

Sadness and hostility in reaction to situational crises were the most characteristic symptoms. Thus, suicidal behavior most likely represents an impulsive reaction to crises, superimposed on pre-existing recurrent depression.

Table 3 presents a comparison of major characteristics which differentiated suicide completers from attempters.

TABLE 3
MAJOR CHARACTERISTICS OF SUICIDE COMPLETERS
VERSUS ATTEMPTERS

| Characteristics | Completers | Attempters |
| --- | --- | --- |
| Gender | Mostly boys | Mostly girls |
| Mean age | 20 | 15 |
| Primary method | Firearms | Drugs |
| Nature of relationships and goals | Stable | Unstable |
| Antecedent illness | Psychiatric | Physical |
| School experience | Success | Failure |

SUMMARY

Completed and attempted suicide by young persons were studied, the former by review of forensic reports throughout the province of Ontario, and the latter by review of emergency-room records of a Toronto pediatric hospital. The studies revealed the following trends:

*Completed Suicide*

1. The number of suicides by 10- to 24-year-olds in Ontario during

January 1971 through August 1978 was at least 10% greater than reported in the official statistics.

2. The rate of suicide, adjusted for changes in population, increased 32% from 1971 to 1977.

3. The rate showed seasonal and regional variations: it was highest in fall and winter and during June, and in rural counties in northwestern Ontario.

4. The choice of method appeared influenced by the subject's age, sex, urban or rural residence, occupation, and social forces of the time. Guns were the most common means of suicide by subjects aged 16 and over. Violent methods were used increasingly by females.

5. Significant personal factors included presence of psychiatric illness, sex, and developmental stage. Suicide by preadolescents was rare, the rate increasing dramatically from about age 16 to a peak at 20 years, then remaining level until 24 years. The overall male:female ratio was 4:1. Psychiatric conditions, including suicide attempts, were noted in 25% of cases.

*Attempted Suicide*

1. Thirty-seven percent of the patients had made at least one previous attempt.

2. The rate showed seasonal and temporal variation, being highest in fall and winter and between 6 p.m. and midnight.

3. Drugs were the choice of method in the large majority of patients.

4. One in every 10 attempts was of moderate to high risk with low to moderate likelihood of rescue.

5. The female:male ratio was 3:1; the average age was 15 years.

6. Psychosocial problems were identified in 94% of cases. Conflict with parents, family, or a boy- or girlfriend had precipitated the event in about 75%.

7. More than half of the attempters were experiencing failure at school or were dropouts.

Comparison with a matched (control) group of patients attending the same emergency department revealed the following significant differences.

1. Attempters were less likely to have parents nearby at the time of the emergency or to be accompanied to the hospital by their parents. They were six times more likely to be accompanied by a professional.

2. Self-inflicted injury required more extensive and prolonged treatment, and more frequent admission to hospital, referral, and investigation.

3. Psychiatric presenting symptoms, chiefly of sadness, isolation or withdrawal, or aggression, were 4.5 times more common.

4. Protestants were overrepresented, and Roman Catholics and Jews were underrepresented.

5. A history of psychiatric or social-service involvement was three times as frequent; and more than half of the attempters had had psychiatric treatment.

6. Gastrointestinal complaints were twice as common, and pregnancy and gynecologic conditions were three times the control rate.

7. Breakdown of the family structure was prevalent. The father was absent in more than 50% of cases as compared to 14% in the control group; and group-home placement was eight times as common. Twice as many fathers were unemployed; and 1.5 times as many mothers worked outside the home.

8. Medical problems were recorded for significantly more of the attempters' fathers and mothers; the fathers were more likely to have chronic, more limiting conditions.

9. Psychiatric illness was identified in 52% of the families, in comparison to 16% for the control group. The most common conditions in family members were alcoholism and drug abuse.

10. The recorded rate of a family history of suicide or attempted suicide was more than seven times the control rate.

*Differentiation of Attempters from Completed Suicides*

1. More girls attempted suicide, but far more boys completed it.

2. The majority of attempters used drugs, whereas most of the suicides killed themselves with guns.

3. Few of the attempters, but the majority of the suicides, had maintained apparently stable relationships and the pursuit of educational and vocational goals.

4. Physical illness, family conflicts, and problems at school were recorded for between 54% and 95% of the attempters, but were noted for less than 5% of the suicides.

5. Severe adult forms of psychiatric illness (schizophrenia and depression) were much less prevalent in attempters than suicides.

## DISCUSSION

The present studies differentiated suicide and attempted suicide into two fairly discreet clinical entities, revealing significant differences in relation to age, sex, character structure and personal background, symptoms, precipitating events, and methods used. Attempters had experienced a significantly increased rate of family discord and breakdown, indicating that attempted suicide reflects a growing relationship between self-injury and the wider gulf between youth and their elders. Bronfenbrenner (15) has graphically described the isolation associated with a declining influence of traditional and social values, and the parallel increase in emotional disturbances, crises, and suicidal behavior in adolescence.

Every child needs a responsive, supportive, and understanding adult to follow the course of his development, and offer help with problems as they arise. Developmentally, adolescents are striving for autonomy: in contrast to childhood, when they were more dependent on family and immediate community, in adolescence they reject many values of parents, teachers, and others in attempts to establish their separate identity. A child who has limited personality resources has difficulty coping with the stresses of functioning alone which accompany this developmental phase. If parents, teachers, or peers are absent, troubled, or in conflict with the adolescent, he cannot get the help he needs particularly when a specific conflict results in crisis. Witnessing marital discord and family breakdown may limit an adolescent's ability to seek support and guidance from adults. Discontinuous care, and particularly absence of the father, appears to be a significant causal factor of suicide attempts by adolescents; and placement in a group-home denies both biologic parents the ability to provide continuous support and care.

Both suicide and attempted suicide demonstrate the failure of others to provide support, guidance, values, and problem-solving models for the person at risk. Specifically, completed suicide reflects isolation, social disorganization, and limited availability of persons who could help (as noted on Indian reservations and in rural communities), whereas attempts result from chronic lack of support from within the family, in many cases associated with the absence of the father.

Typically, an adolescent who commits suicide has maintained superficially stable adjustments at home, school, and work; and there is little evidence of prolonged or repeated maladjustment before the onset of a major affective disorder or psychotic episode in adolescence. He is likely to have been viewed by adults and peers as functioning adequately in work and relationships; to them, his suicide is an unexpected, unaccountable catastrophe.

However, suicide does appear to be related to the development of major psychiatric illness. The young people we studied had experienced a high incidence of severe depression and schizophrenia, conditions that commonly emerge during mid- to late adolescence. Adolescence is normally a period of re-formation of personality structure and coping mechanisms. An adolescent who has limited ability to weigh alternatives and develop more adaptive strategies to cope with severe stress may feel overwhelmed when confronted with psychiatric illness, and choose death as an end to unbearable anxiety and sadness.

By contrast, attempted suicide is often simply the most recent expression of a long history of conflict in multifarious life situations. It is seldom completely unexpected, and in many cases can be anticipated, as the child encounters increasing frustration and disappointment. Unlike completed suicide, the self-destructive behavior indicates considerable impulsivity, poor planning, and weakness of purpose; thus, the conscious wish to die is incompletely and/or inaccurately translated into the attempt. As a result, most ensure their survival by choosing methods of low lethality in circumstances that engender a high likelihood of rescue.

However, it is important to view suicide attempts not just in terms of differences in lethality of method, but to include examination of historical differences and antecedent conditions. Teicher and Jacobs (51) suggested that a young person's attempt at suicide may represent the final alternative after exhausting all perceived solutions to cope with cumulative physical and emotional burdens and deprivations.

The young person whose attempt at suicide is unsuccessful has been chronically deprived of effective guidance. Because he has had limited opportunities to incorporate values and problem-solving strategies, his personality has developed fewer strengths. Compared with the normal adolescent he began with fewer familial and social models. Thus, his suicidal act does not constitute an immediate reaction to crisis alone; it also reflects others' chronic failure to support development of the adolescent's capacity to adapt to and cope with life.

The present study identified paternal absence as a major factor of this deprivation. Both historically and at the time of the attempt, many of the fathers were absent or experiencing medical, emotional, economic, or marital stress, indicating an association between the absence of a responsive, attentive, emotionally available father and adolescent suicidal behavior. For both females and males, there was a trend to a subordinate role for the mother compared with absence or unavailability of the father.

The predominant clinical impression of the attempter is one of chronic and pervasive anguish. Behaviorally, the suicide attempt represents the cumulative expression of continual distress and turmoil, usually resulting from difficulties with physical health, relationships outside the home, scholastic performance, and family members, specifically the parent-child relationship. In the study of attempts, the precipitating crises were principally difficulties at school, family conflicts, and loss of a significant peer relationship. This finding underscores the importance of an adolescent's social, family, and scholastic milieu.

Ironically, the severity of the attempt correlated with the degree of scholastic *success*, and concurs with the comparable finding that most of those who had committed suicide had been industrious and productive. This may reflect the ingenuity of those who have a greater capacity to translate suicidal thoughts and feelings into a serious life-threatening event, a clearer appreciation of the gravity of their problems, or a greater dread of the effect of their problems on their ambitions.

A subgroup of attempters were identified who tended to show less pervasive disturbance and maladjustment (and were scarcely distinguishable from those whose attempt was successful). Many of these were among the 10% whose attempts were highly lethal with little likelihood of rescue, and whose survival depended on chance alone. Thus this group appears to reflect the transition from attempt to completion in the spectrum of suicide.

The patient's sex was the factor that most clearly distinguished suicides from attempters. Significantly more girls than boys attempted suicide, but more boys than girls completed the act. This may indicate that for girls the self-injury represents a less-organized, more ambivalent manifestation of inner pain, whereas for boys, it is intended as a decisive, committed end. Other distinguishing features between completers and attempters included the subject's age, the method chosen to accomplish the act, and illness of the person or other family members. Suicide increased dramatically from about 16 years of age and peaked at 20 years, whereas the attempters' average age was 15 years. The choice of method, also, clearly distinguished the groups: even though the intention of all was to die, overall the attempters' methods were much less lethal.

Psychiatric illness was significantly higher in the suicides and their families, and chronic debilitating illness was more prevalent in attempters' than in controls' fathers.

The steep increase in incidence of suicides beginning at about age 16 may result from the following factors:

1. The greater ability to formulate self-destructive thoughts and feelings into organized, highly dangerous behavior, resulting from developments in perception and cognition during adolescence.

2. The increase in significant psychiatric illness, such as schizophrenia and affective disorder, during late adolescence and early adulthood.

3. Significant challenges, such as choice of career and the formation of close relationships, which are associated with late adolescence.

4. The diminishing stability of the family, school, and community, and their lessening involvement in daily life, which threatens young people who are not ready to handle everyday problems alone.

5. The less high regard and less frequent availability of adults' influence as the young person develops a psychological and social identity distinct from his immediate family.

6. The inability of the young person to utilize the intervention of others, with whose guidance and counsel he is not familiar.

Like all similar studies, the present ones showed a desperate need for delineation of suicidal individuals and implementation of more effective communication with the person at risk. Significantly, suicide attempts were treated as a severe medical emergency more often than other acute states, required longer observation, and resulted in more hospital admissions. The prolonged observation and treatment, which may indicate the emergency-room pediatricians' caution in dealing with self-inflicted injury, and a wariness of problems not exclusively physical, placed a heavy load on the health-care service. In 1961 it was reported that 12% of all admissions of adolescents to a Brooklyn hospital during a 2-year period were because of attempted suicide (49); and a 1978 report (64) stated that suicide attempts accounted for 24% of visits by females and 11% of visits by males to the emergency departments of four general hospitals in Edmonton, Alberta. Thus, suicide attempts constitute a significant proportion of emergency caseloads. This, added to the frequent need for inpatient treatment and referral to psychiatric and other services, results in a huge burden on the social and health-care services.

## CONCLUSIONS

The increasing rates of suicide and attempted suicide appear to reflect the prevalence of serious individual and family pathology and the inability to receive or utilize external support. In addition to causing a tragic degree of human suffering, suicidal behavior is placing an ever-heavier burden on social and health care services. Programs of prevention are urgently needed.

## REFERENCES

1. Farberow, N. L. & Neuringer, C. (1971), The social scientist as coroner's deputy. *J. Forensic Sci.*, 16:15–39.
2. Esquirol, J. E. D. (1845), *Mental Maladies: A Treatise on Insanity*, trans. E. K. Hunt. New York: Hafner, 1965.
3. Durkheim, E. (1897), *Suicide: A Study in Sociology*, trans. J. A. Spaulding & G. Simpson. Glencoe, Ill.: Free Press, 1951.
4. Zilboorg, G. (1937), Considerations of suicide with particular reference to that of the young. *Am. J. Orthopsychiatry*, 7:15–31.
5. Hendin, H. (1956), Suicide. *Psychiatr. Q.*, 30:267–282.
6. Halbwachs, M. (1978), *The Causes of Suicide,* trans. H. Goldblatt. London: Routledge & Kegan Paul.
7. Shneidman, E. S. & Farberow, N. L. (1961), Statistical comparisons between attempted and committed suicides. In: *The Cry for Help*, ed. N. L. Farberow & E. S. Shneidman. New York: McGraw Hill, pp. 19–47.
8. Bergstrand, C. G. & Otto, U. (1962), Suicidal attempts in adolescence and childhood. *Acta Paedopsychiatr.*, 51:17–26.
9. Weissman, M. M. (1974), The epidemiology of suicide attempts, 1960 to 1971. *Arch. Gen. Psychiatry*, 30:737–746.

10. Jacobziner, H. (1960), Attempted suicides in children. *J. Pediatr.*, 56:519-525.
11. Jacobziner, H. (1965), Attempted suicide in adolescents by poisoning. *Am. J. Psychother.*, 19:247-252.
12. Garfinkel, B. D., Chamberlain, C., & Golombek, H. (1979), Completed suicide in Ontario youth. In: *Proceedings of the 10th International Congress on Suicide Prevention and Crisis Intervention*, Ottawa, June 17-20, 1979. Ottawa: International Association for Suicide Prevention, pp. 126-131.
13. Garfinkel, B. D., Froese, A., & Golombek, H. (1979), Suicidal behavior in a pediatric population. In: *Proceedings of the 10th International Congress on Suicide Prevention and Crisis Intervention*, Ottawa, June 17-20, 1979. Ottawa: International Association for Suicide Prevention, pp. 305-312.
14. Frederick, C. J. (1978), Current trends in suicidal behavior in the United States. *Am. J. Psychother.*, 32:172-200.
15. Bronfenbrenner, U. (1974), The origins of alienation. *Sci. Am.*, 231:53-61.
16. Sanborn, D. E., III, Casey, T. M., & Niswander, G. D. (1970), Suicide: seasonal patterns and related variables. *Dis. Nerv. System*, 31:702-704.
17. Lester, D. (1971), Seasonal variation in suicidal deaths. *Br. J. Psychiatry*, 118:627-628.
18. Eastwood, M. R. & Peacocke, J. (1976), Seasonal patterns of suicide, depression, and electroconvulsive therapy. *Br. J. Psychiatry*, 129:472-475.
19. Morris, J. B., Kovacs, M., Beck, A. I., & Wolffe, A. (1974), Notes toward an epidemiology of urban suicide. *Compr. Psychiatry*, 15:537-547.
20. Holinger, P. C. (1978), Adolescent suicide: an epidemiological study of recent trends. *Am. J. Psychiatry*, 135:754-756.
21. Shaffer, D. (1974), Suicide in childhood and early adolescence. *J. Child Psychol. Psychiatry*, 15:275-291.
22. Liberakis, E. A. & Hoenig, J. (1978), Recording of suicide in Newfoundland. *Psychiatr. J. Univ. Ottawa*, 3:254-259.
23. Myers, D. H. & Neal, C. D. (1978), Suicide in psychiatric patients. *Br. J. Psychiatry*, 133:38-44.
24. Kehoe, J. P. & Abbott, A. P. (1975), Suicide and attempted suicide in the Yukon Territory. *Can. Psychiatr. Assoc. J.*, 20:15-23.
25. Sanborn, D. E., III, Sanborn, C. J., & Cimbolic, P. (1973), Two years of suicide: a study of adolescent suicide in New Hampshire. *Child Psychiatr. Hum. Dev.*, 3:234-242.
26. Dizmang, L. H., Watson, J., May, P. A., & Bopp, J. (1974), Adolescent suicide at an Indian reservation. *Am. J. Orthopsychiatry*, 44:43-49.
27. Jacobs, J. (1971), *Adolescent Suicide*. New York: Wiley Interscience.
28. Rook, A. (1959), Student suicides. *Br. Med. J.*, 1:599-603.
29. Hawton, K., Crowle, J., Simkin, S., & Bancroft, J. (1978), Attempted suicide and suicide among Oxford University students. *Br. J. Psychiatry*, 132:506-509.
30. Bagley, C., Jacobson, S., & Rehin, A. (1976), Completed suicide: a taxonomic analysis of clinical and social data. *Psychol. Med.*, 6:429-438.
31. Weinberg, S. (1970), Suicidal intent in adolescence: a hypothesis about the role of physical illness. *J. Pediatr.*, 77:579-586.
32. Balser, B. H. & Masterson, J. F. (1959), Suicide in adolescents. *Am. J. Psychiatry*, 116:400-404.

33. Eastwood, M. R. & Peacocke, J. E. (1975), Suicide, diagnosis, and age. *Can. Psychiatr. Assoc. J.*, 20:447–449.
34. Connell, H. M. (1972), Attempted suicide in schoolchildren. *Med. J. Aust.*, 1: 686–690.
35. Kreitman, N. (1976), Age and parasuicide ("attempted suicide"). *Psychol. Med.*, 6:113–121.
36. Wexler, L., Weissman, M. M., & Kasl, S. V. (1978), Suicide attempts 1970–1975: updating a United States study and comparison with international trends. *Br. J. Psychiatry*, 132:180–185.
37. Leonard, C. V. & Flinn, D. E. (1972), Suicidal ideation and behavior in youthful nonpsychiatric populations. *J. Consult. Clin. Psychol.*, 38:366–371.
38. Lukianowicz, N. (1968), Attempted suicide in children. *Acta Psychiatr. Scand.*, 44:415–435.
39. Rohn, R. D., Sarles, R. M., Kenny, T. J., Reynolds, B. J., & Heald, F. P. (1977), Adolescents who attempt suicide. *J. Pediatr.*, 90:636–638.
40. Tuckman, J. & Connon, H. E. (1962), Attempted suicide in adolescents. *Am. J. Psychiatry*, 119:228–232.
41. Haider, I. (1968), Suicidal attempts in children and adolescents. *Br. J. Psychiatry*, 114:1133–1134.
42. Leese, S. M. (1969), Suicide behaviour in twenty adolescents. *Br. J. Psychiatry*, 115:479–480.
43. Bigras, J., Gauthier, Y., Bouchard, C., & Tassé, Y. (1966), Suicidal attempts in adolescent girls. *Can. Psychiatr. Assoc. J.*, 11(suppl.):s275–s282.
44. Weisman, A. D. & Worden, J. W. (1972), Risk-rescue rating in suicide assessment. *Arch. Gen. Psychiatry*, 26:553–560.
45. Barter, J. T., Swaback, D. O., & Todd, D. (1968), Adolescent suicide attempts. *Arch. Gen. Psychiatry*, 19:523–527.
46. Mattson, A., Seese, L. R., & Hawkins, J. R. (1969), Suicidal behavior as a child psychiatric emergency. *Arch. Gen. Psychiatry*, 20:100–109.
47. Toolan, J. M. (1962), Suicide and suicidal attempts in children and adolescents. *Am. J. Psychiatry*, 118:719–724.
48. White, H. C. (1974), Self-poisoning in adolescents. *Br. J. Psychiatry*, 124:24–35.
49. Schneer, H. I. & Kay, P. (1961), The suicidal adolescent. In: *Adolescents: Psychoanalytic Approach to Problems and Therapy*, ed. S. Lorand & H. I. Schneer. New York: Hoeber, pp. 180–201.
50. Parnell, R. W. & Skottowe, I. (1957), Towards preventing suicide. *Lancet*, 1: 206–208.
51. Teicher, J. C. & Jacobs, J. (1966), Adolescents who attempt suicide: preliminary findings. *Am. J. Psychiatry*, 122:1248–1257.
52. Marks, P. A. & Haller, D. L. (1977), Now I lay me down for keeps: a study of adolescent suicide attempts. *J. Clin. Psychol.*, 33:390–400.
53. Schneer, H. I., Perlstein, A., & Brozovsky, M. (1975), Hospitalized suicidal adolescents: two generations. *J. Am. Acad. Child Psychiatry*, 14:268–280.
54. Stanley, E. J. & Barter, J. T. (1970), Adolescent suicidal behavior. *Am. J. Orthopsychiatry*, 40:87–96.
55. Teicher, J. D. (1970), Children and adolescents who attempt suicide. *Pediatr. Clin. N. Am.*, 17:687–696.
56. Schrut, A. (1968), Some typical patterns in the behavior and background of

adolescent girls who attempt suicide. *Am. J. Psychiatry*, 125:69-74.
57. Otto, U. (1965), Suicidal attempts made by children and adolescents because of school problems. *Acta Paediatr. Scand.*, 54:348-356.
58. Dorpat, T. L., Jackson, J. K., & Ripley, H. S. (1965), Broken homes and attempted and completed suicide. *Arch. Gen. Psychiatry*, 12:213-216.
59. Ackerly, W. C. (1967), Latency-age children who threaten or attempt to kill themselves. *J. Am. Child Psychiatry*, 6:242-261.
60. Cantor, P. (1972), The adolescent attempter: sex, sibling position, and family constellation. *Suicide & Life Threatening Behavior*, 2:252-261.
61. Crook, T. & Raskin, A. (1975), Association of childhood parental loss with attempted suicide and depression. *J. Consult. Clin. Psychology*, 43:277.
62. Brenner, M. H. (1973), *Mental Illness and the Economy*. Cambridge, Mass.: Harvard University Press.
63. Dabbagh, F. (1977), Family suicide. *Br. J. Psychiatry*, 130:159-161.
64. Watson, G. D. (1978), Utilization of emergency departments for psychiatric treatment. *Can. Psychiatr. Assoc. J.*, 23:143-148.

PART FOUR

# FORMS OF
# INTERVENTION

## INTRODUCTION

# PART FOUR:
# FORMS OF INTERVENTION

### CLIVE G. CHAMBERLAIN

In previous parts, the major themes presented have been concerned with the nature of adolescence and its peculiar burdens and troubles. The discussion has taken us from culture and context to an examination of the complexities of adolescent mood disorders, where the process of development makes questions of form and cause more difficult. However intrinsically fascinating, it is well to remember that the purpose of such reflections is to promote understanding which will facilitate health, growth, and healing.

This final section is devoted, therefore, to action. Since it is fashionable to be modest and self-critical, terms like cure and remedy are avoided, and the more antiseptic "intervention" or the less embarrassingly optimistic "management" are preferred. Such humility is appropriate. While support and comfort can be offered to all patients, the efficacy of treatment is often uncertain and difficult to evaluate. In a climate where nihilism comes easy, those who continue to invest energy and talent in the pursuit of improved therapies must possess moral courage. Four authors, each drawing upon a rich background of experience "in the trenches," utilize different points of view in order to explain their recommendations for action.

In the first paper of this section, Dr. Farberow, long associated with the study of suicide, reviews patterns of self-destructiveness in adolescence. He outlines findings regarding causal factors, and more important, examines selected programs of prevention. This author is sailing in difficult waters and he knows it. Existing epidemiological knowledge is often unreli-

221

able and overgeneralized. What passes for knowledge in the study of causal relationships is often clinical or sociological hunch; consequently, the pursuit of solutions proceeds mostly on the basis of random innovation (however creative or energetic). There is a need for more accurate data and greater epidemiological sophistication in the identification of population subgroups. Trend and rate comparisons for self-destructive behavior are notoriously difficult across jurisdictions and over time, because of reporting differences. For example, overall suicide rates for a state, province, or small country often mask great variation between geographic, sociological, or ethnic subgroups; thus more focused studies are necessary.

Similarly, clinical and sociological hunches must be tested against epidemiological models and data, and treatment modalities need to be evaluated. Otherwise, clinical practice can be dominated by fashion, and hard-won experience can fail to enter the domain of public knowledge. This is not to devalue current and past programs, but merely to insist upon learning from experience. The history of medicine is filled with examples of remedies that enjoyed vogue until put to rigorous testing. Prevention programs are no exception; belief in the urgent need for active intervention does not mean that we can deliver.

Where Dr. Farberow's chapter deals with the "forest," the three succeeding chapters deal with the "trees." Dr. Klein discusses, in a personal way, the evolution of his individual clinical perspective. He tells us of his experience in attempting to sort out the relative utility of various clinical paradigms, and in particular, contrasts the dynamic and descriptive models. In doing so, he demonstrates the powerful impact that clinical models have upon our processing of information, and even upon which phenomena we notice.

Adopting what he calls, with tongue in cheek, a "superficial" approach, Dr. Klein identifies two clusters of troubled young patients, and suggests different management and treatment approaches. He takes the risk of seeming casual in his discussion of the subject, but the reader will not fail to discern that honesty, not lightheartedness, directs this choice of style. He refuses to dress up his experience in pseudo-precision, and gives us much of value to ponder and pursue. He invites further controlled trials and more precise definitions.

Drawing upon Heinz Kohut's work on narcissistic personality disorders, Dr. Newman uses the characters in the film "Harold and Maude" to develop a paradigm for understanding and treating a group of severely disturbed adolescents. As with Dr. Klein's paper, this is not merely academic play, but an effort by an experienced and thoughtful therapist to organize and convey his understanding of a new theoretical position and its implications for treatment. Careful and repeated reading will prove worthwhile for the clinician who struggles with adolescents with severe character pathology.

In the last paper, expanding the focus from an individual to a systems perspective, Dr. Guttman draws upon her experience with family therapy for adolescents to discuss the use of this modality with mood disorders. The paper, written in a clear, deceptively simple style, offers practical advice in treating adolescents within the context of their families, whether the mood disturbance is regarded as "endogenous" or as a response to difficult relationships.

All four authors in this section expound their points of view in an effort to organize their experience, without for a moment insisting upon universality. Taken as a group, these papers remind us that we are far from a satisfactory, comprehensive paradigm for understanding disorders of behavior and emotion. We must regard the many models that we have as special tools, each with specific applications and limitations. Tool makers often overvalue the tools they know best and try to extend their applications, whereas practical craftsmen, with a mixture of skepticism and hope, will pick over all available tools, always seeking more effective means to improve their work.

To read these last chapters is to admire and wonder at the conceptual diversity of our field, held together, sometimes tenuously, by the not always compatible contributions of science and humanism.

# CHAPTER FOURTEEN

# SUICIDE IN ADOLESCENCE: PREVENTION AND TREATMENT

## Norman L. Farberow

A rock song a few years ago lamented: "It's the same thing every day, well, I can't get out of bed/Too many questions that's confusing up my head." Chorus: "I got that teen-age depression, and that's what I'm talking about/If you don't know what I mean, then you better look out." The song was entitled *Teen-age Depression* and went on to deplore, with liberal use of four-letter words, the problems of family, school, and drugs.

This song reflects an alarmingly common international phenomenon of depression and suicide among the young, which is apparent in the suicide statistics for adolescents and young adults, aged 15 to 24, in many parts of the world. In Finland, for example, suicide by adolescents increased 128% between 1965 and 1973, while the rate for the entire population rose only 19% (1). During the same period, in Israel, suicide among all ages was down 3%, but 15% more young people took their own lives (1). In Japan, suicides by youth climbed 32% between 1968 and 1974, while the rate for the total population increased 24% (1). The U.S.A. saw a 70% rise from 1966 to 1974 for 15- to 24-year-olds, while the rate for the total population increased only 18% (2). Similarly, between 1965 and 1974, Canada reported a 156% increase in rate for the young group, in contrast to a 47% increase for the total population (1).

## CHARACTERISTICS OF THE SUICIDAL ADOLESCENT

Who and why are the young killing themselves so readily? A search of the literature since 1970 yields at least 120 references to published reports and papers presented about suicide by young people. Assuming that this is an incomplete record of the actual number published, we can estimate that between 150 and 200 articles about suicide among the young were written during the past decade—an impressive number, averaging 17 to 22 publications annually, signifying the great concern about this problem.

I reviewed 35 reports from all parts of the world: 19 from the U.S.A., 3 from France, 2 each from Britain, Canada, and Japan, and 1 each from Australia, Germany, India, Norway, Poland, Sweden, and Yugoslavia. These articles (which are listed on pages 234–237) reported studies of adolescents and children whose suicide had been recorded in coroners' offices or who had appeared in hospitals, clinics, and schools as a result of having attempted or threatened suicide. The characteristics most frequently noted were summarized and tallied to identify the young people who are most at risk.

FEELING STATES

The most frequently mentioned feeling state was depression and hopelessness (in *12* reports),* along with emotional and physical symptoms such as sleep disturbances, changes in eating habits, trouble concentrating, fatigability, apathy, agitation, and anxiety. Aggression and hostility were noted frequently *(7)*, along with low frustration tolerance and low impulse control *(3)*. Each of the other emotional reactions, such as guilt, anger, fear, embarrassment, shame, and the general term "emotional disturbance," was cited at least once.

HISTORY

A suicidal history, of attempts or threats or suicidal ideas, was considered especially significant *(10)*. This confirms our experience that use of a suicidal mode in response to critical situations and severe interpersonal problems is likely to be repeated, often with increased potential lethality (3). A history of psychotherapy and/or hospitalization seemed significant *(5)*, but more as an indication of emotional disturbance with behavior so deviant that professional attention had been required. Suicidal behavior in the family or among friends was mentioned only once as an important identifying factor.

SOCIAL ASPECTS

The social behaviors most frequently mentioned were withdrawal and isolation, accompanied—as might be expected—by poor personal relation-

---

* The numbers in italics indicate the number of articles in which the characteristic was noted.

ships *(12)*. The subjects had few contacts with their peers, and even less communication with them. They had fewer sexual contacts than is usual *(3)*, and felt uncomfortable and uneasy with the opposite sex. Their achievement in school was poor *(11)*, and they expressed frequent worries about performance in class and on examinations *(9)*. Special note was made of drug abuse and/or heavy use of alcohol, but these were reported as significant by only three investigators and apparently were not considered highly important factors in the *suicidal* activity of the young. There were infrequent mentions of a low rate of church affiliation *(2)* and membership in a low socioeconomic class *(3)*.

INTERPERSONAL AND DYNAMIC ASPECTS

Parental and family interaction had the greatest number of significant factors. This area of disturbed relationships with the parents, including loss or threatened loss of a parent, was considered crucial by most of the authors *(20)*. Parental discord *(11)* and even assault by and between the parents *(3)* were mentioned, along with alcoholism in the family *(4)* and parents' projecting themselves on their children *(3)*. As mentioned earlier, disturbance of this relationship affects school performance and leads to severe social and interpersonal difficulties.

Both the family and the school have thus been identified as playing major roles in the suicidal behavior of young people today.

FAMILY AND SCHOOL ROLES

The past two or three decades have seen great changes in the family and its role in society. Helen Frank commented (4): "The family reflects the cultural trend towards replacing commitment, involvement, and tenderness with self-aggrandizement, exploitativeness and titillation. The stimulation of unlimited expectations and the impossible need to validate oneself through fulfillment of them have helped change individualism to egocentricism to the detriment of the family" (p. 91). Etzioni (5) described a continually expanding divestiture of missions from the family to other institutions: education has been invested in the school, meals are obtained at fast-food outlets, economic dependence has been broken by the equal-rights movement, and the care of children has been delegated to day-care centers. Marriage is considered less important than formerly, and second marriages are touted as better than the first. The emotional bonds between husband and wife have been belittled. Shorter stated (6): "A fundamental change in family life is under way, a transition from the 'nuclear family' of the 1940s and '50s to the 'couple family' that is rapidly emerging today..." (p. 10).

The family thus seems to have abrogated its responsibility for preparing the child for appropriate functioning in adult society. The resulting vacuum, unfilled by other social institutions and ignored or denied by schools, has been filled instead by peers. One consequence has been a shift in emphasis to self rather than society, with responsibilities and obligations to others subordinated to gratification of self. Self-focus, self-exploration, self-expression, self-fulfillment, self-awareness, all summed up in the phrase "doing your own thing," have become not only acceptable, but desirable. Parents not only have approved this marked shift in values in their children, but in many instances have adopted the new values for themselves. Separation and detachment from and by the children have left the latter with a sense of alienation, lack of continuity, and instability. The feeling of security that comes from a sense of belonging to a nurturing family environment within which supportive learning could take place has been lost. The affluent society has contributed to this state by providing financial and social independence before youth is ready and can handle them. The family role has been further changed by the women's-liberation movement, as increasing numbers of women have moved out of the home and back into the work force. Although this adjustment is seen as long overdue, there have been no compensatory movements to make up for the loss of the mother in the home. Adjustment to this shift is still in process, with many more changes undoubtedly yet to come.

Repschitz (7) listed several features of today's society that contribute to the alienation and loneliness characterizing our youth. He noted how parents have provided an unfortunate example by their ready use of drugs to alleviate any anxiety or stress, and by behaving as if these were feelings to be avoided at all costs. Drugs of many kinds, especially analgesics, tranquilizers, and soporifics, can be found in most households, their easy availability facilitating impulsive ingestion. Repschitz deplored the lack of inhibitions and discipline that characterize communication today in what he calls an erroneous interpretation of free expression. He stated that the young have seized upon what they consider the right, if not the obligation, to express themselves when the impulse occurs, regardless of time, place, and appropriateness. The result is narcissism and an uncontrolled release of instinctual drives. This tendency has served to drive the wedge even further between youth and adult, since the adults were educated to inhibit and control their free expression, whereas today's young are not.

It is also believed that excessive sexual license has further increased alienation among the young (7). As sexual intimacy has lost its sense of warmth and tenderness, under the bombardment of advertising, television, "pop stars," pornography and X-rated films, mechanized sex has become a bore. Increased rates of separation and divorce, especially among teenagers, support this conclusion. Along with loss of meaning in life has been the feeling that life at present is uncertain and tenuous in the extreme. The young have had to deal with the nuclear age and its potential for instant termination, with a callousness for life exemplified by extermination camps and indifference to "the boat people," and to a marked increase in violence and murders, all leading to a feeling of living on the brink of disaster; life has become cheap and readily expendable.

Repschitz (7) and Weissman (8) feel that physical changes too have contributed to the increase in suicides by youth. Physical development occurs earlier today, as a result of improved nutrition, medical care, social services, and economic conditions. At the same time, the age of entrance into gainful employment and independence has been delayed. The speed of attainment of physical maturity has not been paralleled by emotional growth, however, causing increasing disparity between physical capability and the emotional maturity required to appreciate the consequences of one's actions. Suicide among children below 15 years of age is also reported to have increased, although the numbers remain comparatively small, and their validity probably is even more tenuous than the numbers and rates for any other age group (9-11).

The schools also are not meeting the needs of today's youth. Difficulties in learning lead to self-defeat and frustration, resulting in poor achievement, thus creating a vicious cycle (12). Rohn, Sarles, Kenny, Reynolds, and Heald (13) reported that of 65 young people who had attempted suicide, 75% had poor scholastic records, 35% were truants, 35% had chronic discipline problems, and 19% failed one or more grades. Although the school's immediate responsibility is to impart information on specified subjects, it is also a primary source for models of social adaptation. Introduction of the primarily youth-centered problem of drug abuse caused frantic panic reactions on campuses as the schools tried to cope. The problem of drugs and alcohol brought in by a relatively small proportion of students produced an atmosphere of massive chaos and confusion, suspicion and mistrust; undercover agents, deception, and trickery were introduced, and violence and cheating became common experiences of school life. The students became confused, bitter, and resentful.

In short, suicide by the young is a major, increasingly visible problem that is highly influenced by problems in the family, school, community, and society.

## TREATMENT PROGRAMS

Glaser's assertion (14) that treatment of suicidal adolescents requires an eclectic, flexible approach, using all available methods and resources separately, sequentially, and in conjunction, is unquestionably fitting. A comprehensive program should be widespread, made up of several special programs. It should include not only crisis intervention, "the secondary area" in public-health terminology, but also primary care activities aimed at preventing the event; and tertiary care, with follow-up, hospitalization when necessary, and rehabilitation to help the person recover from the suicidal behavior and adjust better to his environment.

Primary prevention requires removal or modification of causes or precipitants so that the condition does not occur; this means getting at the basic structure of social and family life (8). To be effective, it should aim appropriately at educating parents in mental-health principles of child-rearing, with special emphasis on the development of identity, self-esteem, basic trust, and feelings of self-worth, and in the need for responsibility to others as well as oneself. Social changes, such as reducing the divorce rate, re-emphasizing the family as a nuclear unit, increasing communication between family members, and re-establishing the family as a primary support, are further desirable goals, but their achievement will require major cultural reorganization.

Other more immediate, primary preventive methods should include programs that focus on early identification of potential suicides within high-risk groups, and then intervention with information, modeling, involvement, close and repeated association, and continued evidence of caring. Psychiatric and delinquent youth are examples of groups within which the potential for suicide needs to be assessed constantly, and programs of prevention initiated (10, 15).

Both primary and secondary efforts are necessary in the schools. A comprehensive program of prevention directed toward teachers as well as students should aim at educating both groups to serve as "gatekeepers." They should be trained to recognize the various guises in which suicide might appear, and to reduce the taboos around the event; thus the usual reactions (i.e., denial, embarrassment, and shame) need not prevent a distressed child from expressing his wish for help, or potential rescuers from responding to his communications. Any form of deviant behavior should be investigated immediately and followed up (16).

One such program has been initiated successfully in the Suicide Prevention and Crisis Intervention Center at San Mateo, near San Francisco. Ross and Lee (17) wrote two brochures, one directed to school guidance personnel and teachers, the other to students. For the students, the authors included six warning signs: suicide threats, statements revealing a desire to die, previous suicide attempts, sudden changes in behavior, depression, and making final arrangements. In visits to schools, professionals from the Center meet the staff and students to present information on suicide, reasons for concern, and what to do about it. The critical points are emphasized many times: listen, without being judgmental; do not help the person deny problems; indicate interest and concern; enlist help; re-establish communication with significant others; and use professional help, if necessary, for evaluation. A film, *Suicide at 17*, has been produced especially for school personnel; it details the case of a school student who became suicidal and killed himself.

The principles and procedures developed for school personnel are also useful for most other gatekeeper groups, such as physicians, police, and clergy, and social organizations. It is most helpful to reassure such groups that they are not asked to be therapists or to assume full responsibility for helping, which is often a frightening obligation; rather, their primary purpose should be early identification, support through evidence of caring, and referral to trained persons when necessary.

Secondary prevention services, aimed at reducing any disability as soon as possible after its onset, are provided by suicide-prevention centers, crisis centers, community mental-health centers, and hospital emergency rooms; adolescents may use these services directly or be referred by others in the community. Physicians, clergy, teachers, police, and other individual or group gatekeepers play a major role in this phase, serving as first contacts with the community's social services.

Many adolescents identify themselves as suicidal through a suicide attempt or threat, or through severe depression, withdrawal, hopelessness, and other disturbed behavior. The first objective of treatment is survival beyond the crisis. Principles of treatment to cope with a crisis experienced by an adolescent are the same as those applied to any other age group: establishing rapport and trust, focusing, assessing the potential for suicide, evaluating resources, and making recommendations for disposition and treatment. Details of development for each step are included in the Los Angeles Suicide Prevention Center Manual (18).

"Hot lines" and "crisis lines" for youth are useful in encouraging direct contact from distressed persons. A special feature of these may be the use of workers who are young themselves; they are carefully selected, usually from among university graduates, or from colleges where psychology, nursing education, premedical, and other such courses credit the experience. Training is by professionals, with emphasis on the principles of interviewing, including establishing rapport, genuineness, and empathy, and the recognition of severe disturbances that require professional help. The extent of personal involvement is carefully monitored to avoid the common pitfall of doing too much, e.g., the Magna Mater Complex ("I shall take care of all your problems") and the Jehovah Complex ("I'm the only one who can handle this difficult case") are described as reactions to be avoided. Youthful personnel of suicide-prevention and crisis centers are also excellent representatives in work with schools and other youth organizations.

Tertiary prevention with suicidal youth involves long-term rehabilitation, and usually requires the full range of therapeutic modalities. Toolan (11) feels that every young person who attempts or threatens suicide should be evaluated thoroughly. Pfeffer (19) stated that the psychiatric hospital treatment of suicidal young children is lengthy, and requires the participation of the family. If a child cannot return home because of insufficient changes in the family and environment, it may be necessary to arrange for residential care elsewhere. Other outpatient and inpatient therapies may involve group, family, and psychopharmacologic techniques. However, no one method can be preferred over all others, for, as Pfeffer pointed out (10), there have been few systematic long term prospective studies of children who, initially suicidal, have been followed up through adolescence into adulthood for the purpose of evaluating the benefits of various therapies.

No matter what the treatment modality—individual, group, or family, inpatient or outpatient, prolonged or brief—the therapist's primary objective is to save the person's life, and then to help him change his feelings (and his environment, where feasible) so that he can function comfortably and productively. Severe personality disturbance makes the task much harder.

Suicidal behavior in youth is nearly always a sign of poor communication with parents, and opening the lines of communication is fundamental (20). Glaser (14) emphasized the need to analyze the child's self-image carefully, to help separate those elements that are alterable from those that are not. If medications are used, they must be carefully monitored to ensure they are taken correctly, and the patient must be warned of any possible side-effects, such as dryness of the mouth or drowsiness.

Family therapy seems especially useful, judging by the extensive contribution to suicidal behavior that has been attributed to the family. Richman (21), reporting his use of family therapy in the treatment of many suicidal persons, described the tight defense a family develops against the anxiety produced by suicidal behavior of one of its members. This "closed family system" is characterized by four features: disruption of ties to other institutions by constriction and isolation, forcing its members to rely on each other for satisfying their needs; prohibition of intimacy with non-family members by treating any outside encroachment as an enemy; emotional isolation of the suicidal person by alienating that person both from outside contacts and within the family; and domination by a fragile family member, as in the case of parents who are weak, in need of protection, or even potentially suicidal themselves. The family may not be closed at all times; it may vary between open and closed states according to conditions of stress and crisis.

Pluzek (22) uses a direct social-modification approach in her program in Cracow, Poland. Youth (mostly between 15 and 20 years old) who have attempted suicide are invited to join a club, and are seen in group treatment. There are at least five kinds of groups, depending on the patient's needs: insight therapy, learning work habits, organizing leisure time, stimulation of interests, and relaxation therapy, including sports. She reported success with all of the procedures, but admitted there are some chronic patients with a long history of maladjusted behavior who remain at high risk long after the attempt at suicide. Here crisis intervention is not enough: treatment must be continued to help these young people not only through the suicidal situation, but also through the complicated process of developing a more mature personality.

## CONCLUSION

Although the long-range goals of altering society and schools are slow in arriving, change in secondary and tertiary processes for suicide prevention can be initiated at any time. Treatment takes many forms, the basic ingredients being the attitudes and motivations of professionals and the public. With society alerted to the fact that the young are killing themselves at an alarming and ever-increasing rate, both the motivation and the opportunity emerge for wide-ranging programs of prevention and treatment.

The objective common to all such programs would be to overcome the lethal combination of feelings of worthlessness, helplessness, and hopelessness; thus, the essential ingredient of all approaches is the development of interest and caring for each youngster who despairs, a factor proven fundamental and effective in preventing suicide.

## REFERENCES
(*see also* Studies Reviewed, pages 234–237)

1. World Health Organization (1968–78), *World Health Statistics Annual, 1965–76*, Vol. 1: *Vital Statistics and Causes of Death*. Geneva: W.H.O.
2. U.S. National Center for Health Statistics (1968–78), *Vital Statistics of the United States, 1966–74*, Vol. 2: *Mortality*, part A. Washington, D.C.: U.S. Govt. Printing Office.
3. Worden, J. W. (1976), Lethality factors and the suicide attempt. In: *Suicidology: Contemporary Developments*, ed. E. S. Shneidman. New York: Grune & Stratton, pp. 139–162.
4. Frank, H. (1977), Survival tactics. *J. Curr. Social Issues*, 14:86–92.
5. Etzioni, A. (1977), The family: is it obsolete? *J. Curr. Social Issues*, 14:4–9.
6. Shorter, E. (1977), Changing from nuclear nest to intimate couple. *J. Curr. Social Issues*, 14:10–13.
7. Repschitz, D. H. (1978), Correlation between generation gap and self-aggression in the young. In: *Aspects of Suicide in Modern Civilization*, ed. H. S. Winnick & L. Miller. Proceedings of the 8th International Congress on Suicide Prevention and Crisis Intervention, Jerusalem, Israel, Oct. 1975. Jerusalem: Academic Press, pp. 193–198.
8. Weissman, M. M. (1976), Self-destructive youth: a problem in primary prevention. *Curr. Concepts Psychiatry*, 2:2–4.

9. Aleksandrowicz, M. K. (1975), The biological strangers: an attempted suicide of a 7½-year-old girl. *Bull. Menninger Clin.*, 39:163-176.
10. Pfeffer, C. R. (1979), Unanswered questions about childhood suicidal behavior: a review. In: *Proceedings of the 10th International Congress on Suicide Prevention and Crisis Intervention*, Ottawa, June 17-20, 1979. Ottawa: International Association for Suicide Prevention (Canada), pp. 430-434.
11. Toolan, J. M. (1978), Therapy of depressed and suicidal children. *Am. J. Psychother.*, 32:243-251.
12. A-Davidson, R. (1979), Public interest: private grief. The case of adolescent suicide. *J. Curr. Adolesc. Med.*, 1:28-35.
13. Rohn, R. D., Sarles, R. M., Kenny, T. J., Reynolds, B. J., & Heald, F. P. (1977), Adolescents who attempt suicide. *J. Pediatr.*, 90:636-638.
14. Glaser, K. (1978), The treatment of depressed and suicidal adolescents. *Am. J. Psychother.*, 32:252-269.
15. Paulson, M. J., Stone, D., & Sposto, R. (1978), Suicide potential and behavior in children ages 4 to 12. *Suicide Life Threat. Behav.*, 8:225-242.
16. Sartore, R. L. (1976), Students and suicide: an interpersonal tragedy. *Theory into Practice*, 15:337-340.
17. Ross, C. P. & Lee, A. R. (1977), *Suicide in Youth—A Guide for School Personnel.* West Point, Fla.: Merck, Sharp & Dohme.
18. Farberow, N. L., Heilig, S. M., & Litman, R. E. (1968), *Techniques in Crisis Intervention: A Training Manual.* Los Angeles, Calif.: Suicide Prevention Center.
19. Pfeffer, C. R. (1978), Psychiatric hospital treatment of suicidal children. *Suicide Life Threat. Behav.*, 8:150-160.
20. Glaser, K. (1971), Suicidal children—management. *Am. J. Psychother.*, 25:27-36.
21. Richman, J. (1979), Suicide and the closed family system. In: *Proceedings of the 10th International Congress on Suicide Prevention and Crisis Intervention*, Ottawa, June 17-20, 1979. Ottawa: International Association for Suicide Prevention (Canada), pp. 329-332.
22. Pluzek, Z. (1978), Efficacy of the treatment program of attempted suicide among youth. In: *Proceedings of the 9th International Congress on Suicide Prevention and Crisis Intervention*, Helsinki, June 20-23, 1977, ed. V. Aalberg. Helsinki: Finnish Association for Mental Health, pp. 114-118.

## STUDIES REVIEWED

### AUSTRALIA

Connell, H. M. (1972), Attempted suicide in school children. *Med. J. Aust.*, 1: 686-690.

### BRITAIN

Shaffer, D. (1974), Suicide in childhood and early adolescence. *J. Child Psychol. Psychiatry*, 15:275-291.

White, H. C. (1974), Self-poisoning in adolescents. *Br. J. Psychiatry*, 124:24-35.

CANADA

Garfinkel, B. D., Chamberlain, C., & Golombek, H. (1979), Completed sui-
cide in Ontario youth. In: *Proceedings of the 10th International Congress on
Suicide Prevention and Crisis Intervention*, Ottawa, June 17-20, 1979. Ottawa:
International Association for Suicide Prevention (Canada), pp. 126-131.
Garfinkel, B. D., Froese, A., & Golombek, H. (1979), Suicidal behavior in a
pediatric population. In: *Proceedings of the 10th International Congress on Suicide
Prevention and Crisis Intervention*, Ottawa, June 17-20, 1979. Ottawa: Inter-
national Association for Suicide Prevention (Canada), pp. 305-312.

FRANCE

Davidson, F. & Choquet, M. (1976), (Epidemiological study of suicide by ado-
lescents: comparison between primary suicide and repeated attempts.
English abstract.) *Rev. Epidemiolog. Sante Publ.*, 24:11-26.
Duché, D. J. (1974), (Attempts at suicide by adolescents. English abstract.)
*Rev. Neuropsychiatr. Infant.*, 22:639-656.
Moullembe, A., Tiano, F., Anavi, G., et al. (1973-74), (Essay on suicide: a
theoretical and a clinical approach. English abstract.) *Bull. Psychol.*,
27:804-943.

GERMANY

Hartmann, K. (1970), (Contribution to the psychopathology of minors with
suicidal tendencies. English abstract.) *Prax. Kinderpsychol. Kinderpsychiatr.*,
19:168-170.

INDIA

Sathyavathi, K. (1975), Suicide among children in Bangalore. *Indian J.
Pediatr.*, 42:149-157.

JAPAN

Iga, M. & Ohara, K. (1967), Suicide attempts of Japanese youth and Durkheim's concept of anomie: an interpretation. *Hum. Org.*, 26:59-68.
Ishii, K. (1972), Backgrounds and suicidal behaviors of committed suicides
among Kyoto University students. *Psychologia*, 15:137-148.

NORWAY

Madland, N. (1972), (Problems concerning suicide amongst psychiatric patients in childhood and adolescence. English abstract.) *Tidsskr. Nor. Laege-
foren.*, 92:1190-1193.

POLAND

Pluzek, Z. (1978), Efficacy of the treatment program of attempted suicide
among youth. In: *Proceedings of the 9th International Congress on Suicide Prevention and Crisis Intervention*, Helsinki, June 20-23, 1977, ed. V. Aalberg.
Helsinki: Finnish Association for Mental Health, pp. 114-118.

SWEDEN

Otto, U. (1978), Suicidal behavior in childhood and adolescence. In: *Proceedings of the 9th International Congress on Suicide Prevention and Crisis Intervention,* Helsinki, June 20–23, 1977, ed. V. Aalberg. Helsinki: Finnish Association for Mental Health, pp. 119–126.

UNITED STATES

Cantor, P. (1976a), Frequency of suicidal thought and self-destructive behavior among females. *Suicide Life Threat. Behav.,* 6:92–100.

Cantor, P. (1976b), Personality characteristics found among youthful female suicide attempters. *J. Abnorm. Psychol.,* 85:324–329.

Corder, B. F., Page, P. V., & Corder, R. F. (1974), Parental history, family communication and interaction patterns in adolescent suicide. *Fam. Therapy,* 1: 285–290.

Hendin, H. (1976), Growing up dead: student suicide. In: *Suicidology: Contemporary Developments,* ed. E. S. Shneidman. New York: Grune & Stratton, pp. 317–334.

Knott, J. E. (1973), Campus suicide in America. *Omega: J. Death Dying,* 4:65–71.

Korrella, K. (1972), Teen-age suicidal gestures: a study of suicidal behavior among high school students. *Dissert. Abstr. Int.,* 32(9-A), March, p. 5039.

Marfatia, J. C. (1975), Suicide in childhood and adolescence. *Child Psychiatry Q.,* 8:13–16.

McIntire, M. S. & Angle, C. R. (1975), Evaluation of suicide risk in adolescents. *J. Fam. Pract.,* 2:339–341.

Peck, M. L. & Litman, R. E. (1974), Current trends in youthful suicide. In: *Suicide and Blacks: A Monograph for Continuing Education in Suicide Prevention,* ed. J. Bush. Los Angeles, Calif.: Charles R. Drew Postgraduate Medical School.

Peck, M. L. & Schrut, A. (1971), Suicidal behavior among college students. *Health Serv. Ment. Health Adm.,* 86:149–156.

Pfeffer, C. R. (1979), Unanswered questions about childhood suicidal behavior: a review. In: *Proceedings of the 10th International Congress on Suicide Prevention and Crisis Intervention,* Ottawa, June 17–20, 1979. Ottawa: International Association for Suicide Prevention (Canada), pp. 430–434.

Ross, C. P. & Lee, A. R. (1977), *Suicide in Youth—A Guide for School Personnel.* West Point, Fla.: Merck, Sharp & Dohme.

Sanborn, D. E., III, Sanborn, C. J., & Cimbolic, P. (1973), Two years of suicide: a study of adolescent suicide in New Hampshire. *Child Psychiatry Hum. Dev.,* 3:234–242.

Sartore, R. L. (1976), Students and suicide: an interpersonal tragedy. *Theory into Practice,* 15:337–340.

Schneer, H. I., Perlstein, A., & Brozovsky, M. (1975), Hospitalized suicidal adolescents: two generations. *J. Am. Acad. Child Psychiatry,* 14:268–280.

Stanley, E. J. & Barter, J. T. (1970), Adolescent suicidal behavior. *Am. J. Orthopsychiatry,* 40:87–96.

Teicher, J. D. (1972), Children and adolescents who attempt suicide. In: *Self-destructive Behavior: A National Crisis,* ed. B. Q. Hafen & E. J. Faux. Minneapolis: Burgess, pp. 119–129.

Toolan, J. M. (1975), Suicide in children and adolescents. *Am. J. Psychother.*, 29:339-344.

Weissman, M. M. (1976), Self-destructive youth: a problem in primary prevention. *Curr. Concepts Psychiatry*, 2:2-4.

YUGOSLAVIA

Šojleva, M. (1974), (Psychological examination of adolescents with suicidal attempts.) *Socijalna Psihijatrija*, 2:145-150. English summary (1975), *Psychol. Abstr.*, 54:687-688.

# CHAPTER FIFTEEN

# A PERSONAL VIEW OF PSYCHOPHARMACOLOGY FOR NONPSYCHOTIC ADOLESCENTS

## DONALD F. KLEIN

### HISTORICAL SETTING

My first experience in psychopharmacology was in 1959 when I went to Hillside Hospital, New York, as a budding psychiatric researcher. Hillside was a 200-bed hospital. It was then run by Lewis Robbins, M.D., an eminent psychoanalyst who had been at the Menninger Foundation Hospital for many years, and the major form of treatment was psychoanalytic psychotherapy. At that time the New York City authorities paid all medical bills for the indigent patients however long their stay, which averaged about 10 months, and in some cases was well over a year. (In view of the City's present financial status, it is not surprising that this system is no longer in effect!) Hillside was originally utilized for the treatment of adolescent girls, and in 1959 most of the patients had character disorders or were depressive or schizophrenic.

Like Dr. Robbins, I was much interested in analytic thinking; in fact, I was a candidate at the New York Psychoanalytic Institute. One of my aims was to determine whether knowledge of such issues as the patient's dynamics and intrapsychic conflicts would aid in the proper prescription of medication.

In 1959, those in the forefront of psychiatry believed that descriptive diagnosis was a waste of time and the hallmark of a superficial mind. This was based on the belief that symptoms were simply the manifestation of intrapsychic conflict, and that whether the patient was anxious, depressed, delusional, or drug-addicted was immaterial. Phenomenology depended upon the configuration of drives and defenses one was experiencing; in brief, what really mattered was that the patient had a specific unconscious conflict to work out. Thus, if one paid attention to such superficialities as symptoms, one was obviously barking up the wrong tree.

The trouble came when I tried to apply this thinking to medication. Drugs were not prescribed lightly because their use was interpreted as a sign of incompetence; if one knew what one was doing, one would not have to give drugs. Furthermore, medication was often viewed as a sort of sadistic assault upon the patient, necessitated by unresolved negative counter-transference — and *that* had to be worked through with one's supervisor. This resulted in remarkably few prescriptions for drugs early in treatment. (If the patient's condition had not improved by 8 or 9 months, and discharge was looming, medication was prescribed.)

It was also assumed that the basic problem of every patient was anxiety, either manifest or covert. Therefore, chlorpromazine must be working on anxiety; what else could it be working on? It followed that everyone who was refractory to psychotherapy got chlorpromazine, because he was assumed to be anxious. For some who were obviously very ill (and therefore very anxious), who were delusional and hallucinated, chlorpromazine did remarkable things. But there were others who were simply moderately anxious, phobic, and compulsive, for whom the drug did not allay their anxiety; in fact, they felt worse. It seemed odd, if all patients were suffering from anxiety, and the drug worked well on hyperanxious psychotics, that chlorpromazine did not help patients who were only mildly anxious.

This was the first time I questioned the validity of the theory that psychopathology is a continuum, the various forms representing different degrees of severity on a single scale. In fact, of course, the medication was showing that mental illnesses are more like respiratory illness. For example, pneumonia is a more severe respiratory illness than a cold; yet penicillin can cure pneumonia, but does not affect a cold. The reason is that they are two different illnesses, both respiratory, but they do not reside on a continuum: bacteria that cause pneumonias do not cause colds but are sensitive to penicillin, whereas viruses that cause colds are completely insensitive to penicillin. This is not to say that psychiatric illnesses can be as neatly differentiated as infectious diseases. However, there are qualitative differences, and unless differential diagnostic evaluation is adequate, one is very likely to give the patient the wrong treatment.

I also found it impossible to relate dynamic formulations to the effects of medication, possibly because these evaluations appeared to be more a function of those creating the formulation than they were descriptive of the patient. For example, certain supervisors saw ubiquitous urethral fixation; others saw retroflexed rage; and yet others, latent homosexuality. Currently, it is known that diagnostic evaluation relevant to medication prescription brings us back not to Freud, but to Kraepelin, the investigator who emphasized the phenomenology of syndrome and course.

## EMOTIONALLY UNSTABLE CHARACTER DISORDERS

One group of patients at Hillside Hospital consisted chiefly of adolescents who, in the early 1960s, had identity diffusion. They kept saying contradictory things about themselves and their goals, and could change from liking you to hating you two or three times within one session. Within one day they could be running around, laughing, unable to tolerate any frustration, and showing complete disregard for the rules, then retreat to their rooms, hostile, discontented, giving you the back of the hand and refusing to be jollied out of their mood, and then be up and flying again. When asked why they were behaving this way, they would usually reply in the terms they had been trained in, which were intrapsychic, dynamic, and interpersonal.

I labeled these patients as having "emotionally unstable character disorders" (1, 2). They were predominantly adolescent girls. They did not display any of the usual signs of schizophrenia, but were all termed schizophrenic. Yet, they had no delusions, hallucinations, or loosening of associations, only this extraordinary lability of mood.

The so-called drug culture came into being in the U.S.A. about the middle 1960s. When I first saw these patients in 1959, they were not heavily into cannabis, LSD, or promiscuity, but when the drug culture arrived they moved into it *en masse*; therefore, their behavior was often attributed to participation in these pursuits. I think that interpretation wrong; rather, poly-drug abuse is a secondary manifestation of a particular sort of reckless, labile psychopathology.

Some of these patients who had not responded to intensive psychotherapy were entered in a controlled trial of chlorpromazine. Every week I saw all of the patients (not knowing whether they were taking drug or placebo), their ward personnel, psychotherapist, and supervisor, and compared notes from these four sometimes quite disparate perspectives. All the staff agreed that the drug-treated patients were pleasanter, friendlier, more compliant and more tolerant of frustration, related more easily with others, did not talk suicidally or retreat into their rooms, and worked harder at various milieu and interpersonal tasks.

Strangely, the only people who clearly liked the improved state of affairs were the ward personnel. The psychotherapists complained that terrific discussions about important emotional material had been replaced by a bland involvement with the trivia of social life. The patients didn't like it because it made them "feel bad"; they couldn't be more specific. Their dislike of the drug was so strong that most of them had persuaded their psychotherapists to discontinue the medication. Usually this resulted in prompt relapse, but reinstitution of the medication was refused because the patients in some way preferred the unmedicated state.

One hypothesis for the patients' reaction is that they were suffering from akinesia (3), a subtle extrapyramidal disorder that impairs spontaneity. Akinesic patients may not have tremor or rigidity, but are less spontaneous and enthusiastic, and talk less than usual. It is conceivable that the action-oriented adolescents I was studying regarded the drug's effect as a negative strangulation of their vim and vigor. They seemed quite active, but this may have been less than they wanted. Another possibility is that the patients were addicted to their "high" periods, and that anything which leveled their affect engendered dislike because it deprived them of an emotional lift. In any event, chlorpromazine was useless, despite its efficacy, because the patients wouldn't take it.

Then lithium therapy was introduced. There was sufficient resemblance of these patients to those with affective disorders to merit trying this drug; and in fact, in his book on manic-depressive insanity (4), Kraepelin described "irritable temperament" in terms that portrayed these patients exactly:

The irritable temperament, a further form of manic-depressive predisposition, is perhaps best conceived as *a mixture of the fundamental states*, which have been described, in as much as in it manic and depressive features are associated. As it was demonstrable in about 12.4 per cent of the patients here taken into account, it appears to be still a little more frequent than the depressive predisposition. The patients display from youth up extraordinarily great fluctuations in emotional equilibrium and are greatly moved by all experiences, frequently in an unpleasant way. While on the one hand they appear sensitive and inclined to sentimentality and exuberance, they display, on the other hand, great irritability and sensitiveness. They are easily offended and hot-tempered; they flare up, and on the most trivial occasions fall into outbursts of boundless fury. "She had states in which she was nearly delirious" was said of one patient. . . . It then comes to violent scenes with abuse, screaming and a tendency to rough behaviour. . . [The patients] easily fall into disputes with the people round them, which they carry on with great passion. . . . In consequence of their quarrelsomeness the patients are mostly very much disliked, have frequently to change their situations and places of residence, never come well out of anything. . . . In the family also they are insufferable, capricious, threaten their wives, thrash their children, have attacks of jealousy.

Mood—The coloring of mood is subject to frequent change. In general the patients are perhaps cheerful, self-conscious, unrestrained; but periods are interpolated in which they are irritable and ill-humored, also perhaps sad, spiritless, anxious; they shed tears without cause, give expression to thoughts of suicide, bring forward hypochondriacal complaints, go to bed. At the time of the menses the irritability is usually increased.

Intellectual endowment is often very good; many patients display great mental activity, and they feel keenly the necessity for further culture. But they are mostly very distractible and unsteady in their endeavours. Sometimes they are considered to be liars and slanderers, because their power of imagination is usually very much influenced by moods and feelings.

In conversation the patients are talkative, quick at repartee, pert. In consequence of their irritability and their changing moods their conduct of life is subject to the most multifarious incidents, they make sudden resolves, and carry them out on the spot, run off abruptly, go travelling, enter a cloister.

We conducted both an open clinical trial and a double-blind placebo-controlled cross-over trial of lithium carbonate on our population of adolescent girls (5). The lithium dramatically stabilized the patients' mood, and their resistance to it was so much less than to chlorpromazine that some continued the medication as outpatients. Overall the patients did not like lithium either, so perhaps both of my hypotheses for their resistance to medication are correct: first, phenothiazines produce an unpleasant extrapyramidal akinesia, which these patients find too confining; second, both phenothiazines and lithium carbonate may banish brief periods of elation, which are missed.

By the time of our follow-up study (6), 3½ to 4 years after their discharge from hospital, most of the patients were young adults. About one third were perfectly asymptomatic; they had friends and their careers were going well. Roughly another third were doing reasonably well in regard to career and socialization, but were bothered by occasional fleeting moodiness, often premenstrual. The lives of the remainder were still seriously disrupted by continual fluctuations in mood: these people were unable to make a career or achieve good social or sexual relationships, but none had become psychotic or experienced long hospitalizations and clearly were not truly schizophrenic. A search for relevant historical features in all the cases revealed disorders compatible with hyperkinetic impulsiveness in childhood in an unusually high proportion (about one third), and a distinctly increased amount of affective disorder in their families. Thus, there seemed to be at least two risk factors: personal and familial.

In a further study (7), we sought neurologic soft signs in several hundred psychiatric patients. The neurological examinations were made without knowing the psychiatric diagnosis, and the psychiatric diagnoses were made without the neurologic findings. It was hypothesized there would be a greater occurrence of these signs in the emotionally unstable character disorders, than in patients of comparable age who had hysterical or passive-aggressive character disorders. The findings confirmed the hypothesis: it appeared that the central nervous system in the former patients was compromised in some way, as shown by a high prevalence of soft signs, that resulted in extreme affective lability and over-reactivity. Unfortunately a systematic trial of stimulants of the type Wender (8) is doing was not undertaken, and no one has replicated this study.

There is a certain difference between our findings and Wender's. We found lithium useful in treating emotionally unstable patients, which is contrary to results achieved by Wender (9), who has done the only systematic work on lithium treatment for hyperactive children. However, his study sample was atypically refractory to treatment. Also, it may be simply that there is heterogeneity within the emotionally unstable, some patients being closer to the hyperkinetic syndrome and others closer to affective disorders.

Anyone who has worked with adolescents has encountered some who are emotionally unstable. These patients are usually treated with psychotherapy, but overall are not very responsive to it. It is worth trying lithium therapy in refractory cases.

## HYSTEROID DYSPHORIA

The proper role of medication in the management of this condition is even more unsettled. Here I am speaking from clinical experience, as I have not completed a controlled study.

The syndrome consists of an inordinate sensitivity to rejection. It affects females predominantly, and many of the patients are labeled as hysterical. I term it hysteroid dysphoria (10-12) to reflect the reactive dysphoria that is the underlying pathology: whenever rejection occurs or is felt imminent, the patient reacts with histrionic, seductive, provocative displays that are designed to elicit approval, and obviate the possibility of rejection.

None of us likes being rejected, and all of us like being applauded — which makes good evolutionary sense, because as social animals we are concerned about our fellows' opinions of us. There is a psychobiologic tendency to seek approval, which usually results in conformism. Like any other built-in control mechanism, however, this can malfunction, rendering the person oversensitive.

People who are hypersensitive to rejection are also applause addicts.

In their usual state they are voluble, bright, alert and dramatic, and most of them think and react faster than less sensitive people; many of them choose careers as theatrical performers. When brought down by being rejected, they crash into a phase that brings stereotyped vegetative signs of over-sleeping and overeating. On the other hand, these patients do not have autonomous depression; personal attention, applause, and interest improve their mood.

The first signs of difficulty usually appear at the time of puberty, approximately 13–15 years of age, when the girls "go boy-crazy." The focus of attention shifts entirely from the usual concerns of students (e.g., progress in school and being liked by parents, peers, and teachers) to the beginning of a romantic roller-coaster where central gratifications are from someone being in love with them, or feeling that they are in love with that person. This is accompanied by extreme hypersensitivity to rejection. Naturally, it results in the need to avoid rejection, which unfortunately is very difficult for these patients to do; and the difficulty is compounded by their use of intrusive and demanding types of behavior that generate rejection.

A typical example is as follows. The patient is told by her boyfriend: "I'll call you at 8 o'clock"; but the call comes at 8:15. The girl's first words are: "I've been waiting here for 15 minutes."

"Well, you know, dear, I was delayed in the subway."

"Yes, but do you know how bad I feel? If you were going to call me at 8 o'clock, you could have been at the phone at 7:45, so you could be sure this wouldn't happen." This goes on and on.

This relentless, demanding, intrusive aspect of the patient's personality renders stable relationships virtually impossible, and inevitably there is a crash. Then the period of overeating and oversleeping begins, when the patient is temporarily unable to carry out mundane tasks. If you ask these patients, "Why do you go to bed?" they say, "Well, I'm retreating from reality," and pull the covers over their head. Again, a psychologic explanation is given for what seems to be a physiologic shift.

Most of these patients do not come to a therapist's attention until their early twenties. This is because adolescence is the time for getting to know many people; the development of long-term, psychosocial, psychosexual relationships is not expected. Therefore, an adolescent who is flitting from person to person is not obviously peculiar. Only the realization that romance has become the narrow focus of the child's life, that nothing else is of any importance, might cause one to think of the possibility of "hysteroid dysphoria."

This syndrome initially seems to be the type for which medication is contraindicated: the depressions are clearly reactive, and the emotional vulnerability appears to be blatantly psychogenic. However, because psychotherapy alone is of little use, various pharmacologic agents have been tried. Imipramine and the phenothiazines were failures because the patients felt groggy and stupid. But better results have been obtained with monoamine oxidase inhibitors (e.g., Nardil and Parnate), which seem to reduce reactions to rejection until they are temporary, fairly normal responses, and lessen the likelihood of the paralyzing wave of lethargy and fatigue that forces the patients to bed.

Hysteroid dysphoric patients are in need of a great deal of guidance, discussion, clarification, as well as someone they can identify with; yet in my experience psychosocial interventions alone have been a failure. Therefore, these particular patients may do best with a combination of both pharmacotherapy and psychotherapy.

## SUMMARY

The current psychopharmacologic literature is replete with reports of schizophrenia and psychotic depressive disorders in adolescence (12, 13), but contains few references to nonpsychotic disorders that result in marked shifts in affect and labile behavior. However, the latter disorders, which I have referred to as "emotionally unstable character disorders" and "hysteroid dysphoria," can give rise to severe problems, and we should be alert to their detection. Pharmacologic management should be attempted as early as possible. In the latter condition in particular, combined treatment with psychotherapy (but not psychotherapy alone) is recommended.

## REFERENCES

1. Klein, D. F. & Fink, M. (1962), Behavioral reaction patterns with phenothianizes. *Arch. Gen. Psychiatry*, 7:449–459.
2. Klein, D. F. (1967), Importance of psychiatric diagnosis in prediction of clinical drug effects. *Arch. Gen. Psychiatry*, 16:118–126.
3. Rifkin, A., Quitkin, F., & Klein, D. F. (1975), Akinesia: a poorly recognized drug-induced extrapyramidal behavioral disorder. *Arch. Gen. Psychiatry*, 32: 672–674.
4. Kraepelin, E. (1921), *Manic Depressive Insanity and Paranoia*. Edinburgh: Livingstone. Reprint ed. New York: Arno, 1976.
5. Rifkin, A., Quitkin, F., Carrillo, C., Blumberg, A. G., & Klein, D. F. (1972), Lithium carbonate in emotionally unstable character disorders. *Arch. Gen. Psychiatry*, 27:519–523.
6. Rifkin, A., Levitan, S. J., Galewski, J., & Klein, D. F. (1972), Emotionally unstable character disorder—a follow-up study. I. Description of patients and outcome. II. Prediction of outcome. *Biolog. Psychiatry*, 4:65–79, 81–88.
7. Quitkin, F., Rifkin, A., & Klein, D. F. (1976), Neurologic soft signs in schizophrenia and character disorders: organicity in schizophrenia with premorbid asociality and emotionally unstable character disorders. *Arch. Gen. Psychiatry*, 33:845–853.

8. Wood, D. R., Reimherr, F. W., Wender, P. H., & Johnson, G. E. (1976), Diagnosis and treatment of minimal brain dysfunction in adults. A preliminary report. *Arch. Gen. Psychiatry*, 33:1453–1460.

9. Greenhill, L. L. Rieder, R. O., Wender, P. H., Buchsbaum, M., & Zahn, T. P., (1973), Lithium carbonate in the treatment of hyperactive children. *Arch. Gen. Psychiatry*, 28:636–640.

10. Klein, D. F. & Shader, R. I. (1975), The borderline state: psychopharmacologic treatment approaches to the undiagnosed case. In: *Manual of Psychiatric Therapeutics: Practical Psychopharmacology and Psychiatry*, ed. R. I. Shader. Boston: Little, Brown, pp. 281–293.

11. Klein, D. F. (1977), Psychopharmacologic treatment and delineation of borderline disorders. In: *Borderline Personality Disorders: The Concept, the Syndrome, the Patient*, ed. P. Hartocollis. New York: International Universities Press, pp. 365–383.

12. Klein, D. F. & Davis, J. M., Eds. (1969), *Diagnosis and Drug Treatment of Psychiatric Disorders*. Baltimore: Williams & Wilkins.

13. Klein, D. F. (1976), Diagnosis and differential use of antianxiety drugs. In: *Drug Treatment of Mental Disorders*, ed. L. L. Simpson. New York: Raven, pp. 61–72.

CHAPTER SIXTEEN

# PSYCHOTHERAPY OF NARCISSISTIC DISORDER IN ADOLESCENCE: A PARADIGM FROM *HAROLD AND MAUDE*

KENNETH NEWMAN

## INTRODUCTION

The Freudian structural model of the mind is most efficacious in the therapy of persons whose system for regulating tension and self-esteem is relatively consolidated, and in whom conflicts between drives and established, excessively rigid structures (superego, ego) have led to pathologic defenses, maladaptive character traits, and affective symptoms. A newer theoretical model, "the psychology of the self" in the treatment of narcissistic disorders (1), is based on the thesis that in some patients the core pathology is a deficit in psychic structure. The deficit results in fixation on a self that is insufficiently cohesive (and therefore vulnerable to fragmentation) and depends on external objects for functions it has not internalized. The principal source of these patients' anxiety stems not from conflicts over internal drives, but from the breakup of a weakly cathected self. This is especially so when the latter has lost connections with external objects (or their substitutes) upon which the organization of the self relies.

In adolescents who have developed a fairly firm self, psychopathology relates to reactivation of unresolved conflicts over infantile drives and objects, and to the maturing self's need to relinquish them, as well as to the pressures of external demands and major internal bodily changes. For those with chronic deficits in their psychic structure, late adolescence — with its demands for autonomy which necessitate giving up old supports — brings additional dangers. These include the revival of experiences in not finding needed selfobjects, and the reawakening of crippling anxiety emanating from defective self-experiences. These are accompanied by vague fears of inner emptiness, depression and even feelings of deadness or dread of psychic dissolution.

In order to dramatize the experience of stalemate or failure in some cases when using traditional treatment models and concepts, and the value of therapeutic interventions derived from the psychology of the self, I have borrowed liberally from the main character in a so-called "cult" film, *Harold and Maude*. First I shall review the treatment of "Harold," in which traditional concepts were applied. Then I shall reformulate the problem in terms of psychology of the self.

## HAROLD AND MAUDE: A PARADIGM

Harold was brought to me by his mother after prolonged therapy with a Dr. Strawman had ended in failure. Treatment of this 19-year-old youth had been initiated a year or so earlier, when his major problem was the repeated dramatization of suicidal attempts, apparently staged to horrify his widowed mother. The phony suicides, all witnessed by his mother, included theatrical wrist-slashing in the bath, hanging, decapitation, drowning, and a creative self-immolation from which he emerged phoenix-like, unscathed. Harold seemed to have little purpose, nor could he find sufficient meaning in life to guide him toward a career. He had little interest in girls, especially those chosen for him by his mother.

In his first interview with me Harold gave additional personal history. His father had committed suicide when Harold was 6 years old, leaving the child alone with his mother, a wealthy, socially active, intrusive, and seductive woman. She had outlined for her son a series of ambitious pursuits viewed as leading to success for him and applause for herself. Harold remembered that he had been able to hold her interest in his earlier attempts to meet her fantasies, but she was not interested or even deprecatory over activities he felt were important. Harold had masturbated quite frequently since the age of 6 or 7, and the precursors of his self-destructive behavior had arisen in these masturbation-induced fantasies. Also, from an early age he had had many somatic complaints and worries and frequent dreams in which his body parts seemed separate from himself.

Over the next few months Harold described his therapy with his former therapist. Despite his flippant and cynical demeanor he demonstrated a great capacity to recall details of the treatment, and was distressed that it had failed. He outlined most perceptively his therapist's diagnosis of his symptoms, dynamic working formulations, and therapeutic posture and technique.

Based on Harold's presenting complaints and overly close relationship with his mother, Dr. Strawman had seen the symptoms as catalyzed by the turmoil of adolescence and resulting from severe inner conflicts. These had activated a psychic regression away from anxiety-ridden, phallic-aggressive activities and fantasies toward a sado-masochistic, passive, highly erotic, exhibitionistic attachment to the mother. He had viewed this defensively regressive behavior as a classic neurotic compromise between the demands of a primitive superego and infantile incestuous longings. He had likewise thought that guilt over hostile competitive fantasies toward the dead father, and fear of phallic narcissistic humiliation at the hands of the powerful and potentially rejecting mother, had caused Harold to regress to a form of exhibitionism and masochism which appeased his superego and reduced castration anxiety, but maintained his extreme attachment to his mother. Harold sensed that Dr. Strawman had aimed to use this working hypothesis to interpret his drives and defenses, and to reveal the nature of the pathologic conflict that had been aggravated by the resurgent forces of adolescence.

Harold then described the treatment process and how he and Dr. Strawman had worked together. He remembered that, initially, he had begun to talk about himself and some of the fantasies he had held since childhood. In telling me about this, he revealed contempt for many values he felt had been imposed on him, specifically the phoniness of his uncle (a career army officer) and the local minister, both of whom had been pressed into service to try to guide him. Harold also recalled a dream he had had several times in childhood in which he was on a stage, talking, with the feeling that people were listening in the background—a sort of Greek chorus. His former therapist had interpreted this dream and others like it as representing Harold's unconscious presumption of specialness, and related it to his close tie to his mother.

As Harold had evidenced little interest in these interpretations, and because he seldom made specific reference to Dr. Strawman, Dr. Strawman had initiated discussion of Harold's resistance to examining feelings developing in the transference. Dr. Strawman had interpreted both the absence of anyone else on stage and Harold's self-centered posture on the couch as a massive narcissistic regression to avoid facing conflicting attitudes, drives, and feelings he had toward his therapist; Harold had reacted to these interpretations by becoming even more silent, sullen, and withdrawn. In ensuing dreams, Harold had witnessed physical attacks on himself, and even had a nightmare that parts of his body were disintegrating;

these had been viewed as reactions of guilt due to unconscious destructive fantasies toward males.

At times, Dr. Strawman also had reacted critically to Harold's increasing negativism and apathy by suggesting that his own critical attitude was caused by the projection of Harold's punitive superego; in effect, he said that he was using his own countertransference reactions as a guide to the nature of Harold's inner world and tensions. Dr. Strawman had further suggested that Harold was also subtly rendering useless every insight he was offered. He was unconsciously gratifying his narcissistic fantasies of omnipotence, but by suffering and failing to be helped, was simultaneously submitting to and appeasing his unduly harsh superego.

Apparently the treatment had foundered over the interpretation of specific dreams and the meaning of Harold's new friendship with an 80-year-old woman. The suicide-dramatics had continued. At that time, Harold's stated solaces were masturbation (which included fantasies of the suicidal gestures he made in his mother's presence), viewing the demolition of cars and buildings, converting his car to a hearse, and almost daily attendance at funerals for persons unknown to him. It was at one of these funerals that Harold had met a spry old lady named Maude.

Maude made her appearance during treatment in a series of dreams. Harold's relationship with her had intensified through the sharing of interests, including playful cavortings that seemed to have breathed life into the boy in a way completely new to him. Harold claimed that Maude showed an appreciation of him he otherwise lacked, having the capacity to listen to him as an individual and take interest in his uniqueness and liveliness. When he told Dr. Strawman that Maude resembled a specific actress (Ruth Gordon), his response was that this tryst with a nonsexual woman represented yet another attempt on Harold's part to find and maintain a wish-fulfilling regressive fantasy. Dr. Strawman had further maintained that it was designed to preserve infantile fantasies and escape anxiety over growing up and confronting masculine aggressive strivings. Harold had resisted these interpretations, repeating that Maude provided something he needed, confirmation of him as an individual; he had even coined a term for his relationship to her, calling Maude his own special "selfobject." But Dr. Strawman had persisted in regarding Harold's behavior as a retreat to a defensive position, and had urged him to relinquish these attachments and face adult-type conflicts.

Finally, in the face of Harold's increasing sullenness and lack of cooperation, Dr. Strawman had claimed failure in the necessary therapeutic alliance, and insisted that progress could be achieved only if the relationship with Maude were forsaken. Harold chose Maude, and left his therapist.

## PSYCHOLOGY OF THE SELF
## IN RELATION TO NARCISSISTIC DISORDERS

During the several months it took Harold to relate this information, I became interested in Kohut's work on psychology of the self in the treatment of narcissistic disorders (1); and I began to consider the application of these concepts and treatment recommendations for Harold.

The major tenet of psychology of the self is that there is a separate, narcissistic line of development whose basic unit is a self-selfobject relationship. Progress along this line commences with the infant as a virtual self to the pregnant mother, and it continues to the establishment of an increasingly autonomous and self-regulating, cohesive self. This occurs through step-by-step internalizations whereby the selfobject's function (e.g., the maternal function of mirroring, self-confirming, tension-regulating) becomes part of the self's matrix as a result of gratification and optimal frustration.

Kohut has emphasized two major forms of selfobject needs: for mirroring, echoing, and self-enhancing responses to the phase-appropriate claims of the infant's exhibitionistic needs; and for an idealized parent. Initially, the latter serves to soothe and regulate tension by merging with the infant's sense of omnipotence, and later, will be an object of admiration who can provide goal-setting values and ideals to the child's ambitions, and give meaning and direction to his actions. Implicit in the theory is that the selfobjects' (i.e., parents') availability to provide these functions (and the parents' empathic recognition when a break in availability causes temporary fragmentation) aids in the gradual processes of internalization and consolidation of the self.

Persistent failure of the selfobject, in either its mirroring or its idealizing function, arrests development of the psyche and results in narcissistic disorders. The developmental arrest is characterized by:

1. *A chronic deficit in the cohesiveness of the self,* rendering it diffusely vulnerable to fragmentation. The feeling of impending breakup of the self engenders feelings of emptiness and/or unbearable tension states.

2. *Unconscious fixations to the unfulfilled need for the selfobject,* which motivate a search for a responsive substitute that will restore the self's integrity. Children and adolescents thus affected may display many manifestations of drive activity designed to provide sexual substitutes and to counteract inner feelings of deadness.

3. *Behavioral disturbances and maladaptive character traits.* The meaning of these, and transference reactions that arise in therapy, differ markedly from those found in classical neuroses (i.e., in patients who have achieved sufficient self-cohesion, autonomy, and self-differentiation, along with adequate psychic structure).

In classical neuroses, harsh conflicts between unneutralized infantile drive fixations and a severe superego lead to signal anxiety and distorted defensive operations. Defenses to ward off this anxiety include the development of clinical transferences that defend against and yet partly gratify the underlying infantile object-libidinal strivings.

By contrast, in narcissistic disorders the anxiety experienced by those whose self is disturbed concerns the danger of fragmentation, especially if the needed selfobject has been lost or has failed. Early frustrations along this narcissistic line of development fix the need for external objects to provide the missing functions. Resultant character formation and behavior represent admixtures of a search for the requisite selfobject, a substitute for its function, and/or defenses against acknowledging the full depth of this transference need. Thus, these transference expressions are *not* defenses against object-directed instinctual conflicts.

Acting-out and pathologic variants of the narcissistic character are attempts to contain or ward off psychic fragmentation or dreaded states of self-depletion and emptiness. They reflect an inability to sustain feelings of purpose, strength, or liveliness. A large number of our child and adolescent patients constitute a contemporary group who present with bizarre and/or reckless behavior (e.g., compulsive seeking out of daredevil stunts, or competition in auto "chicken" races), indiscriminate sexual acting-out, drug-taking, and other forms of self-stimulating addictive activities that reflect structural deficits rather than structural conflicts. Complaints may include boredom and lack of purpose as well as the frantic pursuit of actions that may appear drive-motivated. Deeper analysis reveals that the basis of these disturbances is the sense of missing something needed to feel whole and alive, to correct low self-esteem, or to soothe and regulate tension.

With these concepts in mind, let us return to the case of Harold. Gradually it became clear to me that Harold's creatively staged, near-erotic, faked suicides were an attempt to dramatize his feelings about his self-experience. Specifically, he was portraying a subjective sense of a chronically deadened self whose independence (Winnicott's "true self" [2]) had been smothered in his mother's narcissism. The stimulation of acting-out these masochistic fantasies provided some outlet, however distorted, for his self-assertive claims. His emergence unscathed from the threat of annihilation represented confirmation of his right to exist, despite inner feelings of chronic emptiness and inability to maintain feelings of continuity and self-validation. These had resulted from early and persisting failures in his mother's empathic mirroring function.

We might also speculate that Harold's symptoms reflected both his unconscious fear of dying and his chronic hypochondriasis, which related to a deeper concern about the vulnerability of his self and a continuing dread of fragmentation or disintegration (3). The faked suicides* gave Harold the repeated feeling of mastery over his greatest anxiety — the fear of psychic death. For Harold, the price of gaining responses from his narcissistic mother and continuing their bond meant the subordination of claims for satisfaction of his own needs and performing as an extension of her.

The major benefit of viewing Harold's primitive, almost perverse, suicidal preoccupations as desperate efforts to ward off frightening self-experiences of a deficient psyche, is that it directs the therapist to an understanding that archaic states are the primary source of anxiety, and that the pathologic expressions of drive are restitutional. The symptoms and drive fragments are remnants of developmental deficits and arrests (3, 4), rather than derivatives of object-directed instinctual conflicts. Thus treatment rests not on interpretations of conflicts and drives the patient is trying to ward off, but on interpretations of chronic feelings of self-depletion and what the patient is trying to achieve through his distorted behavior. In part, the pathologic activity represents a substitute for, and a statement about, failure in the original selfobject. Harold's exhibitionistic displays, so obviously tinged with depression and despair, were attempts to dramatize his continuing search for an audience to satisfy his mirroring needs, attempts that betrayed his hopelessness that these needs could be met.

Acceptance of the concept of a separate, narcissistic line of development with its own progressive and regressive forms of needs (object relations), reactions, and frustrations, shifts the emphasis away from the nature of narcissistic transferences. Accepting the self-model as an alternative also forces us to reconsider the technical approach to our patients; it requires us to re-examine the basic components of treatment, therapeutic alliance, analysis of resistance, transference, negative therapeutic reactions, countertransference, and working through. How one views the patient is important, for it significantly influences therapeutic technique: it determines whether one considers transference as defensive or related to primary need states, one's view of countertransference, sudden regressive shifts, and other phenomena of treatment.

Major interferences in a child's early selfobject needs for mirroring, echoing, and self-confirming responses, set the child on an external search for selfobject functions to correct the imbalance. Harold's transference needs were revealed most dramatically in his dreams, thoughts, and feelings about the woman he called Maude. However, as long as Dr. Strawman continued to apply classical formulas, particularly in regard to Maude's role, the treatment failed. More specifically, the point that ultimately was

---

* Suicide can also be viewed as one of the ways a person may try to preserve his true self from being taken over by a false self-existence (2).

responsible for the treatment's failure was that, contrary to Dr. Strawman's interpretations, Maude did not represent an object that would ward off conflicts, but was a person who could provide the needs of Harold's unmirrored self to gain responses to rehabilitate itself.

In practice, at this stage one would offer confirmation that Harold's relationship with his mother had been faulty, particularly that there had been no empathy with the needs of his developing nuclear self. A striking example, which might be viewed as a summary of their involvement since the boy's infancy (the telescoping of genetically analogous events [1]), concerned the mother's attempts to find a prospective wife for Harold through a computer dating service. Harold had complied with his mother's request to sit near her while she completed the personal questionnaire for him. He noted that initially his mother had asked him for the answers, but almost immediately had shifted to "we" (e.g., "We like tall girls"), and then, imperceptibly, to discussing the answers only with herself, ending with "I" — speaking for herself as if she were Harold. Finding himself first preempted and then ignored, Harold had fantasized the sudden appearance in his hands of a gun, which at first he had directed at himself and then at his mother.

Remembrance of this incident opened up for Harold a lifetime of memories that revealed how often he had sensed the crushing of his independence in an atmosphere dominated by his mother. This in turn called up a hundred other similar incidents when he had felt dwarfed by his mother's needs or had been required to focus attention on her. He now recalled it was in the context of such interactions that, as a little boy, he would retreat to his room: there began his lonely masturbation practices which included fantasies of joyless submission to a powerful woman. These were the precursors of suicidal fantasies with him defiantly triumphant over the woman's protest.

Gradually it became clearer that, in the figure of Maude, Harold was creating his own transference object, not out of defense but of need. Further, he was communicating a prescription for treatment. If I could understand the meaning of his need, I could permit him to use me as a transference object in the way he had used Maude; i.e., if I did not misinterpret this need as a defense, the transference could unfold spontaneously and would lead to establishment of a stable and gradually stronger self-selfobject unit.

From this point, the therapy would differ markedly according to whether complete reconstruction or a smaller repair process was the aim. In extensive psychoanalytic therapy, eventually my significance as a substitute selfobject would become paramount, and the need for this mirror of the nuclear self could be understood. There would be periods of disillusionment with my abilities, but frustrations optimally experienced and empathically understood would lead to constructive internalization. Failures on my part, such as frequent separations or lack of proper empathy, would catalyze shifts in Harold's self-experience, and might activate old symptoms and regressive solutions; but in time they would be understood by both of us. In a more limited therapy, noninterpretative use of my confirming presence, and attempts to discuss empathically the relationship between Harold's symptomatic acts and his underlying anxiety and fragile sense of self, might afford him the selfobject experience he so desperately needed. Most important in therapy of either kind is the therapist's recognition that, for the patient, the search for an appropriately responsive selfobject is an essential quest; it represents a rare substance for which the self hungers to provide a sense of pleasure in existence, and feelings of continuity and solidarity from which one's talents and skills can emerge.

## TOWARD A FURTHER UNDERSTANDING OF NEGATIVE THERAPEUTIC REACTIONS

In the earlier treatment, as Harold had become increasingly lethargic and resistant to all interpretations, his apparent negativism had been interpreted first as latent hostility, then as self-punishment, and finally as maintenance of a sadomasochistic tie to his mother and an unconscious wish to triumph over his therapist. Dr. Strawman had regarded these as a "negative therapeutic reaction," and stated that its continuation would render treatment impossible. In my treatment with him, Harold ultimately realized that Dr. Strawman was wrong and that, in fact, this had been simply a negative reaction—a repetition of typical earlier experiences with his mother that had left him with a profound sense of rage and despair; in short, his sullen withdrawal had been motivated by his failure once more to gain a sense of connectedness and to find a needed selfobject.

Harold's insight pointed out the necessity to re-evaluate the concept of "negative therapeutic reaction." In the past we have attributed such stalemates in therapy to the patient's unconscious envy and need to defeat us or himself because of the untamed nature of his omnipotent destructive impulses. However, now it is clear that, at least in some cases, this clinical reaction represents despair, and is caused by a misunderstanding of the patient's central pathology and transference need. When a therapist interferes prematurely with the establishment of the narcissistic transference, interpreting the reaction as resistance and urging his patient to relinquish it in favor of object-directed instinctual conflicts, the patient may experience this as being in the presence of a self-absorbed narcissistic mother who requires her child to deflect his energies and attentions onto her.

Nearly every aspect of the treatment is influenced by the therapist's concept of the nature of narcissistic transference, and the requirement that he become, at least temporarily, part of the complex self-selfobject unit. The patient's denial of the therapist's independent existence may be the primary cause of intense countertransference reactions; the therapist's understanding of his own reaction to this depends on his theoretical persuasion.

According to Kernberg (5), absence of an object-directed instinctual cathexis reflects an unconscious tendency to control and devalue the therapist in order to defend against feelings of envy and rage. The latter are feared because they activate old, dreaded internal persecutors. This theoretical position, which stems from Kleinian roots, determines the strategy of therapeutic conduct. When the therapist feels impatient or critical of his patient's posture or at being denied autonomy, he can interpret this attitude as a complementary identification (6) with the patient's introjects (for example, the feeling of being hated). Then he can use this experience to identify unconscious emotional attitudes, and help the patient recognize the reasons for his rage, envy, and destructive aims, and his inner world of terrifying, guilt-inducing introjects.

From the viewpoint of psychology of the self, however, nonrecognition of the therapist as psychologically separate can be considered the consequence of arrested psychic development (7). It may be recognized, even in its most extreme form, as a signal that narcissistic structures in need of activation before their gradual rehabilitation, are being engaged. Even in the early stages of treatment when some patients may seem to be ruthlessly controlling, we may empathically sense that we are witnessing in the transference the absolute need for mirroring, and for the availability of a responsive selfobject. The intensity and near-sadistic quality of the patient's control does not necessarily mean that the patient has destructive intentions; rather, it may signify the powerful force of his need to reconstitute a self-selfobject matrix. The search for this response, together with the character defenses against re-experiencing the danger of traumatic disappointments, may be the most relevant data the patient can give us.

The therapist's attitude to the patient's narcissism is of utmost importance to the outcome of treatment. This is especially true for adolescents, in whom narcissistic factors are paramount. But more often, a deeper form of suffering emanating from a self-disorder is the basis for the adolescent patient's intensity and clamor for recognition, concern for self-stimulation and addiction-like drive in seeking outlets, periodic profound lethargy, hypochondriacal depression, and preoccupations. When faced with such avid demands for attention and praise as well as the lack of object-directed instinctual transference, therapists thus deprived of libidinal gratification may feel bored or irritated. The temptation may be to explain these seemingly immoderate demands as part of a regressive transference, and to relegate the excessive pursuits of self-stimulating activities as infantile drives that need taming. A further tendency may be the therapist's attempts to persuade these youngsters to give up their cultural narcissism and accept the limitations imposed by life's realities.

The cruder expressions of sexuality, perverse activities, and addictions represent attempts to use drive-fragments to counteract feelings of emptiness, or to find some form of heightened sensory experience to substitute for the missing function the patient, when a child, assigned to the parent. Even when an adolescent assumes an arrogant posture, boasts about his abilities, and insists that the therapist bear witness to his greatness, this is not the essence of his narcissistic disorder. Rather, unfulfilled narcissistic needs reside in a repressed, walled-off state, buried beneath the facade of archaic grandiosity. Once these needs are uncritically explained, the therapist will witness the gradual mobilization of the truer childhood needs for a selfobject's joyful acceptance, and will be part of the rehabilitation of his patient's self.

Thus, this concept of cure suggests that the dominant psychologic problem of our time concerns central disturbances in the self, and the individual's efforts to re-establish self-cohesion and find meaning for his nuclear needs. Self-assertiveness, and the capacity to work meaningfully and embrace ideals and goals, emanate from a firm sense of self and the resultant ability to enjoy the feeling of wholesomeness that comes from a stable self-selfobject matrix.

There is also the possibility of an alternative therapeutic pathway for Harold that also might have circumvented the development of a negative therapeutic reaction. The boy had lost his father when 6 years of age, and he showed little evidence of a completed mourning process. Therefore, another therapist might have considered the principal aim as the provision of an atmosphere that would promote an idealizing transference (8) to a male figure. He might have argued that the untimely interruption of the boy's relationship with his father prematurely deprived Harold of the libidinal and idealizing functions needed for gradual internalization of a reliable set of guiding ideals and values. This could have provided Harold with a selfobject that was an alternative to his mother, who was so obviously suffering from a narcissistic disturbance of her own that she could not provide self-enhancing responses. A course of therapy to achieve this aim would permit Harold to use his male therapist to form a stable idealizing transference, and thereby rehabilitate his defective psychic structure. Through this identification, Harold might find a source of strength and support for his self-experience, as well as direction and purpose for his nuclear goals and skills.

## PSYCHOSOCIAL INFLUENCES
## ON THE PSYCHOPATHOLOGY OF THE SELF

The changing form of psychopathology, from classical neuroses to disturbances within the self, may be at least partly a consequence of psychosocial changes, especially those that influence stability of the family, parents' roles and their emotional availability, and the stresses of modern technology.

For various reasons (best detailed by a social psychologist), many of today's children experience parental remoteness and/or vagueness as to parents' roles. A common outcome of materialistic indulgence coupled with barren psychological nurture is the development of clinical disorders characterized by an addiction-like search for stimulants to relieve loneliness and fill a void. In those already vulnerable to problems of low self-esteem, the isolating effects of modern technology can exaggerate the understimulation of the self that results from parental remoteness. Woody Allen's *Manhattan* (9), which depicted some pathogenic effects of a culture based in trendiness and artificiality, illustrated that the attraction of immediate gratification reflects a shift in the emotional diet from authentic nourishment in human relationships to a "fast-food" mentality.

However, our appreciation of these changes and stresses in modern life should not cause us to overlook their interplay with personality disturbances in parents that can lead to pathology of the self in their children. Some parents who have a defective self may unwittingly induce similar pathology in their children by overcloseness, enmeshing them in a narcissistic nexus. Deprived of wholesome responses to their nuclear (1) or true (2) selves, children may be seduced through selective parental responsiveness into becoming a narcissistic extension of the parent. This may correspond to the form of pathologic bond described by Winnicott (2) as "the false self." Many variants of this type of disorder seem to be emerging as a major source of our clinical practice. In Harold's case, his suicides can be interpreted as desperate paradoxical attempts to assert his right to live his own life, to confirm his true self and destroy his false self-existence.

## CONCLUSION

The treatment of Harold by the symbolic presence of Maude marks a significant departure from the traditional methods of therapy for those who have neurotic disorders. The aims of treatment toward the resolution of conflict neurosis are to interpret resistances and thereby uncover latent drive fixations, and to attempt modification of superego attitudes that have set up crippling defenses and/or caused symptoms. However, the major focus of treatment of narcissistic disorders, so prevalent in adolescent patients today, is the amelioration of the central disturbance, the structurally deficient self.

In the latter therapy, based on the psychology of the self, the therapist must understand that the presenting character and behavioral disturbances are communications about missing psychic structures, and are attempts (however bizarre or maladaptive) at self-cure. When the patient reveals his needs for selfobject responses to provide the support and self-enhancing enthusiasm essential for firming the self, they must be recognized and accepted as they emerge in treatment. The therapist must avoid premature interpretation in order to allow for the development of a stable idealizing transference that can rehabilitate a narcissitically defective psychic structure.

In a final scene (10) in the film, *Harold and Maude*, when Harold is playing his guitar and dancing a jig which he now presumes is, at long last, to his own tune, it is suggested that his psychic structure has developed, and a distinctive self has emerged.

## REFERENCES

1. Kohut, H. (1971), *The Analysis of the Self: A Systematic Approach to the Psychoanalytic Treatment of Narcissistic Personality Disorders.* New York: International Universities Press.
2. Winnicott, D. W. (1960), Ego distortion in terms of true and false self. In: *The Maturational Processes and the Facilitating Environment: Studies in the Theory of Emotional Development.* London: Hogarth Press, 1965, pp. 140–152.
3. Stolorow, R. D. (1979), Defensive and arrested developmental aspects of death anxiety, hypochondriasis, and depersonalization. *Int. J. Psychoanal.*, 60: 201–213.
4. Stolorow, R. D. (1979), Psychosexuality and the representational world. *Int. J. Psychoanal.*, 60:39–45.
5. Kernberg, O. (1974), Further contributions to the treatment of narcissistic personalities. *Int. J. Psychoanal.*, 55:215–240.
6. Racker, N. (1968), *Transference and Countertransference.* New York: International Universities Press.
7. Ornstein, P. (1974), Discussion of O. F. Kernberg. *Int. J. Psychoanal.*, 55:241– 247.
8. Kohut, H. (1977), *The Restoration of the Self.* New York: International Universities Press.
9. Allen, W. (1979), *Manhattan.* Cinescript. Hollywood: United Artists.
10. Higgins, C. (1971), *Harold and Maude.* Cinescript. Hollywood: Paramount Pictures Corp.

# CHAPTER SEVENTEEN

# FAMILY THERAPY IN THE TREATMENT OF MOOD DISTURBANCE IN ADOLESCENCE

## HERTA A. GUTTMAN

To consider an adolescent family member as the locus of a problem designated as a "mood disturbance" negates an important concept of family therapy. For better or worse, family therapists have always tended to focus on the system of which the individual is an integral member, and to formulate that person's problem in terms of the system's malfunctioning (1, 2). As we all know, this switch to an "ecologic" perspective has dramatically enlarged the possibility of describing, understanding, and effectively intervening in many situations, particularly those involving young children and adolescents.

Despite this "systems" tradition, not every psychological problem of every child can be defined as stemming from maladaptive family interaction or unhealthy parental projections. This may be true of those mood disorders, usually mild, that are reactive; but in many cases of major mood disorder, there is an endogenous component that seems independent of upbringing, which occurs with or without evidence of familial transmission. In any event, major mood disorders in adolescents — whose incidence probably has been underestimated (3, 4) — can affect other family members, even if not caused by them.

Whether a mood disorder in an adolescent is considered a cause or a result of familial malfunctioning is immaterial: the entire family system is ultimately involved, and family intervention is indicated. To decide on the role and type of family treatment in any given case, one must evaluate the extent to which family psychopathology is contributing to the child's condition, and the extent to which the child's plight is affecting the family. With this in mind, I shall consider several relatively common presentations in which family intervention is a potent and perhaps essential ingredient in treatment.

## FAMILY THERAPY IN MINOR AFFECTIVE DISORDER

Adolescents are frequently saddened to various degrees as they traverse individuation, a phase that inevitably involves losing and giving up something before gaining anything. They lose the security of their dependent relationship with their parents, the certainty that their parents' view of the world is the correct one, and the reassurance that their parents will generally approve of and accept whatever they choose to do. Until this stage in life, many adolescents have experienced a relative balance between autonomy and dependence, and their self-image has been relatively positive. Parents ordinarily have enough in their lives to be able to tolerate individuation without perceiving it as abandonment or rejection. Therefore, most adolescents can grope through these years with some discomfort but without despair, and are able to try out, cast off, and finally integrate those life solutions that seem most appropriate. However, such is not always the case: less harmonious development can result in low self-esteem, with depressed mood, feelings of inadequacy, inability to detach oneself from the family satisfactorily, and failure to achieve one's potential (5).

When is family therapy the best approach? First, it is always necessary to acquaint oneself with the family situation and to assess the following factors at first hand:

1. *The extent to which the adolescent is experiencing and living out a parent's intrapsychic conflict.* The very fact of a child's adolescence revives in the parents all their unfinished business (6); for instance, an adolescent may represent freedom or potential never realized by the parent(s). Therefore, the child may be expressing the parent's dissatisfaction with his or her lot in life, with missed opportunities, and depression may be a mechanism of guilt, serving to prevent the child from realizing ambitions to a greater extent than the parent. The parent may also unconsciously thwart the adolescent's goals: "If I didn't have/do it, neither can you." In other cases, the adolescent may be reacting with despair at the prospect of measuring up to a parent's fantasied expectations or actual achievements. This is often a triadic process, in which parents and child play both initiating and reactive roles.

2. *The immutability of roles in a given family.* Many families cannot negotiate the life crisis of adolescence because the parents are overcommitted to their

role as parents — they cannot "survive" without the children, so they cling to the children's continued existence as 10- or 12-year-olds. This is especially true of child-centered couples who have little positive feeling or involvement with each other in the absence of their children. In family terms, the child's depression represents an attempt to "save" the parents by serving as a detour for their conflict or their having to face the fact of a devitalized marriage. Another common reason for an adolescent's depression is that he has filled the role of a surrogate parent, and the family's stability depends on it; this situation is particularly common in one-parent families or in those in which one parent does not or cannot fulfill the parental function properly (7). In such cases the adolescent's depression represents unexpressed anger, which is really directed against parents who have expected him to play an inappropriate, parental role.

3. *The fixedness of the parents' relationship to one another and with their child.* Family therapy can result in rapid gains to the extent that the parents are amenable to intrapsychic and interactional change; indeed, in many cases, this therapy alone is a potent activator of change.

4. *The extent to which the adolescent's depression represents conflicts that have become part of his or her character* (and no longer fluctuate directly with the parent-child relationship). This situation, which is probably more frequent with older than with younger adolescents, militates against family therapy as the primary or exclusive approach to the depression.

Family therapy is probably the treatment of choice if evaluation of the above factors has shown that the adolescent's depression represents both an individual and a collective attempt to cope with a stalemate in family development. Family loyalty often dictates that any possible gains by the child through individual therapy must be sacrificed for the good of the family unless another family member takes over the "sick" role (8); this especially occurs where there are destructive processes of projective identification between parent and child, or where the child's present role is a condition of familial stability. In such cases, family therapy both liberates the adolescent from overtight bonds of family life and gives other family members new developmental potential.

For example, a tearful, depressed, apathetic 15-year-old girl was seen with her parents and two siblings — an older sister and a younger brother. The girl was not nearly as scholastically gifted as her brother nor as physically attractive as her sister. She became depressed as high-school graduation examinations approached, being afraid she would not do well enough for her own or her parents' satisfaction. The situation changed as we began focusing on her allegedly perfect siblings' defects, and the heavy price they felt they had to pay for their favored positions in the family. In fact, it emerged that the older sister often felt left out of the family, because the father favored his younger daughter, and the mother favored her son. The sister was also burdened by her "mission" of being the only attractive female in the family, compensating for her mother and younger sister, who were tolerated even though they were unattractive. The brother lived in fear of displeasing his father, and served as a detour for tensions between the parents; the father would attack his son verbally in lieu of his wife. The 15-year-old daughter's depression lifted quickly as family therapy progressed and these dyadic and triadic problems were revealed and worked through.

Family therapy is particularly effective in cases of depressive reactions (with or without acting-out) that constitute a response to chronic illness, such as juvenile diabetes. There can be several reasons for this reaction: the parents may be overconcerned and overinvolved with the child's condition, and find it difficult to allow the child greater control over the management of his illness. The parents and the child may share both realistic and unrealistic fears and feelings of despair regarding the long-term prognosis of the illness. In such cases, their shared hopelessness and wish to give up are expressed in the adolescent's lack of self-care and depressed affect. If the illness cements the family and covers over possible splits between the parents (10), the adolescent's depression consolidates the parents in their mutual concern for their child.

Individual therapy for the adolescent, concomitant with or subsequent to family therapy, is advisable in some cases. However, the curative effect of realigned family relations alone is striking; it is almost as if a new potential, once released, can flourish and expand on its own. Framo's work has indicated that the presence and example of change in a parent is of special importance to a child, no matter what the child's age (9). It suggests that our original developmental models remain the most compelling ones throughout life; even for the adolescent in the midst of rebellion, change and development in his parents not only relieve him of a burden, but also are models for his own further development.

Until now I have discussed family therapy mainly as a method of facilitating the adolescent's individuation and separation, and thereby increasing self-esteem, energy, and resourcefulness, by working through symbolic rather than real losses. There are also many cases in which adolescent depression is at least partly a reaction to the actual loss of an intact, seemingly normal, functioning family. As we all know, the divorce and separation rate is rapidly rising, not the least among parents of teenage children. In Canada in 1975, 30%–35% of divorcing men and women were between the ages of 35 and 50 (11); presumably, many of them had teenage children.

A rationale commonly expressed by parents for separating at this point is that the adolescent "already has one foot through the door" and can survive without them. The parents' separation, however, results in a premature loss for the teenager. It is far easier to detach oneself gradually at one's own pace than to precipitously lose one's parents and the image of a fairly happy family life at such a vulnerable period (12). I have seen several such children of divorce when they had reached their early or middle twenties. A characteristic pattern seems to be that an adolescent thus bereft casts about for someone else to whom he becomes attached, and commits himself prematurely to an intense love relationship that sooner or later ends in disappointment. This pattern may be repeated several times, and can lead to chronic dissatisfaction and despair.

Family therapy at the time of separation can help all concerned to work through such a loss, to try to maintain respect for family bonds and reduce vindictiveness as much as possible. Some of the issues such families must face are the parents' anger and resentment of each other, their guilt and sadness over the failure of their relationship, and the children's sadness and anger at losing a family. Family therapy, sometimes combined with couple sessions or with individual therapy of one or more members, can help them live through the stages of separation, and later, conciliation toward new, continuing, relationships between the parents, the children, and between the children and their parents. It can also enable the parents to cooperate as parents while relinquishing their connection as spouses, and can prevent the children from making precocious and unsatisfactory romantic choices.

Another area of real loss in which family therapy is helpful is in cases in which the adolescent's depression is a mourning equivalent, often many years later, for a dead parent who has never been adequately mourned by the family. In some instances the adolescent has been the living representative of the dead parent; by symbolically replacing this parent, the adolescent has "saved" the family from complete mourning and detachment from the deceased. The child's budding individuation and incipient separation trigger the dormant mourning process, and the adolescent then introjects the family's depression. The child's depression may be masked by conversion symptoms that indicate his or her identification with the dead parent through symptoms of that parent's physical illness. For example, a 15-year-old girl complained of headaches which were identical to those experienced by her father, who had died of a brain tumor 2 years earlier. Family therapy may be the most effective way of releasing both the family and the identified parent from the burden of mourning.

## FAMILY THERAPY IN MAJOR AFFECTIVE DISORDER

Family sessions are often therapeutic for families in which an adolescent member is in the throes of, or has recovered from, a major affective episode. Such illnesses often begin suddenly and quite dramatically. This is especially so when a bipolar mood disturbance first presents as mania, which is most often the case with adolescents (3). In such situations the other family members are understandably shocked, overwhelmed, guilt-stricken, puzzled, and in need of help.

During the acute phase of the illness, it is counterproductive to have long, insight-producing therapy sessions involving the adolescent patient. Family meetings should be short and highly directive, whether the patient is at home or in a hospital. Their main purposes should be to present and interpret the patient's behavior to the family in a way that allows them to accept the need for treatment; and to support and reassure them that he will eventually recover. This involves drawing the family's attention to the patient's defective judgment, distractibility, and agitation, and providing any necessary supportive measures (such as sedation or other medication, seclusion, or hospital admission) to control the symptoms. These interviews may help the family maintain the adolescent at home rather than hospitalizing him. Family meetings may also give the therapist some insight into the family dynamics likely to prolong the episode or precipitate future attacks, but their main goal should be to mobilize the family's strengths and resources in understanding and managing the shock of the illness.

During the acute phase it is usually advisable to meet with family members in the patient's absence, to allow them to ventilate their feelings, reiterate anxious questions as to course or prognosis, blame themselves or others, and so on. In my experience, the patient's presence during the expression of such feelings intensifies the psychotic symptoms that are his only defense against the anxiety engendered by the family's concern (13, 14).

Once the adolescent has recovered sufficiently, it is important to have family therapy sessions with the following goals:

1. To help the patient and the family assimilate the traumatic events leading up to the illness, and the illness itself, *without* keeping the adolescent permanently in the role of scapegoat or "sick" family member.

2. To explore some of the unconsciously shared fantasies and assumptions that may serve as a nucleus for the psychotic ideas elaborated by the patient. Such exploration will help control renewal of the patient's symptoms.

3. To help other family members — particularly siblings — regain a comfortable position within the family, which they may have lost as a result of the family's response to the stress of one member's illness.

4. To help the patient and the family make a realistic assessment of their expectations of the patient, so that they can avoid further stresses, and appropriately alter their expectations.

5. Finally, to help the family members change maladaptive interaction patterns and relationships that have been a problem, but which by

themselves would not have engendered a need for family therapy.

The "Smith" family illustrates these goals. The family comprised a father, mother, 22-year-old married daughter no longer living at home, 19-year-old son ("Leon"), 13½-year-old son ("Brian"), and a 10-year-old daughter. Leon had first become overactive and uncontrollable 2 years earlier, at age 17, before his sister's wedding. He had taken his parents' credit cards and run up vast bills, and his reckless driving resulted in a car accident. He had been admitted to a psychiatric ward and there his behavior was attributed to an antisocial personality disorder, a diagnosis unchanged at the time of discharge. Soon afterwards Leon went West and started to look for a summer job, but further antisocial behavior led to imprisonment; it was several months before a prison psychiatrist recognized the boy's condition as mania, and recommended psychiatric inpatient therapy. Leon was to be transferred to his home town for treatment in time for his younger brother's Bar Mitzvah, but arrived after the ceremony had taken place. During hospitalization his condition responded to lithium and phenothiazines, and he was discharged home after 3 months. The family was seen once while Leon was in the hospital, and was referred for family therapy after his discharge.

Leon had been a fairly good student, and his father had had great hopes for him. From the boy's point of view, his father had begun treating him differently and had lost faith in him since his illness. From the father's point of view, his promising son had become first a jailbird, then a psychiatric patient. For all family members, the highly disturbing events of the last two years had to be reviewed many times before they could acquire a perspective on the psychiatrists' mistaken diagnoses, and the resultant bewilderment, anguish, frustration, and feeling of betrayal they had experienced.

Second, therapy had to be directed toward allowing some expression of the father's disappointment in his son, and Leon's disappointment in himself and his father, who he felt did not accept him. The father had to be encouraged to talk of his former hopes for Leon — that he would be successful and make a lot of money, and would do so by using his intelligence. In this way, Mr. Smith probably had expected to vindicate his own long-standing feelings of intellectual and financial inadequacy. However, these fantasies of power and wealth may also have fed Leon's manic behavior, and made the return to reality all the more painful.

Mrs. Smith, by preaching and exhorting the family members to look on the bright side of things, had not been helpful; rather, she seemed to have driven both her husband and Leon deeper into depression, apathy, and withdrawal from one another. This had been relieved periodically by arguments, which had increased after Leon's return home. Mrs. Smith had to learn to keep herself out of the interaction between her husband and son, so they could engage in more productive and pleasurable activities together.

As his depressed feelings lifted, Leon, who previously had been almost inert in his sadness and depression, became more active socially and acquired the energy to find himself a job.

At this point, Brian became vociferous, paradoxically complaining that family therapy was useless. It emerged that he felt trapped in the role of an uncomplaining child. His father often verbally attacked and belittled him in the need to vent on someone else feelings of frustration over Leon; Brian, a nervous perfectionist, had become the scapegoat. Brian resented that his Bar Mitzvah had not been the ultra-happy occasion he had anticipated because of the emotional preoccupation and financial straits Leon's problems and illness had created for the parents; in particular, he felt cheated because his parents had not been able to afford a gold ring for him. Brian at first violently rejected the therapist's interpretation that he resented the importance of Leon's position in the family. However, with his mother's support he could gradually express these feelings, and state his need for validation from his father.

These therapeutic steps enabled the parents, particularly the father, to come to a more realistic assessment and acceptance of their older son's problems and potential. Mr. Smith could face the fact that Leon might suffer manic attacks in the future, but that in all likelihood, with medication he could live a normal life. The final focus was the relationship between the parents. Mr. Smith had always been overshadowed by his wife, who tended to tell him what he should do and feel; he had accepted this because of feelings of inadequacy and because his mother had treated him similarly. The Smiths had always interacted in this manner, and probably would have continued doing so but for the fortuitous therapeutic contact provided by Leon's illness. By focusing on the couple's interaction and encouraging a more symmetrical and mature interchange between them, the therapist helped Mr. Smith become more assertive with his wife. He could thus make some inroads into one of the longest-standing maladaptive relationships within the family.

This case description illustrates the possibility of achieving the goals indicated, and that treatment for the family of an adolescent who has a major mood disorder is a mixture of support and intervention. One is greatly aided, however, by the fact that most such families have no severe pathology, and can respond fairly quickly to family intervention.

## FAMILY THERAPY IN THE VALIDATION OF DEVELOPMENTAL HYPOTHESES

Family interviewing gives the clinician a unique opportunity to validate many hypotheses concerning personality development. In particular, several useful concepts have been derived from or deepened by observation during treatment of families with adolescent children. Observation of families provides better documentation of parental involvement in the mechanisms of projective identification, introjection, and identity formation (15). It also permits delineation of the family's role in creating a depressive climate, modeling depressive or manic defenses, and designating an adolescent member as a bearer of depressive symptoms for the entire family. The role of the family in the development of narcissistic personality disorders (16) and the genesis of antisocial acting-out (17) has been confirmed with data most readily available through continuing involvement with families. The work of Paul (18), Berkowitz and colleagues (19), and Jensen and Wallace (20) is a beginning; much remains to be done.

## CONCLUSION

Family therapy of mood disturbances in adolescents can be both supportive and curative. In milder disorders attributable to objective or subjective losses, insight- or task-oriented family therapy can significantly alter mutually stunting processes of projective identification between parent and child. Family intervention alone may be sufficient to promote further development of the adolescent and his parents, but in some cases it should be combined with, or followed by, individual therapy of the adolescent.

In major mood disturbance, family intervention must be supportive and cathartic as well as interpretive and insight-producing. Major mental illness is a significant stress; it can have a profound impact on the structure of the family, with deleterious effects on all family members. The therapy should permit all family members to assimilate and understand what has happened, facilitate the acute treatment of the adolescent, and restore family functioning.

Aside from its curative aspects, family therapy permits observation of adolescents within families. This experience enables us to formulate, validate, and expand hypotheses concerning the familial source of mood disorders in adolescence.

## REFERENCES

1. Haley, J. (1971), Approaches to family therapy. In: *Changing Families: A Family Therapy Reader.* New York: Grune & Stratton, pp. 227–236.
2. Greenberg, G. S. (1977), The family interactional perspective: a study and examination of the work of Don D. Jackson. *Fam. Process*, 16:385–412.
3. Hudgens, R. W. (1974), Affective disorders. In: *Psychiatric Disorders in Adolescents.* Baltimore: Williams & Wilkins, pp. 38–89.
4. Loranger, A. & Levine, P. M. (1978), Age at onset of bipolar affective illness. *Arch. Gen. Psychiatry*, 35:1345–1348.
5. Evans, J. (1975), Depression in adolescents. *Proc. R. Soc. Med.*, 68:565–566.
6. Rashkis, H. A. (1968), Depression as a manifestation of the family as an open

system. *Arch. Gen. Psychiatry*, 19:57-63.

7. Kreider, D. G. & Motto, J. A. (1974), Parent-child role reversal and suicidal states in adolescence. *Adolescence*, 9:365-370.

8. Boszormenyi-Nagy, I. & Sparks, G. M. (1973), *Invisible Loyalties: Reciprocity in Intergenerational Family Therapy.* Hagerstown, Md.: Harper & Row.

9. Framo, J. L. (1976), Family of origin as a therapeutic resource for adults in marital and family therapy: you can and should go home again. *Fam. Process*, 15:193-210.

10. Minuchin, S., Rosman, B. L., & Baker, L. (1978), *Psychosomatic Families: Anorxia Nervosa in Context.* Cambridge, Mass.: Harvard University Press.

11. Government of Canada. (1977), *Vital Statistics, 1975, Vol. 2: Marriages and Divorce.* Ottawa: Statistics Canada (Health Division).

12. Wallerstein, J. S. & Kelly, J. B. (1974), The effects of parental divorce: the adolescent experience. In: *The Child in His Family*, Vol. 3: *Children at Psychiatric Risk*, ed. E. J. Anthony & C. Koupernik. New York: Wiley, pp. 479-505.

13. Guttman, H. A. (1973), A contraindication for family therapy. The prepsychotic or postpsychotic young adult and his parents. *Arch. Gen. Psychiatry*, 29:352-355.

14. Anderson, C. M. (1977), Family intervention with severely disturbed inpatients. *Arch. Gen. Psychiatry*, 34:697-702.

15. Stewart, R. H., Peters, T. C., Marsh, S., & Peters, M. J. (1975), An object-relations approach to psychotherapy with marital couples, families, and children. *Fam. Process*, 14:161-178.

16. Berkowitz, D. A., Shapiro, R. J., Zinner, J., & Shapiro, E. J. (1974), Family contributions to narcissistic disturbances in adolescents. *Int. Rev. Psychoanal.*, 1:353-362.

17. Singer, M. (1974), Delinquency and family disciplinary configurations. An elaboration of the superego lacunae concept. *Arch. Gen. Psychiatry*, 31:795-798.

18. Paul, N. L. (1967), The role of mourning and empathy in conjoint marital therapy. In: *Family Therapy and Disturbed Families*, ed. G. H. Zuk & I. Boszormenyi-Nagy. Palo Alto: Science & Behavior Books, pp. 186-205.

19. Berkowitz, D. A. (1977), On the reclaiming of denied affects in family therapy. *Fam. Process*, 16:495-501.

20. Jensen, G. D. & Wallace, J. G. (1967), Family mourning process. *Fam. Process*, 6:56-66.

# Index

suicide and, 197, 213
Aggression, in depression, 173, 183, 203, 209, 226
  agoraphobia, 104, 105, 108, 110, 111
  akinesia, drug-induced, 242, 243, 246
Alcohol(ism), 80, 173
  suicidal behavior and, 197, 198, 203, 207, 208, 227
Alienation, sense of, 38, 43, 54, 73–82, 156, 228; case-reports, 74–76, 78–79
  antidotes, 19, 20, 77–80
  apathy: end-stage of, 74, 77, 269
  attention-deficit disorder, in, 96
  definitions, 20, 73–74
  epidemiology, 75, 76, 79
  ethical standards lacking, 18, 48, 49
  historical contexts destroyed, 39, 42–45, 47–48
  management, 78, 80
  normal adolescence in, 75, 76, 80
Allen, Woody: *Manhattan*, 260
American (North) youth/society
  alienation in, 18–19
  Indians: suicidal behavior, 43, 196, 211
  new mythology, 38–39
  sociocultural factors. *see* Historical forces; Socio-economic factors
  scholastic problems, 62, 66, 80, 203, 209, 229
*Amok*, 56
Anomie, 77
  historical contexts destroyed, 38, 43, 44
  suicide and, 43
Anorexia nervosa, 124, 125–126, 136
  abandonment depression and, 141–142
  bulimia in, 126
  medication, 125, 126
  suicide, timing of, 126
Anthony, E. J.
  adolescence comparable to emigration, 148
  classification and depressogenic sequence of mood disorders, 156
  depression in adolescence: psycho-

dynamic approach to nosology, 151–165
  ego-psychology cycle, 160, 161
Antisocial behavior. *see* Behavioral disturbances
Antisocial personality in adulthood, 91
Anxiety, 60–62, 66, 74, 77, 105, 107, 108, 131, 240
  anticipatory, 111
  'anxious attachment,' 106
  archaic states as source, 255
  castration, 251
  chronic physical illness and, 131
  depression and, 131, 152, 163, 168, 171, 173, 211
  differentiation from fear, 105
  narcissistic disorders and, 250, 251, 254, 257
  separation, 111
  social, 107, 108, 110, 118
Anxiety neurosis, 105
Anxiety state, phobic symptoms in, 105, 107, 108
Attention-deficit disorder, 85, 89–102;
  clinical experience, 92–93. 94–96
  attentional deficits, 89, 95, 96, 98
  conduct disorders, 89, 91–94, 95, 98
  definition and differential diagnosis, 89, 96–97
  epidemiology, 90–94, 101
  hyperactivity, 89, 91, 92, 94, 95; paradoxical response to stimulant medication, 92
  lability of affect, 93, 95–96
  management: education, 98–99; medication, 92, 93, 95, 97, 99–100, 101; psychotherapy, 100–101
  natural history, 89–92
  neurological signs/tests, 92, 93, 94
  pre-adolescence, in, 89–95, 98, 101
  psychological tests, 92, 93, 94, 97
  psychopathology in adulthood, 91
  *see also* Learning difficulties

Beck, A., 'cognitive triad' in depression, 160, 162
Behavioral disturbances, 77, 79, 269